Pain Management in Interventional Radiology

As interventionalists become more involved with patients as care providers rather than solely as proceduralists, understanding and treating pain is a vital part of daily practice. This book provides an overview of the multiple techniques used in the management of pain in interventional radiology suites. Topics include techniques for the treatment and prevention of pain caused by interventional procedures, as well as minimally invasive techniques used to treat patients with chronic pain symptoms. Approximately half of the book is dedicated to the diagnosis and treatment of spinal pain; other chapters focus on intraprocedural and post-procedural pain management, embolization and ablation techniques used to treat patients with uncontrollable pain, and alternative treatments for pain relief. This book is a practical resource for anyone looking to acquire skills in locoregional or systemic pain control and wishing to improve the quality of life for patients undergoing procedures or suffering from disease-related pain.

Charles E. Ray, Jr., MD is Professor of Radiology, Co-Director of Research (Clinical), and Associate Residency Program Director at the University of Colorado Health Sciences Center, Aurora, Colorado.

To C. Eugene and Virginia L. Ray

Pain Management in Interventional Radiology

Charles E. Ray, Jr., MD

Professor of Radiology
Co-Director of Research (Clinical)
University of Colorado Health Sciences Center
Aurora, Colorado

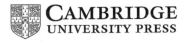

CAMBRIDGE UNIVERSITY PRESS
Cambridge, New York, Melbourne, Madrid, Cape Town, Singapore, São Paulo, Delhi

Cambridge University Press
32 Avenue of the Americas, New York, NY 10013-2473, USA

www.cambridge.org
Information on this title: www.cambridge.org/9780521865920

First published 2008

Printed in the United States of America

A catalog record for this publication is available from the British Library.

Library of Congress Cataloging in Publication data

Pain management in interventional radiology / [edited by] Charles E. Ray Jr.
   p. ; cm.
Includes bibliographical references and index.
ISBN 978-0-521-86592-0 (hardback)
 1. Interventional radiology. 2. Analgesia. I. Ray, Charles E.
   [DNLM: 1. Pain–therapy. 2. Pain–prevention & control. 3. Radiology, Interventional. 4. Spine–physiopathology. WL 704 P146591 2008]
RD33.55.P35 2008
616'.0472–dc22   2007052022

ISBN 978-0-521-86592-0 hardback

Contents

PART II. SYSTEMIC PAIN CONTROL

Contributors

Iftikhar Ahmad, MD
American Access Care
Pittsburgh, Pennsylvania

Jason R. Bauer, MD, RVT
Director, Interventional Radiology
   Clinic
ICON, Interventional Consultants
Legacy Good Samaritan Hospital
Portland, Oregon

George Behrens, MD
Department of Radiology
Rush University Medical Center
Chicago, Illinois

James Choi, MD
Staff Radiologist
Iowa Radiology
Clive, Iowa

Felipe Birchal Collares, MD
Department of Radiology
Harvard Medical School
Beth Israel Deaconess Medical
   Center
Boston, Massachusetts

Blaze Cook, MD
Department of Radiology
University of Colorado
   Health Sciences Center
Aurora, Colorado

Kirkland W. Davis, MD
Associate Professor of Radiology

University of Wisconsin School of
   Medicine and Public Health
Madison, Wisconsin

Anthony P. Dwyer, MD
Department of Radiology
Denver Health Medical Center
Denver, Colorado

Salomao Faintuch, MD
Interventional Radiologist
Department of Radiology
Harvard Medical School
Beth Israel Deaconess Medical
   Center
Boston, Massachusetts

Frances D. Faro, MD
Department of Orthopaedics
Denver Health Medical Center
Denver, Colorado

Hector Ferral, MD
Professor of Radiology
Rush University Medical Center
Chicago, Illinois

Michael Fleisher, MD
Department of Radiology
Denver Health Medical Center
Denver, Colorado

Curt Freudenberger, MD
Department of Orthopedic Surgery
Cedars-Sinai Medical Center
Los Angeles, California

Jennifer R. Huddleston, MD
Department of Radiology
University of Wisconsin Medical Center
Madison, Wisconsin

Stephen P. Johnson, MD
Department of Radiology
University of Colorado Health
    Sciences Center
Aurora, Colorado

Elvira V. Lang, MD
Associate Professor of Radiology
Harvard Medical School
Director Nonpharmacologic
    Analgesia Program
Beth Israel Deaconess Medical Center
Boston, Massachusetts

Keira P. Mason, MD
Associate Professor of Anesthesia
    (Radiology)
Harvard Medical School
Director, Radiology Anesthesia and
    Sedation
Children's Hospital
Boston, Massachusetts

Frank Morello, MD
West Houston Radiology Associates
Houston, Texas

Jan Namyslowski, MD
Clinical Associate Professor of
    Radiology
University of Illinois College of
    Medicine at Peoria
Interventional Radiologist
Methodist Medical Center of Illinois
Peoria, Illinois

Nilesh H. Patel, MD, FSIR
Medical Director, Vascular and
    Interventional Program
Central DuPage Hospital
Winfield, Illinois

Vikas V. Patel, MD
Assistant Professor of Orthopaedic
    Surgery
University of Colorado Health
    Sciences Center
Chief Orthopaedic Spine Surgery
The Spine Center

University of Colorado
Aurora, Colorado

Brian D. Petersen, MD
Assistant Professor of
    Radiology and Orthopaedics
Director Musculoskeletal Radiology
University of Colorado Health
    Sciences Center
Aurora, Colorado

Charles E. Ray, Jr., MD
Department of Radiology
University of Colorado Health
    Sciences Center
Aurora, Colorado

Leo J. Rothbarth, MD
Radiology Specialists of Denver, PC
Denver, Colorado

Gloria Maria Martinez Salazar, MD
Department of Radiology
Harvard Medical School
Beth Israel Deaconess Medical Center
Boston, Massachusetts

Mitchell T. Smith, MD
Department of Radiology
University of Colorado Health
    Sciences Center
Aurora, Colorado

Nick Stence, MD
Department of Radiology
University of Colorado Health
    Sciences Center
Aurora, Colorado

David T. Wang, DO
Department of Radiology
University of Colorado Health
    Sciences Center
Aurora, Colorado

Derek L. West, MD
Department of Radiology
University of Illinois at Chicago
    Medical Center
Chicago, Illinois

Stan Zipser, MD, JD
Attending Radiologist
Santa Clara Valley Medical Center
San Jose, California

Preface

Everyone feels pain. Everyone feels physical pain, to one degree or another. Pain, or simply the thought of being in pain, often changes our actions as no other physical sensation can. While often a necessary physical response to keep us out of harm's way (touching the hot handle of a pot, for example), pain becomes its own entity when it is associated with an underlying disease process.

Why is pain associated with disease? From an evolutionary perspective, was pain necessary for some reason to let the individual know that something was amiss (even though nothing could be done about it)? Was disease-associated pain used for some other, perhaps subconscious, purpose? Perhaps understanding the "why" is not all that important in today's world; after all, the bottom line is that pain simply hurts! And disease-associated pain can hurt most of all. We as health care providers should be able to do something about it – shouldn't we?

From one perspective, medicine (traditional or "Western" medicine in particular) has done relatively little to abate pain. Most of the major advances in pain control over the past 150 years have been in the field of pharmacology; general anesthesia is the prime example of pain control. With the exception of medications, however, little progress has been made in managing disease-associated pain over the past few decades. More work – much more work – remains. Shouldn't minimally invasive techniques spearhead this effort?

The goal of this book is simple. It is to provide the appropriate tools to the interventional radiologist, anesthesiologist, surgeon, or whoever else is interested in minimally invasive techniques to control pain before, during, or after procedures. Its intent is to provide an overview of multiple techniques used in pain management, to review the currently available literature regarding these techniques, and hopefully to act as a springboard to motivate practitioners and researchers alike to develop the next better mousetrap to care for our patients in pain. It is my sincere hope that someone, somewhere, will have an improved quality of life stemming from the reading of this book by their health care provider.

Charles E. Ray, Jr., MD
Denver, CO

Acknowledgments

Many individuals are secondarily involved in the publication of a book. Unfortunately, those who are most affected are often those with the least interest in the project. It is only through the support of those that surround us that an undertaking such as this is finished – or, for that matter, even begun. My sincerest thanks (a small token if ever there was one) to Bob Allen, MD, and my colleagues at Radiologic Specialists of Denver, Denver Health Medical Center, and the University of Colorado for providing whatever time and support they could during the generation of this text. Thanks are also extended to Beth Barry at Cambridge University Press, who has guided me through this book as well as another. I would also like to thank artist Stacy Erickson for her illustrations accompanying this book. The staff at the Society of Interventional Radiology, most notably Joy Gornal and Beverlee Galstan, were remarkably tolerant as their tasks were put on hold in order to meet another deadline related to this book.

Finally and foremost, my thanks and love are extended to my wife, Kris, for her endless support and unequaled patience during this project.

Pain Management in Interventional Radiology: An Introduction

Jason R. Bauer and Charles E. Ray, Jr.

THE PROBLEM OF PAIN

The management of pain continues to be one of the most vexing of problems for health practitioners worldwide. The pain response is difficult to manage for multiple reasons: responses vary widely in their mechanism of action as well as anatomic location; individual responses to pain are variable; secondary gains can be had by individuals falsely claiming to be in pain; cultural differences in description of pain and the willingness to admit to a pain response exist; even responses by the health care provider to a patient in pain varies widely. For these reasons, each and every patient who presents with pain, or in whom we as health care providers are likely to produce a painful response during a procedure, has a widely variable and largely unpredictable pain response.

Traditional medicine (so-called Western medicine) has demonstrated great advances in the management of pain; however, the advances have been relatively few and far between. Opium was cultivated for recreational use by the Sumerians nearly 5,000 years before it was first introduced specifically for medicinal purposes (1). It was not until 1680 that opium was introduced in England as Laudanum, a combination of opium, herbs, and sherry, specifically to be used for medicinal purposes. Although likely poorly understood at the time, the pain-relieving effects of opium must have significantly contributed to the use of opium as a medicinal agent. It is amazing, actually, that a plant discovered nearly five centuries ago remains the mainstay for pain relief throughout nearly all cultures and medical systems worldwide.

The next great advance in pain control was the discovery of agents used for general anesthesia during operations. The first public display of the effect of general anesthesia was performed at the Massachusetts General Hospital in 1846 (2). Dr. John Warren, a preeminent surgeon of the day, removed a vascular tumor from the jaw of a patient. This surgery was performed in conjunction with William Morton, a local dentist, serving as an anesthetist, by using an ether-soaked sponge under a glass dome. Upon awaking at the end of the procedure, the patient claimed he had no pain during the operation, to which Dr. Warren proclaimed to the audience (legend has it), "Gentlemen, this (anesthesia) is no humbug!"

One must take note that these two greatest advancements in the history of pain control – narcotics and general anesthesia – occurred a remarkably long time ago. Clearly, advancements have been made since then with regards to pain control, and the adjustments to the use of both narcotics and general anesthesia have allowed significant advancements in pain management. Other advancements, such as postoperative pain control with patient-controlled analgesia [described by Sechzer in 1971(3)] and the administration of intraprocedural sedation and analgesia, are the more recent improvements that have been major factors in pain management. However, if one regards the changes in other fields of medicine that have occurred since 1846 (antibiotics, chemotherapy for cancer, open heart surgery, transplant surgery, etc.), one is struck by the relative paucity of new methods of pain control, particularly long-lasting or "curative" pain control, that have occurred over the past several decades.

Western medicine has had a difficult time throughout its history in dealing with a patient in pain. One needs look no further than the number and types of alternative therapies available to individuals to treat pain. Chiropractic, napropathic, and homeopathic medicine forms largely deal with patients in pain, as does acupuncture, massage therapy, craniosacral therapy, and many others. Are the successes of these alternative medicine systems in treating patients in pain in part due to our failure as traditional medicine providers?

If Western medicine has largely fallen short when dealing with the patient in pain, interventional radiology (IR) has in many ways ignored the problem altogether. Except for giving a touch of sedation and analgesia during our procedures, or occasionally treating the patient in pain with a nerve block, spinal procedure, or embolization, IR provides very little attention to the patient in pain. This is perhaps historical as much as anything; because IR started as a diagnostic modality where our contact with any given patient extended for only an hour or two; the need to understand the pain response and the best way to treat it was underappreciated. It has only been because we as interventionalists have become more involved with patients as care providers rather than proceduralists that the need to understand patients in pain has become more vital to our daily practice.

PAIN IN MEDICINE AND SOCIETY

Pain, and the treatment of pain, is an enormous medical/social issue. From a societal standpoint, the cost of pain is tremendous. One study evaluated nearly 30,000 workers in the U.S. workforce, and estimated that the total cost of lost productivity in the workplace because of common pain conditions (headache, arthritis, back pain, and other musculoskeletal pain) was $61.2 billion per year (4). The same study noted that the majority of the lost productivity was due to reduced performance while at work, rather than taking time off.

The costs (in dollars) associated with pain control are nearly impossible to accurately calculate. One study evaluated 373 cancer patients, nearly 40% of who reported having some sort of cancer-related pain (5). Of these patients, three-quarters incurred a pain-related expense, averaging $891 per month

Table 1. Results from PubMed Search, January 2007	
Search Term	*Number of Articles Returned*
"Pain"	341,298
"Pain," limited to last one year	18,569
"Pain, interventional radiology," limited to last one year	19

related specifically to pain control. Other studies have evaluated common conditions such as low-back pain, which in terms of both direct costs and indirect costs (lost productivity, etc.), is likely the most costly medical problem facing the medical establishment in the United States. In 1991, low-back pain was estimated to cost the United States $25 billion in *direct costs alone* (6,7). It has also been estimated that 80% of all adults at some point in their lifetime will seek medical care of some sort for low-back pain and that a third of all disability costs in the United States are due to the same problem (6,8). Clearly, pain management represents a huge percentage of both the time and dollars spent on health care in this country.

Medically, the search for improvement in pain management is also consuming when one considers the amount of research time (and dollars) spent on pain control. The importance of research into pain and the management of pain are revealed when one considers the attention given to pain by the National Institutes of Health (NIH). The NIH has previously focused attention on pain research with the development of multiple committees, such as the NIH Pain Research Consortium, the NIH Extramural Pain Staff Workgroup, and the NIH Pain Interest Group, specifically charged with attempting to drive more research into pain control (9).

Also illustrative of the research efforts regarding pain management, over twenty journals are dedicated to pain, with such widely varied titles as "Pain," "Journal of Orofacial Pain," and "Molecular Pain" (whatever THAT may be!). At the time of the manuscript preparation, a PubMed search was performed with the single keyword "pain" (Table 1). A total of more than 340,000 articles were returned. When limited to manuscripts published within the past year, nearly 19,000 articles were returned. Amazingly, when the keywords "interventional radiology" were added to the search, only 19 articles were returned for a one-year time period. Clearly, we as interventionalists have some catching up to do with regard to understanding the importance of pain management for our patients.

IR AND PAIN MANAGEMENT

The role of IR in pain management varies widely from institution to institution, from practice to practice, and from operator to operator. To try to define pain management as a major or minor player in the field as a whole is impossible, and each individual practitioner must determine the needs of the patient, the referral patterns for their individual practice, and their own desire to become involved with pain management to decide what amount of time and effort will be spent on the management of pain. At one of the authors' (CER) institutions, for instance, the number of pain procedures we have performed over the past two years has increased by a factor of 2.7, largely due to increased involvement with low-back pain management. Parenthetically, the number of procedures performed for an indication of pain still only accounts for 5% of all the cases performed at that one institution.

One instance in which we all must be involved in pain management, however, is in controlling the pain (and anxiety) that we specifically cause during procedures performed for other reasons. It is in this management of intraprocedural pain that we all have a common interest. Intraprocedural pain control is important for several reasons. As described by the American Society of Anesthesiologists in their practice guidelines for sedation and analgesia by nonanesthesiologists (10), the goals of intraprocedural sedation and analgesia are twofold. First, it "... allows patients to tolerate unpleasant procedures by relieving anxiety, discomfort, or pain." Second, "... in children and uncooperative adults, sedation-analgesia may expedite the conduct of procedures that are not particularly uncomfortable but that require that the patient not move" (10). Control of intraprocedural pain is important for other reasons as well, particularly if the same patient is going to return to the same interventionalist for repeat procedures. Nothing will dissuade an individual from returning for repeat procedures quite like a previously painful experience!

Pain management in IR has evolved over time. Intially, nearly completely ignored except for the use of local anesthestics at the skin entry site, increasing attention was paid to pain control needed during the procedure itself, with widespread use of intraprocedural sedation and analgesia. Procedures specifically designed to treat a patient's underlying pain, such as embolization or ablation of painful osteolyses, were developed. Finally, again with our increasing involvement in patient care, further attention has been given to postprocedural management of pain. For these reasons, many IR divisions are now considered along with anesthesia, neurology, neurosurgery, oncology, and orthopedic medicine, as one of the "pain services."

The use of intra-arterial injection of local anesthesthetics provides an example of the evolution of pain management in IR – a brief synopsis is given in the following paragraphs.

USE OF INTRA-ARTERIAL LOCAL ANESTHETICS

The use of intra-arterial anesthetics in the management of pain is relegated to few uses today. From a historical perspective, the use of these agents intravascularly was linked to the evolution of angiography and the pain resulting from contrast injections (11,12). There has been a reemergence of intra-arterial analgesia in IR largely as a result of increased interest in transcatheter tumor therapy.

As early as 1939, adjuvant injection of medications to limit pain experienced during peripheral angiography was explored. Procaine hydrochloride (Novocaine) injection was mentioned by Dimitza and Jaegar with apparently improved pain during peripheral angiography (11). In 1982, Cranston performed a double-blinded placebo-controlled trial of thirty-four patients having peripheral angiography (13). Subjective and objective evaluations were performed using verbalization and movement. One milliliter of 2% lidocaine was mixed for each 10 ml of Conray-60 used. Seventeen patients received lidocaine during the first injection of contrast, thirteen during the second injection, and four received two injections without contrast. All patients who received lidocaine in the first injection reported subjective improvement, and there were no associated complications.

The debate regarding effectiveness or need for intra-arterial lidocaine administration during peripheral angiography is now all but moot. With the evolution of digital subtraction angiography (using less contrast at lower rates) and low osmolality contrast agents such as Visipaque (GE Healthcare, Cork, Ireland), few patients experience symptoms so intolerable as to warrant intra-arterial lidocaine.

When considering transcatheter tumor therapy for malignant tumors, such as hepatocellular carcinoma in the liver, or benign tumor management, such as symptomatic leiomyomata in the uterus, pain management strategies have included intra-arterial lidocaine injection. In 1990, Molgaard et al. injected intra-arterial lidocaine in the hepatic artery prior to and during Transcatheter arterial Chemoembolization (TACE) in 45 patients (14). Analgesic requirements during and following the procedure were compared with that in 20 patients previously treated without intra-arterial lidocaine (14). They found a remarkable decrease in the amount of medication required during (98.9% decrease in narcotic dose) and after (75% fewer individuals requiring a patient-controlled analgesia pump) the procedure in those who received lidocaine. Lee et al. evaluated the importance of timing of intra-arterial lidocaine injection (15). In 113 consecutive patients, three groups of patients (no lidocaine, lidocaine just prior to TACE, and lidocaine following TACE) were evaluated by quantifying the mean dose of analgesic and subjective pain score. There was a statistically significant difference in both the amount of analgesics used and the pain score; those patients who received 100 mg of lidocaine prior to TACE used fewer narcotics and reported a lower pain score than those receiving similar treatment administered after delivery of the chemotherapeutic agent. The authors reported few complications, with only one patient experiencing transient hypotension.

Intra-arterial lidocaine has also recently been investigated during the endovascular treatment of uterine fibroids. Embolization in this setting notoriously results in a postembolization syndrome, punctuated by pain and cramping. Postprocedural pain in this setting may extend the length of hospital stay and lead to return visits. Similar to TACE, pain is thought to result from leiomyoma ischemia, spasm, and parenchymal swelling (16). However, uterine arteries do not appear to respond to lidocaine in the same way as hepatic arteries following injection of intra-arterial lidocaine; this may be due to their need to meet the demands of a gravid uterus (17). Keyoung et al. injected 200 mg of lidocaine in 10 consecutive patients (while eight received placebo) prior to uterine artery embolization (UAE) for leiomyomata (17). Lidocaine was found to significantly improve subjective pain reported by patients but not the amount of analgesia required following the procedure. More importantly, moderate to severe vasospasm was noted in seven of ten patients after lidocaine; none of the placebo patients demonstrated such spasm, resulting in early termination of the study. Vasospasm due to lidocaine injection may therefore contribute to a higher treatment failure rate and therefore is not commonly used during UAE.

Intra-arterial lidocaine was once common during peripheral angiography; its safety profile has been supported during years of use for this application. With overall few reported complications, intra-arterial lidocaine injection prior to tumor embolization provides practitioners with a safe strategy to achieve better patient comfort during and after embolization procedures.

CONCLUSIONS

"Pain management continues to be the most difficult problem facing medicine today." This statement is debatable, but arguments against it are largely due to a matter of degree and opinion, not of underlying substance. The patient in pain is ubiquitous, regardless of culture, geographic location, socioeconomic status, sex, race, or any other variable of which we can think.

IR can play a major role in pain management and is unique as a field in that we can be responsible for controlling patients' pain as a primary goal of therapy, or in controlling the pain that we cause during our procedures. This book is organized in such a way, with chapters on intraprocedural and postprocedural pain management, and multiple chapters on procedures performed specifically to treat underlying processes that may be responsible for the pain response. Special attention is given to spinal procedures, although other publications provide a more in-depth overview of spinal procedures. The goal of this book is to provide an overview of pain management in IR and introduce concepts that can be used on a daily basis in the interventional suite to better provide pain management for our diverse group of patients.

REFERENCES

1. opiods.com/timeline – accessed January 2007.
2. http://neurosurgery.mgh.harvard.edu/History/gift.htm – accessed January 2007.
3. Sechzer PH. Studies in pain with the analgesic-demand system. Anesth Analg, 1971;50: 1–10.
4. Stewart WF, Ricci JA, Chee E, Morganstein D, Lipton R. Lost productive time and cost due to common pain conditions in the US workforce. JAMA, 2003;290: 2443–54.
5. Fortner BV, Demarco G, Irving G, et al. Description and predictors of direct and indirect costs of pain reported by cancer patients. J Pain Symptom Manage, 2003;25: 9–18.
6. Bratton RL. Assessment and management of acute low back pain. Am Fam Physician, 1999;60: 2299–308.
7. Frymoyer JW, Cats-Baril WL. An overview of the incidences and costs of low back pain. Orthop Clin North Am, 1991;22: 263–71.
8. Kuritzky, Carpenter D. The primary care approach to low back pain. Prim Care Rep, 1995;1: 29–38.
9. http://www.ninds.nih.gov/find_people/nands/council_minutes_may1998.htm – accessed January 2007.
10. Practice guidelines for sedation and analgesia by non-anesthesiologists. An updated report by the American Society of Anesthesiologists Task Force on sedation and analgesia by non-anesthesiologists. Anesthesiology, 2002;96: 1004–17.

11. Lindbom A. Arteriography of the lower limb in the living subject. Acta Radiol [suppl], 1950;80: 9–15.
12. Bjork L, Erikson U, Ingelman B. Clinical experiences with a new type of contrast medium in peripheral angiography. Am J Roentgenol, 1969;106: 418–24.
13. Cranston PE. Lidocaine analgesia in peripheral angiography: a confirmation of effectiveness. South Med J, 1982;75: 1229–31.
14. Molgaard CP, Teitelbaum GP, Pentecost M, et al. Intra-arterial administration of lidocaine for analgesia in hepatic chemoembolization. JVIR, 1990;1: 81–5.
15. Lee SH, Hahn ST, Park SH. Intra-arterial lidocaine administration for relief of pain resulting from trans arterial chemoembolization of hepatocellular carcinoma: its effectiveness and optimal timing of administration. Cardiovasc Invervent Radiol, 2001;24(6): 368–71.
16. Cibils LA. Response of human uterine arteries to local anesthetics. Am J Obstet Gynecol, 1976;126: 202–10.
17. Keyoung JA, Levy EB, Roth AR, et al. Intra-arterial lidocaine for pain control after uterine artery embolization for leiomyomata. JVIR, 2001;12: 1065–9.

2

Clinical Evaluation of Low-Back Pain

Anthony P. Dwyer, Curt Freudenberger, and Vikas V. Patel

INTRODUCTION

The goal of this chapter is to explain the mindset and thought processes of the clinician evaluating a patient presenting with symptoms of low-back and leg pain.

The accurate clinical evaluation of the symptom of low-back pain is essential to the successful management of patients presenting with this problem, and interventional radiology (IR) plays an important role in the process.

It is vital to recognize that low-back pain is only a symptom and not a diagnosis or a disease entity in and of itself. Unfortunately, the successful management of patients with low-back pain is difficult because of the diversity of the pathologies producing low-back pain. There are many pathologies that can produce the symptom of low-back pain, and its treatment is very difficult or impossible unless one can locate and understand the causative pathology. The key to successful management of patients presenting with low-back pain is to identify and understand the pathological cause of their presenting symptoms of low-back pain, and to direct therapy toward the underlying cause rather than solely relieve the symptom of pain.

Although low-back pain typically arises from spinal causes, it must be remembered that there are pathologies outside of the spinal column that can present with low-back pain. These etiologies are typically considered only after a spinal column abnormality has been excluded.

A useful classification of the causes of low-back pain is the classification scheme described by Macnab et al. (1). These are presented in Table 1.

Another diagnostic hurdle is the difficulty in determining whether the pathologies identified on spinal imaging are the cause of the low-back pain or coincidental to it, as a significant percentage of asymptomatic patients have pathology identified on spinal imaging [especially on magnetic resonance imaging (MRI)] (2). Not infrequently, clinical examinations, patient symptoms, and imaging studies are discordant. Spinal interventions are often requested as a method by which to determine whether or not the pathology

Table 1. Classification Scheme for the Causes of Low-back Pain
Viscerogenic
Vascular
Neurogenic
Psychogenic
Spondylogenic
Traumatic
Infectious
Neoplastic
Metabolic
Source: Macnab et al. (1).

noted on the imaging study is responsible for the patients' pain. This subject is beyond the scope of this chapter and is discussed in the individual, procedurally oriented chapters that follow.

This chapter will concentrate on the clinical evaluation of the more common spinal pathologies that affect the vast majority of low-back pain patients in clinical practice. Oftentimes, regardless of the underlying cause (e.g., traumatic, infectious), the symptom of pain itself is caused only after significant degenerative changes have occurred within the spinal column.

LUMBAR PAIN OVERVIEW

By definition, *somatic* pain occurs with noxious stimuli to musculoskeletal structures, *visceral* pain occurs with noxious stimuli to an organ, and *neurogenic* pain occurs with noxious stimuli to axons and cell bodies. *Referred* pain is felt at a location away from the site of the causative pathology, with the site of pain being innervated by nerves different than the structure causing the referred pain. It must be remembered that virtually any structure receiving innervation is a potential source of pain when it is at the site of pain-producing pathology.

With lumbar pain, the causative pathology usually involves the structures of the disc and facet joints involved in degenerative cascade, as described in depth by Yong-Hing and Kirkaldy-Willis (3). Sources of lumbar pain are outlined in Table 2 (4).

Lumbar pain can be axial (central lumbar) or may radiate from the spine. The latter cause is felt as deep, aching, poorly localized pain usually in the buttocks and thighs. This latter constellation of symptoms is referred to as "somatic referred pain." Radicular pain arises from involvement of the spinal nerves with inflammation, irritation, and compression, producing a sharper pain localized in the radicular distribution of the involved nerve root. Radicular pain is often associated with objective neurological deficits, the most notable of which are sensory change and muscle weakness. Clinical studies have

Table 2. Anatomic Sources of Lumbar Pain
Vertebra
Disc
Facet joints
Sacroiliac joints
Muscles
Ligaments
Dura
Source: Van Akkerveeken et al. (4).

established that nerve root compression alone does not produce radicular pain and that the nerve root must first be inflamed in order for compression to produce pain. These studies also confirmed the outer annulus as the common site of lumbar pain, with the facet joint capsule only occasionally being a cause (Figure 1) (5).

The vast majority of low-back pain is mechanical in nature and is usually related to spinal degeneration, or subclinical episodes of "wear and tear" that are aggravated intermittently by episodes of trauma. This "degenerative cascade," as described by Yong-Hing and Kirkaldy-Willis (3), is ubiquitous; its extent and severity is multifactorial, such as genetic predisposition, smoking, and occupational loads to the lumbar spine. The degenerative cascade produces degenerative joint changes in the articular cartilage of the facet joints, loss of hydration of the intervertebral disks with concomitant loss of stability and resistance to torsion, eventually leading to radial

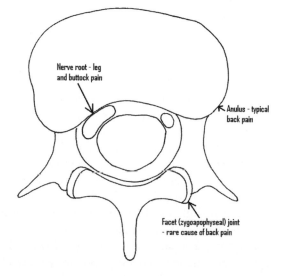

Figure 1. Possible sites of lower back pain. (From Kuslich and Ulstrom (5)).

tears in the annulus. These annular tears allow herniation of the disc material out of the disc into the vertebral canal and onto the adjacent nerve root, causing the symptom of "sciatica" or pain in the distribution of that involved nerve root. The damaged disc also releases neuropeptide, phospholipase A2, and inflammatory peptides, further irritating the nearby neurological structures (6).

The Clinical Evaluation Process

In the initial evaluation of a patient with low-back pain, an initial triage process must occur to determine the need for urgent intervention. One such example of a triage algorithm is given in Figure 2 (7).

Once a surgical emergency has been excluded, a more systematic evaluation of the patient with low-back pain can occur. To illustrate the evaluation process at our institutions, we present the following sample history questions and issues to be resolved from the physical examination.

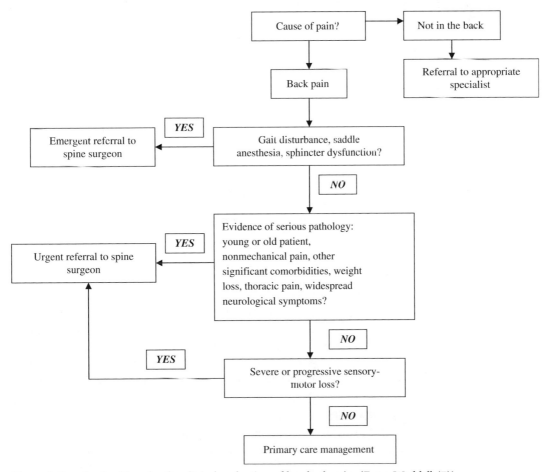

Figure 2. Sample algorithm for the clinical evaluation of low-back pain. (From Waddell (7)).

HISTORY

For the history, the following questions are asked:

- "Where is the pain the worst – the back or leg?"
- "Is the pain *mechanical* (i.e., worse with activity and relieved with rest) OR *nonmechanical* (i.e., having red flag or sinister symptoms of weight loss, fevers, worse at night and at rest)?"
- "Are the leg symptoms '*radicular*' (shooting and bandlike, from irritation of a spinal nerve or root) OR '*referred*' (deep, diffuse, poorly localized and aching, from irritation of the nerves supplying the structures of the vertebral motion segment [e.g., annulus, facet joint])?"
- "If there is claudication, is it *neurogenic* (from ischemia and compression of the nerve roots, arising from a central or lateral spinal stenosis) OR *vascular* (reproducible, relieved by rest, from leg muscle ischemia arising from peripheral vascular disease)?"
- "Are there symptoms of cauda equina syndrome? (bladder and bowel sphincter dysfunction)?"

PHYSICAL EXAMINATION

During the physical examination the examiner will record:

- Spinal deformity
- Spinal range of motion and any symptoms produced
- Hip and knee range of motion and any symptoms produced
- Objective neurological deficit (reflex loss, wasting, weakness)
- Subjective neurological deficit (sensory loss)
- Nerve root irritation (sciatic or femoral nerve stretch test)
- Distal pulses and any ischemic leg skin signs (loss of hair, skin discoloration, "shiny" skin appearance)
- Perianal and rectal examination findings in patients suspected of having cauda equina syndrome

RADIOLOGIC INVESTIGATIONS

Different radiologic modalities provide different data that can be instrumental in the evaluation of a patient with low-back pain. A specific imaging modality may be vital in one clinical scenario and worthless in another, and rarely are all modalities (radiography, nuclear medicine scans, computed tomography (CT), MRI, invasive techniques) necessary (8). In order to best utilize such resources, algorithms that suggest the most appropriate utilization of radiologic studies have been produced. Some general rules of thumb regarding what information can be gleaned from the different imaging modalities follow.

RADIOGRAPHS

Anterior/posterior, lateral, oblique views and flexion/extension radiographs of the lumbar spine provide the following clinically important information:

- Number of normal lumbar levels, the intercristal line, the length of the L5 transverse process, and any thoroco-lumbar or lumbo-sacral anomalies

■ Secondary and primary signs of degenerative disc disease and degenerative facet joint disease
■ Coronal or sagittal deformities of alignment
■ Pars interarticularis defects
■ Stability of the spine on flexion/extension lateral radiographs
■ Evidence of osseus destruction from infection or neoplasm

CT AND MR IMAGES

Cross-sectional imaging studies provide the following clinically important information:

■ Disc space narrowing with loss of T2 signal indicating degenerative disc disease
■ Facet joint enlargement, effusion, and/or cyst formation, indicating degenerative facet joint disease
■ Central stenosis, usually from ligament flavum hypertrophy or inferior facet joint hypertrophy
■ Lateral stenosis, usually from superior facet hypertrophy and medial displacement
■ Disc displacement
■ Vertebral canal tumors
■ Dural cysts

ELECTROMYELOGRAPHY/NERVE CONDUCTION VELOCITIES

Information provided by electromyelography/nerve conduction velocities is vital, particularly as evidence for physiologically significant disease. These physiological studies are particularly effective in diagnosing the following:

■ Peripheral neuropathy
■ Radiculopathology
■ Spinal stenosis

IR REFERRAL

Referrals to IR are not all that frequent when considering the number of patients seen in a spine pain clinic. Select patients, however, may benefit greatly from IR procedures. Evidence-based medicine for IR procedures is distinctly lacking, and there are no widely accepted algorithms for when an IR procedure is indicated. The clinician will consider an IR referral to effect the following:

■ Improve low-back and leg symptoms (the various forms of epidural steroids injections and nerve root blocks)
■ Identify the "pain locator" by placing a needle in a specific anatomic location, first to reproduce the symptoms and second to relieve the symptoms (e.g., discograms)
■ Confirm the specific level and side of the causative pathology (selective nerve root blocks when there is bilateral or multilevel pathology)

The results of these IR procedures are just one piece of the clinical evidence that assist the clinician in deciding what therapy (e.g., spinal decompression, fusion) is indicated, and at what locations and levels.

SELECT IR SPINAL PROCEDURES: A CLINICIAN'S PERSPECTIVE

Discography

The clinical use of discograms remains controversial. The pathogenesis of discography-induced pain reproduction is poorly defined (9–13). Critics describe unsatisfactory sensitivity and specificity rates and the lack of correlation between a positive discogram and successful treatment as evidence that discography should not be utilized in the evaluation of discogenic pain. Conversely, advocates of the technique point out that the accuracy of clinical and radiologic evaluations are just as poor in predicting postoperative clinical outcomes. The authors believe that discography can be helpful in select patient populations when deciding if surgery is indicated, and if so, what levels need to be addressed.

In an attempt to reduce the problem of false-positive or false-negative discograms, the International Spine Injection Society recommends some standardization (14):

- Recording of volume and injection pressure of the injected contrast
- Correlation with the patients' symptoms, to decide if there is clear symptom reproduction (i.e., the pain caused by the discogram is "concordant" or "non-concordant" with the patients' underlying symptoms)
- Description and classification of the contrast injection on postprocedure radiographs and/or CT (15)
- Injection of anesthetic into the disc at completion of a positive discogram, and the keeping of a postprocedure pain diary to determine the duration of any pain relief

Selective Anesthetic Blocks

The philosophy of the successful use of anesthetic blocks has not been based on objective or blinded studies. These procedures have been handicapped by the lack of definitive evidence supporting their use, the very subjective nature of the blocks, and the placebo effect. Some authors maintain that the placebo effect can be minimized if the following injection sequence is followed with the appropriate time interval (e.g., two weeks) between injections:

- Normal saline
- Short-acting local anesthetic (e.g., 1–2% lidocaine)
- Longer acting anesthetic (e.g., 0.25% bupivicaine)

A positive block is one that has symptom reproduction on injection of contrast and shows no relief with the saline injection, short-term relief with the short-acting anesthetic, and longer relief with the longer acting anesthetic. Subjective relief of 50–75% of the patient's underlying pain is considered diagnostic.

Table 3. The Role of various Interventional Spine Procedures: A Clinician's Perspective

Injection/ Procedure	Radiological Confirmation Required	Diagnostic of Pain Locator	Therapeutic Effect	Surgical Decision Making
Discography	++	+++	−	+++
Epidural steroids	++	−	+++	+/−
Facet joint blocks	+/−	+/−	+++	+/−
Median branch blocks	+/−	+/−	+++	+/−
Sacroiliac joint blocks	++	+++	++	++
Nerve root blocks	++	+++	+++	+++

SUMMARY

The clinician's expectations of the various IR procedures presented here are summarized in Table 3. These include:

Discography (16)

■ Finds the pain/symptom source or "pain locator."
■ Determines if the "black disc" on T2 is the pain locator and the source of symptoms
■ Determines what levels need to be included or excluded in the fusion construct, for example, whether L4/5 needs to be included in the fusion of an L5/S1 spondylolisthesis.

Selective Nerve Root Blocks (17)

■ Determine which nerve roots are involved in the symptom production when there are multiple roots involved on imaging studies.
■ Provide a period of symptomatic relief, which may be either short (temporary) or prolonged (definitive). This period of symptom relief may afford the patient an opportunity to derive benefit from physical therapy and other nonoperative treatments.

Epidural Steroid Injections (18,19)

■ Provide symptom and functional improvement (mainly for radiculopathy from disc herniation and spinal stenosis), and allow temporary nonoperative symptomatic improvement.

Facet Blocks (20–23)

- Can determine the source of pain in patients in whom no other source can be identified
- Allow the clinician to stop evaluating other potential sources of spinal pain
- Can provide relief for 3–4 months

Sacroiliac Joint Blocks (24)

- Provide symptomatic and functional relief, either as a standalone method or in combination with other nonoperative treatments
- Determine if the sacroiliac joint is the pain locator
- Allow the clinician to stop evaluating other potential sources of spinal pain

Interventional radiologic procedures play an important role in both the diagnosis and treatment of spinal back pain in select patient populations. Close communication with the referring spine physician is vital to performing the appropriate imaging-guided procedure.

REFERENCES

1. Macnab I, McCullock JA, Transfeldt E. In: Macnab's Backache. Classification of backache. Baltimore: Livingstone Williams Wilkins, 1997, pp. 86–9.
2. Boden S, Davis D, Dina TS, et al. (1990) Abnormal magnetic resonance scans of the lumbar spine in asymptomatic subjects: a prospective investigation. JBJS Am, 72-A(3): 403–8.
3. Yong-Hing K, Kirkaldy-Willis WH. "The Three Joint Complex." In: The Lumbar Spine. Philadelphia: W.B. Saunders Company, 1990, pp. 87–90.
4. Van Akkerveeken P. "Pain Patterns and Diagnostic Blocks." In: The Lumbar Spine (2nd ed.). Philadelphia: W.B. Saunders Company, 1996, pp.105–22.
5. Kuslich SD, Ulstrom CL. "The Origin of Low Back Pain and Sciatica: A Microsurgical Investigation." In: Williams RW, McCulloch JA, Young PH (eds.) Microsurgery of the Spine. New York: Raven Press, 1990, pp.1–7.
6. Saal JS, Franson RC, Dobrow R, et al. (1990) High levels of inflammatory phospholipase A2 activity in lumbar disc herniations. Spine, 15: 674–8.
7. Waddell G. The Back Pain Revolution. New York: Churchill Livingstone, 1998, p. 107.
8. Grossman ZD, Katz DS, Alberico RA, Loud PA, Luchs JS, Bonnaccio E (eds.) Cost-Effective Diagnostic Imaging: The Clinician's Guide (4th ed.). Philadelphia: Mosby Elsevier, 2006, pp. 247–52.
9. Holt EP. The question of lumbar discography. J Bone Joint Surg, 50A: 720 (1968).
10. Simmons JW, Dwyer AP, Aprill CA, Brodsky AE. (1988) A reassessment of Holt's data on: the question of lumbar discography. CORR, 237: 120.
11. Walsh T, Weinstein J, Spratt K, et al. (1990) Lumbar discography in normal subjects: a controlled prospective study. JBJS, 72-A(7): 1081–8.
12. Carragee EJ, Tanner CM, Khurana S, et al. (2000) The rates of false-positive lumbar discography in select patients without low back symptoms. Spine, 25(11): 1373–80; discussion 1381.
13. Carragee EJ, Tanner CM, Yang B, et al. (1999) False-positive findings on lumbar discography: reliability of subjective concordance assessment during provocative disc injection. Spine, 24(23): 2542–7.

14. Derby R, Howard M, Grant J, et al. (1992) The ability of pressure controlled discography to predict surgical and non-surgical outcomes. Spine, 24(4): 364–71.

15. Adams MA, Dolan P, Hutton WC. (1986) The stages of disc degeneration as revealed by discograms. JBJS Am, 68-B: 36.

16. Bogduk N, April C, Derby R. "Discography." In: White A, Schofferman A, eds. Spine Care. Diagnosis and Conservative Treatment. St. Louis: Mosby, 1995, pp. 219–36.

17. Riew K, Yin Y, Gilula L, et al. (2000) The effect of nerve-root injections on the need for operative treatment of lumbar radicular pain: a prospective, randomized, controlled, double-blind study. JBJS Am, 82-A(11): 1589–93.

18. Bogduk N, Aprill C, Derby R "Epidural Steroid Injections." In: White A, Schofferman A, eds. Spine Care. Diagnosis and Conservative Treatment. St. Louis: Mosby, 1995, p. 322.

19. Vad VB, Bhat AL, Lutz GE, et al. (2002) Transforaminal epidural steroid injections in lumbosacral radiculopathy: a prospective randomized study. Spine, 27(1): 11–16.

20. Bogduk N, Aprill C, Derby R. "Diagnostic Blocks of Spinal Synovial Joints." In: White A, Schofferman A, eds. Spine Care. Diagnosis and Conservative Treatment. St. Louis: Mosby, 1995, p. 298.

21. Mooney V. "Facet Syndrome." In: Weinstein JN, Wiesel SW, eds. The Lumbar Spine: The International Society for the Study of the Lumbar Spine. Philadelphia: W.B. Saunders, 1990, pp. 422–41.

22. Schwarzer AC, Aprill CN, Derby R, et al. (1994) Clinical features of patients with pain stemming from the lumbar zygapophysial joints. Is the lumbar facet syndrome a clinical entity? Spine, 19(10): 1132–7.

23. Schwarzer A, Aprill CN, Derby R, et al. (1994) The relative contributions of the disc and the zygapophysial point in chronic low back pain. Spine, 19: 801–6.

24. Fortin JD, Dwyer AP, West S, et al. (1994) Sacroiliac joint pain referral maps upon applying a new injection/arthrography technique. Spine, 19: 1475.

PART I

Locoregional Pain Control

Local Anesthetics

Jan Namyslowski

HISTORY

Ruetsch et al. provide an in-depth review of the history of local anesthesia in their 2001 paper titled "From Rocaine to Ropivacaine: The History of Local Anesthetic Drugs" (1). What follows is a summary of pertinent points in their eloquent historical review.

Cocaine has its linguistic origin in a Peruvian plant, revered by the natives for its stimulating properties. The word *Khoka,* meaning "the plant," evolved into the European *coca* over time. We owe the term *cocaine* to Albert Niemann who isolated the main alkaloid from the coca leaves. A Viennese pharmacologist, Karl Damian Ritter von Schroff, described coca-induced skin insensibility. Samuel Percy was "the first to propose the use of the coca leaves as an anesthetic" in 1856. Carl Koller, in 1884, first used cocaine for ophthalmological anesthesia at the suggestion of Sigmund Freud. Addictive properties of cocaine were soon discovered as well, and many practitioners became affected, Freud and William Halsted among them. The dependency placed a significant damper on the availability of local anesthesia for medical procedures.

Subsequent pharmacological advances have led to the development of several local anesthetic compounds in the late 19th and throughout most of the 20th centuries. The delivery of local anesthetics would not have been possible, were it not for the invention, in 1844, of a hollow hypodermic needle and syringe by an Irishman, Francis Rynd (2). Rynd's clinical contributions, although not arrived at in an FDA-approvable style, allowed for a significant medical progress at the time:

> The subcutaneous introduction of fluids, for the relief of neuralgia, was first practised in this country by me, in the Meath Hospital, in the month of May, 1844. The cases were published in the "Dublin Medical Press" of March 12, 1845. Since then, I have treated very many cases, and used many kinds of fluids and solutions, with variable success. The fluid I have found most beneficial is a solution of morphia in creosote, ten grains of the former to one drachm of the latter. (3)

Charles Gabriel Pravaz and Alexander Wood are also credited with the invention of hollow needle syringe devices, in the 1850s.

BASIC ANATOMY AND PHYSIOLOGY

The cutaneous nerves that are the target of local anesthetics have dermal as well as epidermal endings (4). In addition, pain receptors are also present in the periosteum, arterial walls, and joint surfaces (5). Depending on the site and depth of injection of a local anesthetic, a number of peripheral nerve fibers are affected to a variable degree (6). The nerve fibers that are primarily involved in pain perception belong to Aδ group which are fast fibers, conducting at velocities of 6–30 m/s, and the slow C fibers, conducting at 0.5–2 m/s. Therefore, a dual pain sensation may occur wherein the Aδ fibers are responsible for the instantaneous, often self-defensive reaction to pain, followed by a more chronic pain, carried centrally by the slow C fibers (5).

FUNDAMENTALS OF PHARMACOLOGY

The cellular mechanisms involved in clinical performance of local anesthetics, their pharmacodynamic and pharmacokinetic properties, and the specifics of nerve conduction blockade are all quite complex, and a detailed discussion is beyond the scope of this chapter. Interested readers are referred to an in-depth review by Strichartz and Berde in Miller's Anesthesia textbook (7). Here, pertinent points will be discussed briefly.

Local anesthetics are divided into ester and amide compounds. The most commonly used esters include benzocaine, chlorprocaine, cocaine, procaine, and tetracaine. The common amides are bupivacaine, lidocaine, mepivacaine, prilocaine, and ropivacaine. Selected properties of local anesthetics in common clinical use are listed in Tables 1 and 2.

The basic molecular structure of a local anesthetic is an aromatic ring, which is connected to a tertiary amine by an intermediate ester or amide link. The tertiary amine is hydrophilic and, to some degree, positively charged. The aromatic ring, in contrast, is responsible for the affinity of local anesthetics to tissue membranes, or lipophilicity (7). It is this affinity to tissue membranes that is primarily responsible for the impulse-blocking effect of local anesthetics (8). Anesthetics in solution exist in equilibrium of a positively charged form and a neutral base form. The tissue membranes concentrate the neutral base form to a greater degree than the positively charged form. Within a certain range, more lipophilic drugs exert longer lasting anesthesia and are more potent. Tissue pH may also play a role in the effect of local anesthetics by changing the proportions of the charged and uncharged forms. Such situation exists, for example, in inflamed tissues, which are characterized by low pH. This favors the positively charged form of the local anesthetic to predominate, which in turn impedes tissue penetration of the drug (7). Clinically, this may explain why patients are extremely sensitive to an anesthetic injection into the inflamed tissue commonly surrounding chronically indwelling drains, and why it is difficult to adequately anesthetize such an area. In contrast, alkalinization of an anesthetic solution, for

Table 1. Amide Local Anesthetics

Name	Brand Name	Duration of Action	Adult Without Epinephrine (dose/kg)	Adult Without Epinephrine (max dose)	Adult With Epinephrine (dose/kg)	Adult With Epinephrine (max dose)	Child Without Epinephrine (dose/kg)	Preservative Free	Remarks
Articaine	Septocaine, ultracaine	1–2 hours	7 mg/kg	≤500 mg	N/A	N/A	5 mg/kg (4–12 years)		Primarily for dental use
Lidocaine	Xylocaine	60 minutes	4.5 mg/kg	≤300 mg	7 mg/kg	500 mg	3.3–4.4 mg/kg (>3 years) 5–6 mg/kg	Yes	
Mepivacaine	Carbocaine	45–90 minutes	N/A	400 mg (0.5–1%)	N/A	N/A			
Ropivacaine	Naropin	2–6 hours	N/A	200 mg	N/A	N/A	2.5 mg/kg (0.25%) [epidural only]	Yes	Pediatric safety and efficacy not established
Bupivacaine	Sensorcaine, Marcaine	3.5–8.5 hours	N/A	175 mg (0.25%)	225 mg (0.25%)	N/A	0.5–2.5 mg/kg (0.25–0.5%)	Yes	Not recommended for children <12 years
Levobupivacaine	Chirocaine	7.7–10.7 hours	N/A	150 mg (0.25%)	N/A	N/A	N/A	Yes	Not recommended for children <12 years
Prilocaine	Citanest	2–3 hours	8 mg/kg	600 mg	8 mg/kg	600 mg	6.6–8.8 mg/kg	Yes	Approved for dental and topical use
Ethidocaine	Durarest	4–10 hours	N/A	300 mg	N/A	400 mg	N/A		

Table 2. Ester Anesthtics

Name	Brand Name	Duration of Action	Adult Without Epinephrine (dose/kg)	Adult Without Epinephrine (max dose)	Child Without Epinephrine (dose/kd)	Child With Epinephrine (dose/kg)	Adult With Epinephrine (max dose)
Procaine		60 min		350–600 mg (0.25–0.5%)	15 mg/kg (0.5%)		350–600 mg (0.25–0.5%)
Chlorprocaine	Nesacaine	60 min	11 mg/kg (0.5–3%)	800 mg	11 mg/kg (0.5–1%) [>3 years]	14 mg/kg (0.5–3%)	1000 mg

example, by the addition of sodium bicarbonate ($NaHCO_3$), may hasten the onset of action and result in a more effective impulse blockage (9).

The basic impulse-blocking mechanism of local anesthetic is blockage of sodium channels on neural membranes that, in turn, leads to the cessation of propagation of impulses. Differences exist in susceptibility of nerve fibers to local anesthetics. The least susceptible are small, nonmyelinated C fibers, followed in increasing order of reactivity by the large Aα and Aβ fibers. The most susceptible ones are Aδ sensory Aγ motor fibers (7,10).

Local anesthetics may affect the vascular tone of blood vessels in their surroundings. Vasoconstricting effects may predominate at low concentrations, whereas the vasodilatory properties are evident at higher concentrations. This is drug specific, however. For example, EMLA is initially a cutaneous vasoconstrictor and then becomes a vasodilator after two hours of application (7,11–12).

The addition of epinephrine to a local anesthetic may increase the extent and duration of anesthesia because it decreases the rate of vascular absorption from tissue (13–17). The effect is most pronounced with lidocaine, including markedly dilute solutions (7).

Once they have been absorbed into the bloodstream, local anesthetics are metabolized primarily in the liver (amides), or hydrolyzed in plasma by cholinesterase enzymes (esters) (7). The blood concentration of local anesthetics depends on the amount injected, the rate of absorption, tissue distribution, biotransformation, and excretion. There are also patient-specific factors such as age, and cardiovascular, hepatic, and renal functions (7). For example, the plasma half-life for lidocaine is almost doubled in the elderly population when compared to healthy young adults (18). The relationship of the blood level is usually directly proportional to the volume injected; larger volumes of a correspondingly dilute solution will cause higher blood levels than the same dose in a smaller volume (7).

The primary toxicity of local anesthetics is manifested by neurological and cardiovascular symptoms. The initial symptoms of central nervous system (CNS) toxicity are dizziness and lightheadedness that may be followed by tinnitus and difficulty in focusing. Patients often demonstrate tremors, muscle twitching, and shivering – all eventually leading to tonic-clonic convulsions. Although the initial phase of CNS toxicity is clearly excitatory, the late effects are those of CNS depression leading to respiratory arrest (7). With large doses of anesthetic absorbed into the bloodstream, the excitatory phase of toxicity may be rather short. The decrease in ventilation may lead to hypercapnia, which in turn may worsen the toxicity by dilating the cerebral blood vessels and increasing the delivery of the local anesthetic into the brain (7,19). The cardiovascular effects are due to the anesthetic-induced impairment of the conducting system (19–24). Although beneficial in certain situations (e.g., ACLS protocols), this is obviously undesirable when using local anesthetics for their primary function. Bupivacaine is particularly capable of inducing malignant reentry-type cardiac dysrhythmias. Thresholds for CNS versus cardiovascular toxicity vary depending on the particular drug. For example, a sevenfold higher lidocaine blood level is needed to produce cardiovascular collapse compared to the level needed to induce seizure activity. By contrast, this ratio is less than fourfold for bupivacaine (25). In fact, bupivacaine may potentially stop a patient's heart before it stops their breathing.

TOPICAL ANESTHETICS

A commonly used topical anesthetic in the United States is EMLA (AstraZeneca Pharmaceuticals, Wilmington, DE, USA), an emulsion of 2.5% lidocaine and 2.5% prilocaine. Approved by the FDA in 1992, this preparation has been used extensively in a number of applications, such as prior to venipuncture, infusion port access, local skin excisions, therapeutic injections, circumcision, etc. The maximum depth of penetration is 5 mm (26), and the minimum recommended effective application time is 60 minutes (although shorter effective times have been reported). Its use in infants and neonates is limited because of the possible development of methemoglobinemia (27,28).

ELA-max, or its newer formulation called LMX 4 (Ferndale Laboratories, Ferndale, MI, USA), is a lysosomal-based formulation of lidocaine (4% or 5%), which has a faster onset of action and longer anesthetic effect compared to EMLA (29). LMX 4 has the added benefit of not causing methemoglobinemia. However, LMX 4 is an over-the-counter drug that is not currently FDA approved for the spectrum of use similar to that of EMLA given earlier.

Amethocaine is a 4% tetracaine gel, in use in Europe, Canada, Australia, and New Zealand, although it is not currently FDA approved. Its efficacy may be superior to EMLA in alleviation of pain associated with venipunctures (30). This could be due to its affinity for neuronal receptors and high lipophilicity that allow a rapid onset of action and a lasting effect after small doses (31,32). Iontophoresis takes the topical anesthetic delivery from a passive absorption to an active, low-electrical current administration that relies upon the polar property of anesthetic molecules (33). Although it offers the fastest delivery of topical anesthesia, the delivery device is expensive and provides only small surface area coverage (29). Several reviews of a number of clinical trials summarize the clinical efficacy of EMLA and amethocaine (29,32,34,35).

ALLERGIC REACTIONS

True allergic reactions to local anesthetics are rare, probably less than 1% (36). Symptoms that are thought to represent an allergic reaction are not infrequently a result of an unrecognized intravascular injection, vasovagal reaction, or cardiovascular effects of epinephrine. Of the two groups of local anesthetics, esters are more likely to elicit allergic reactions. These reactions are caused by *p*-aminobenzoic acid, an allergenic metabolite of this group. Although an amide anesthetic might be a safer choice in a setting of proven allergy to an ester compound, rare allergic reactions have also been described with this group. They have been attributed to the presence of a preservative, methylparaben (37), which is hydrolyzed to *p*-hydroxybenzoic acid (38). An additional mechanism responsible for methylparaben's antigenicity is that it may act as a hapten that requires binding with a carrier, typically a protein, to become antigenic (38,39). Another potential allergen may be the latex rubber stop in some of the local anesthetic bottles.

Clinically, when presented with a patient who is allergic to an ester anesthetic, the next best choice is to use a preservative-free amide drug (37,38). Unfortunately, the most commonly encountered problem is history of a reaction to lidocaine, an amide! Because cross-reactivity within the amide group is rare, and given that a prior reaction may have been due to an amide containing methylparaben, one should perform intradermal testing with a different, preferably preservative-free, amide (37). A rather elaborate protocol has been described by Feldman et al. (40). Briefly, it includes intradermal administration of 0.1–0.2 ml of a local anesthetic in decreasing dilution (1:1000, 1:100, 1:10, 1:1, nondiluted) and observing for local signs of allergic reaction. Anecdotally, one of the author's anesthesiology colleagues uses 0.1–0.2 ml of nondiluted anesthetic from the outset – an approach that has worked reliably for more than 15 years of clinical practice. If cross-reactivity to amides is present, then intradermal testing with an ester is appropriate (37).

What if neither an amide nor ester anesthetic is safe to use? Anesthetic properties of antihistamines and antihistaminic properties of anesthetic compounds have been described (41). The anesthetic property of antihistamines is thought to be due to the blockage of sodium channels (42). The anesthetic effectiveness of diphenhydramine hydrochloride has been compared against lidocaine in randomized clinical studies (43–45). Solutions of 1% lidocaine and either 0.5% or 1% diphenhydramine were examined. The latter two are prepared by diluting 1 ml (50 mg) vial of diphenhydramine with 9 or 4 ml of normal saline solution yielding, respectively, 0.5% or 1% solutions. In general, there was no difference in the anesthetic effectiveness between lidocaine and diphenhydramine, with an exception for facial lacerations where lidocaine was more effective. One patient in a particular study developed a superficial skin sloughing after using diphenhydramine as an anesthetic (43).

THE ROLE OF SODIUM BICARBONATE

There are a number of variables associated with pain on administration of local anesthetics. For example, the injection site, speed of injection, intradermal versus subdermal injection, temperature of the drug, presence of any admixtures (epinephrine, $NaHCO_3$), solubility in lipids, and size of the needle may all influence the degree of pain associated with the administration of local anesthetics. As discussed earlier, increasing pH of the solution by the addition of

NaHCO$_3$ should increase the uncharged base form, which has been shown to have better diffusion kinetics in the soft tissues resulting in a more rapid onset of action (9). McKay et al. (46) showed that NaHCO$_3$ reduced pain on cutaneous administration of local anesthetics. The results of randomized clinical trials in this regard are varied. Nakayama et al. (47), in a study of fifty patients, showed the effectiveness of NaHCO$_3$ in decreasing pain sensation associated with the epidural needle insertion. In this study, however, patients were not their own controls. Watts et al. (48) studied sixty-four patients undergoing open carpal tunnel decompression under local anesthesia and showed no statistical difference in pain scores between patients receiving buffered versus plain lidocaine. The size of the needle was not reported. Similar to the Nakayama study, patients were not their own controls. In the remaining studies, discussed below, patients were their own controls. Masters (49) found that the reported pain score was significantly lower in patients receiving lignocaine with epinephrine buffered with NaHCO$_3$ versus without the buffer. A trend, albeit not statistically significant, toward buffered lidocaine with epinephrine causing less pain than a freshly mixed lidocaine with epinephrine but no buffer was found by Burns et al. (50). Palmon et al. (51) studied the effect of needle gauge (25 vs. 30 gauge) and lidocaine pH on pain during intradermal injection and showed that the contribution of NaHCO$_3$ was greater, even though both the needle gauge and the addition of bicarbonate buffer had a role in diminishing pain. And finally, Scarfone et al. (52) reported on the impact of buffering and the rate of administration on pain perception and found that the latter had a greater impact. Buffering ameliorated the pain associated with rapid injection.

TUMESCENT ANESTHESIA

Tumescent anesthesia is used extensively in plastic and reconstructive surgery. The development of percutaneous varicose veins ablation has brought this technique into the interventional radiology practice not only as a pain control tool but also as an important mechanism responsible for the efficacy of this therapy. Infiltration of the tumescent solution allows collapse of the saphenous vein around the laser fiber or RF probe, thus optimizing the contact of the vein wall with the device. Tumescent anesthesia also creates a heat sink effect, which offers protection to the surrounding tissues. Many "recipes" are available for the tumescent solution. For example, as described by Min and Khilnani (53), a 0.1% solution of lidocaine may be created by adding 50 ml of 1% lidocaine to 450 ml of normal saline solution, with an addition of 5–10 ml of 8.4% NaHCO$_3$. An even more dilute (0.05%) lidocaine concentration may be utilized if large volumes of tumescent solution are required, for example, in simultaneous bilateral treatment. The limiting factor is the maximum safe dose of lidocaine, which must not exceed 4.5 mg/kg when administered without epinephrine, or 7 mg/kg with the vasoconstrictor. However, as suggested by Klein (54,55), the maximum safe doses mentioned above may represent a significant underestimate as to what may be applicable in the clinical practice of plastic and reconstructive surgery. Klein's tumescent solution (54) consists of 0.05% or 0.1% lidocaine with 1:1,000,000 epinephrine and NaHCO$_3$. He studied the pharmacokinetics of such mixture, following injections of large volumes (up to 2,000 ml) of dilute anesthetic, in a series of limited clinical experiments involving the total of fourteen patients. It was determined that the maximum safe dose is 35 mg/kg in patients undergoing liposuction. He also reported that the procedure resulted in the decrease of the total amount of lidocaine absorbed systemically as well as the magnitude of the peak plasma concentration (approximately 25–30% each), due to partial removal of the anesthetic with liposuction (54). Klein also suggested that the well-publicized maximum safe lidocaine doses had been arrived at by inference from data available for procaine in the initial application for the FDA, rather than objective data on this compound. More recently, Grossmann et al. (56) studied the pharmacokinetics of articaine hydrochloride, an amide anesthetic, in liposuction. The advantages of articaine include a rapid metabolism in tissue and plasma to an inactive articainic acid, and a lower rate of CNS toxicity than lidocaine (57,58). No side effects were observed following articaine doses of up to 38.2 mg/kg, and similar to the results of Klein, the liposuction procedure reduced the amount of the drug absorbed by approximately 30%. However, contrary to the prior investigations, Ostad et al. (59) found the amount of lidocaine in the liposuction aspirate to be negligible. The applicability of data quoted here to the field of interventional radiology is, at present, limited (54–56,59). This is mostly because highly dilute lidocaine solutions, as low as 0.05%, are hardly expected to produce toxic levels even with a simultaneous bilateral lower extremity varicose vein ablation. The safety of exceeding the recommended lidocaine dose in venous ablation has yet to be defined.

CONCLUSIONS

Familiarity with different local anesthetics is vital to the practice of interventional radiology. Differing clinical situations, as well as patient variables, call for a tailored approach to the type and amount of local anesthetic used.

REFERENCES

1. Ruetsch YA, Böni T, Borgeat A. From cocaine to ropivacaine: the history of local anesthetic drugs. Current Top Med Chem 2001, 1(3):175–82.
2. http://www.patentsoffice.ie/en/student_inventors.aspx (accessed November 2006).
3. http://www.inventnetireland.com/fii.asp (accessed November 2006).
4. Clemente CD. Gray's Anatomy of the Human Body. 13th Edition. Philadelphia: Lea and Febiger, 1985:1350.
5. Guyton AC, Hall JE. Somatic sensations: II. Pain, headache, and thermal sensations (Ch. 48). In: Guyton AC, Hall JE, eds. Textbook of Medical Physiology. 10th Edition. Philadelphia: W.B. Saunders Company, 2001:552–63.
6. Guyton AC, Hall JE. Sensory receptors; neuronal circuits for processing information (Ch. 46). In: Guyton AC, Hall JE, eds. Textbook of Medical Physiology. 10th Edition. Philadelphia: W.B. Saunders Company, 2001:528–39.
7. Strichartz GR, Berde CB. Local anesthetics (Ch. 14). In: Miller RD, ed. Miller's Anesthesia. 6th Edition. Philadelphia: Elsevier, 2005:573–603.
8. Gissen AJ, Covino BG, Gregus J. Differential sensitivities of mammalian nerve fibers to local anesthetic agents. Anesthesiology 1980, 53(6):467–74.

9. DiFazio CA, Carron H, Grosslight KR, Moscicki JC, Bolding WR, Johns RA. Comparison of pH-adjusted lidocaine solutions for epidural anesthesia. Anesth Analg 1986, 65(7):760–4.

10. Gokin AP, Philip B, Strichartz GR. Preferential block of small myelinated sensory and motor fibers by lidocaine: in vivo electrophysiology in the rat sciatic nerve. Anesthesiology 2001, 95(6):1441–54.

11. Johns RA, Seyde WC, DiFazio CA, Longnecker DE. Dose-dependent effects of bupivacaine on rat muscle arterioles. Anesthesiology 1986, 65(2):186–91.

12. Johns RA, DiFazio CA, Longnecker DE. Lidocaine constricts or dilates rat arterioles in a dose-dependent manner. Anesthesiology 1985, 62(2):141–4.

13. Braid DP, Scott DB. The systemic absorption of local analgesic drugs. Br J Anaesth 1965, 37:394–404.

14. Braid DP, Scott DB. The effect of adrenaline on the systemic absorption of local anaesthetic drugs. Acta Anaesthesiol Scand Suppl 1966, 23:334–46.

15. Braid DP, Scott DB. Dosage of lignocaine in epidural block in relation to toxicity. Br J Anaesth 1966, 38(8):596–602.

16. Scott DB, Jebson PJ, Braid DP, Ortengren B, Frisch P. Factors affecting plasma levels of lignocaine and prilocaine. Br J Anaesth 1972, 44(10):1040–9.

17. Moore DC, Batra MS. The components of an effective test dose prior to epidural block. Anesthesiology 1981, 55(6):693–6.

18. Nation RL, Triggs EJ, Selig M. Lignocaine kinetics in cardiac patients and aged subjects. Br J Clin Pharmacol 1977, 4(4):439–48.

19. Englesson S. The influence of acid-base changes on central nervous system toxicity of local anesthetic agents. I. An experimental study in cats. Acta Anaesthesiol Scand 1974, 18(2):79–87.

20. Wagman IH, de Jong RH, Prince DA. Effects of lidocaine on the central nervous system. Anesthesiology 1967, 28(1):155–72.

21. Moller RA, Covino BG. Cardiac electrophysiologic effects of lidocaine and bupivacaine. Anesth Analg 1988, 67(2):107–14.

22. de Jong RH, Ronfeld RA, DeRosa RA. Cardiovascular effects of convulsant and supraconvulsant doses of amide local anesthetics. Anesth Analg 1982, 61(1):3–9.

23. Coyle DE, Sperelakis N. Bupivacaine and lidocaine blockade of calcium-mediated slow action potentials in guinea pig ventricular muscle. J Pharmacol Exp Ther 1987, 242(3):1001–5.

24. Kotelko DM, Shnider SM, Dailey PA, et al. Bupivacaine-induced cardiac arrhythmias in sheep. Anesthesiology 1984, 60(1):10–18.

25. Morishima HO, Pedersen H, Finster M, et al. Bupivacaine toxicity in pregnant and nonpregnant ewes. Anesthesiology 1985, 63(2):134–9.

26. Bjerring P, Arendt-Nielsen L. Depth and duration of skin analgesia to needle insertion after topical application of EMLA cream. Br J Anaesth 1990, 64(2):173–7.

27. Jakobson B, Nilsson A. Methemoglobinemia associated with a prilocaine-lidocaine cream and trimetoprim-sulphamethoxazole. A case report. Acta Anaesthesiol Scand 1985, 29(4):453–5.

28. Elsner P, Dummer R. Signs of methaemoglobinaemia after topical application of EMLA cream in an infant with haemangioma. Dermatology 1997, 195(2):153–4.

29. Chen BK, Cunningham BB. Topical anesthetics in children: agents and techniques that equally comfort patients, parents and clinicians. Curr Opin Pediatr 2001, 13:324–30.

30. McCafferty DF, Woolfson AD, Handley J, et al. Effect of percutaneous local anesthetics on pain reduction during pulse dye laser treatment of portwine stains. Br J Anaesth 1997, 78:286–9.

31. Woolfson A, McCafferty DF. Percutaneous local anaesthesia: drug release characteristics of the amethocaine phase-change system. Int J Pharm 1993, 94:75–80.

32. O'Brien L, Taddio A, Lyszkiewicz DA, Koren G. A critical review of the topical local anesthetic amethocaine (Amethop^{TM}) for pediatric pain. Pediatr Drugs 2005, 7(1):41–54.

33. Maloney JM, Bezzant JL, Stephen RL, Petelenz TJ. Iontophoretic administration of lidocaine anesthesia in office practice. An appraisal. J Dermatol Surg Oncol 1992, 18(11):937–40.

34. Rogers TL, Ostrow CL. The use of EMLA cream to decrease venipuncture pain in children. J Pediatr Nurs 2004, 19(1):33–9.

35. Taddio A, Gurguis MGY, Koren G. Lidocaine-prilocaine cream versus tetracaine gel for procedural pain in children. Ann Pharmacother 2002, 36(4):687–92.

36. Schatz M, Fung DL. Anaphylactic and anaphylactoid reactions due to anesthetic agents. Clin Rev Allergy 1986, 4(2):215–27.

37. Eggleston ST, Lush LW. Understanding allergic reactions to local anesthetics. Ann Pharmacother 1996, 30(7–8):851–7.

38. Soni MG, Taylor SL, Greenberg NA, Burdock GA. Evaluation of the health aspects of methyl paraben: a review of the published literature. Food Cham Toxicol 2002, 40(10):1335–73.

39. Larson CE. Methylparaben – an overlooked cause of local anesthetic hypersensitivity. Anesth Prog 1977, 24(3):72–4.

40. Feldman T, Moss J, Teplinsky K, Carroll JD. Cardiac catheterization in the patient with history of allergy to local anesthetics. Cathet Cardiovasc Diagn 1990, 20(3):165–7.

41. Landau SW, Nelson WA, Gay LN. Antihistaminic properties of local anesthetics and anesthetic properties of antihistaminic compounds. J Allergy 1951, 22(1):19–30.

42. Brown BR Jr. Pharmacology of local anesthesia. In: Clark WG, Brater DC, Johnson AR, eds. Goth's Medical Pharmacology. St. Louis: Mosby-Year Book, 1992: 397–405.

43. Dire DJ, Hogan DE. Double-blinded comparison of diphenhydramine versus lidocaine as a local anesthetic. Ann Emerg Med 1993, 22(9):1419–22.

44. Ernst AA, Anand P, Nick T, Wassmuth S. Lidocaine versus diphenhydramine for anesthesia in the repair of minor lacerations. J Trauma 1993, 34(3):354–7.

45. Ernst AA, Marvez-Valls E, Mall G, Patterson J, Xie X, Weiss SJ. 1% lidocaine versus 0.5% diphenhydramine for local anesthesia in minor laceration repair. Ann Emerg Med 1994, 23(6):1328–32.

46. McKay W, Morris R, Mushlin P. Sodium bicarbonate attenuates pain on skin infiltration with lidocaine, with or without epinephrine. Anesth Analg 1987, 66(6): 572–4.

47. Nakayama M, Munemura Y, Kanaya N, TschuchidaA Namiki. Efficacy of alkalinized lidocaine for reducing pain on intravenous or epidural catheterization. J Anesth 2001, 15:201–3.

48. Watts AC, Gaston P, Hooper G. Randomized trial of buffered versus plain lidocaine for local anesthesia in open carpal tunnel decompression. J Hand Surg [Br] 2004, 29(1):30–1.

49. Masters JE. Randomised control trial of pH buffered lignocaine with adrenaline in outpatient operations. Br J Plast Surg 1998, 51(5):385–7.

50. Burns CA, Ferris G, Feng C, Cooper JZ, Brown MD. Decreasing the pain of local anesthesia: a prospective, double-blind comparison of buffered, premixed 1% lidocaine with epinephrine versus 1% lidocaine freshly mixed with epinephrine. J Am Acad Dermatol 2006, 54(1):128–31.

51. Palmon SC, Lloyd AT, Kirsch JR. The effect of needle gauge and lidocaine pH on pain during intradermal injection. Anesth Analg 1998, 86(2):379–81.

52. Scarfone RJ, Jasani M, Gracely EJ. Pain of local anesthetics: rate of administration and buffering. Ann Emerg Med 1998, 31(1):36–40.

53. Min RJ, Khilnani NM. Endovenous laser ablation of varicose veins. J Cardiovasc Surg 2005, 46(4):395–405.

54. Klein JA. Tumescent technique for regional anesthesia permits lidocaine doses of 35 mg/kg for liposuction. J Dermatol Surg Oncol 1990, 16(3):248–63.

55. Klein JA. Tumescent technique chronicles. Local anesthesia, liposuction, and beyond. Dermatol Surg 1995, 21(5):449–57.
56. Grossmann M, Sattler G, Pistner H, et al. Pharmacokinetics of articaine hydrochloride in tumescent local anesthesia for liposuction. J Clin Pharmacol 2004, 44(11): 1282–9.
57. Oertel R, Rahn R, Kirch W. Clinical pharmacokinetics of articaine. Clin Pharmacokinet 1997, 33(6):417–25.
58. Malamed SF, Gagnon S, Leblanc D. Efficacy of articaine: a new amide local anesthetic. J Am Dent Assoc 2000, 131(5):635–42.
59. Ostad A, Kageyama N, Moy RL. Tumescent anesthesia with a lidocaine dose of 55 mg/kg is safe for liposuction. Dermatol Surg 1996, 22(11):921–7.

4

Functional Lumbar Spine Anatomy: A Review

Anthony P. Dwyer, Curt Freudenberger, Vikas V. Patel, Michael Fleisher, and Charles E. Ray, Jr.

The purpose of this chapter is to provide a brief outline of lumbar anatomy that is relevant to both the clinical evaluation of patients with low-back pain, and the role of interventional radiology (IR) in the investigation and treatment of these patients. This chapter is intentionally superficial; if further anatomical detail is desired, the reader is recommended to look up reference 1 of this chapter.

OSSEOUS STRUCTURES

So-called motion segments exist between two adjacent vertebrae in the lumbar spine. These motion segments articulate through the two posterior

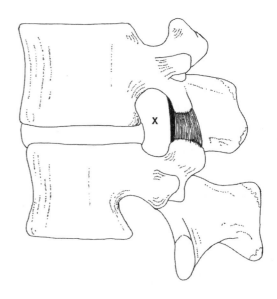

Figure 1. Line drawing demonstrating the neural foramina (X) in a sagittal projection. [Adapted from (1).]

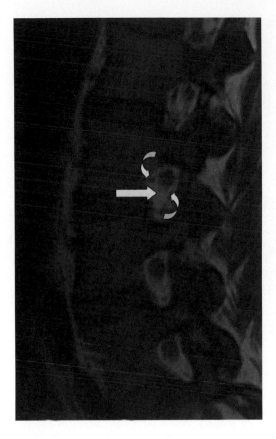

Figure 2. Sagittal T2W magnetic resonance imaging (MRI) demonstrating the neural foramina at multiple lumbar levels. Note the normal amount of fat adjacent to the exiting nerve root (block arrow). The intercostal vein and artery can be seen adjacent to the nerve root (curved arrows).

zygapophyseal (facet) joints and the anterior intervertebral disc. Other than these components of the vertebral column, the spine remains relatively static and immobile due to both osseous and ligamentous structures.

The lumbar vertebra has anterior elements (consisting of the vertebral bodies), middle elements (consisting of the pedicles), and posterior elements (consisting of the facet joints, the lamina, spinous processes, and transverse processes). The anterior elements sustain compressive loads applied to the spine, whereas the posterior elements control spinal motion through the ligaments and muscles attached to these osseous structures. The middle elements connect the anterior vertebrae body to the posterior elements, and transfer loads between these components.

The nerve roots exit the spinal column via the neural foramina, and oval-shaped space surrounded by osseous structures from two adjacent vertebrae (Figures 1, 2).

INTERVERTEBRAL DISC

The intervertebral disc is interposed between the vertebral bodies, and consists of a central gelatinous nucleus pulposis, a surrounding dense annulus fibrosis, and the cartilaginous vertebral end plates capping the adjacent vertebral body

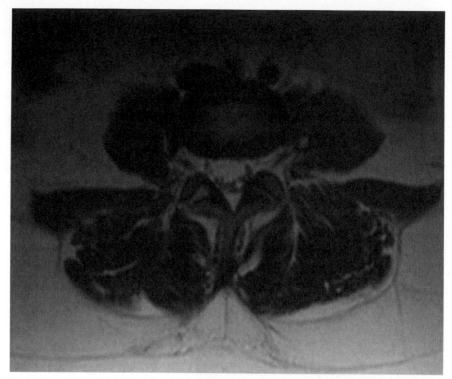

Figure 3. Axial T2W MRI demonstrating the typical appearance of a disc space. Note the higher intensity nucleus pulposus, which is largely composed of a highly fluid-comprised gelatinous material, and the lower intensity annulus fibrosis, composed largely of dense fibrous tissue.

surfaces (Figure 3). The disc is innervated by multiple sources (discussed in the following paragraphs).

LUMBAR LIGAMENTS

The posterior ligaments of the lumbar spine consist of the interspinous, super-spinous, and intertransverse ligaments. Although numerous, these posterior ligaments are not substantial structures and add little to lumbar spine stabilization (Figures 4, 5).

The iliolumbar ligament extends from the transverse process of L5 to the ilium. It is stouter than the other three posterior element groups and, when fully developed, significantly resists sliding, bending, and rotation of L5 on S1.

The ligamentum flavum courses between adjacent lamina, providing some resistance to flexion. The main role of the ligamentum flavum has been described as providing a constant, distinct elastic smooth surface along the dorsal aspect of the vertebral canal (Figure 6).

The posterior longitudinal ligament is a thin and weak ligament that does little to impede separation of the vertebral bodies. In contrast, the anterior longitudinal ligament is more robust and significantly resists hyperextension between the vertebral bodies (Figure 7).

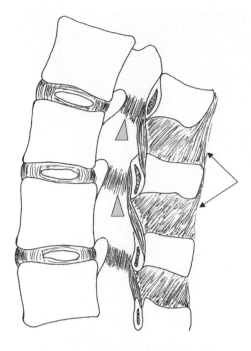

Figure 4. Line drawing demonstrating the interspinous ligaments. Like the remainder of the posterior ligaments, the interspinous ligaments are notoriously weak (arrows – interspinous ligaments; arrowheads – ligamentum flavum). [Adapted from (1).]

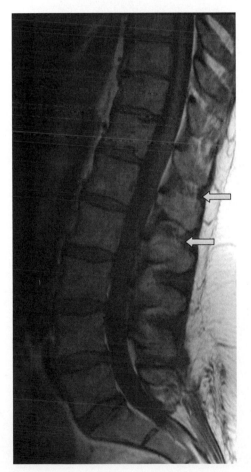

Figure 5. Sagittal T1W MRI demonstrating the fibrous interspinous ligaments (arrows).

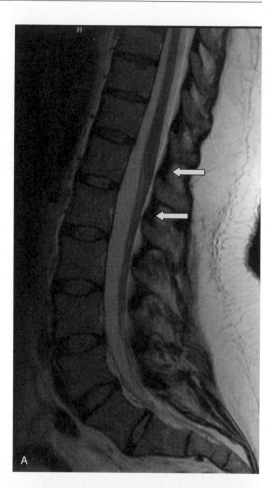

Figure 6. Sagittal (A) and axial (B) T2W MRI demonstrating the dense, lower intensity ligamentum flavum (arrows).

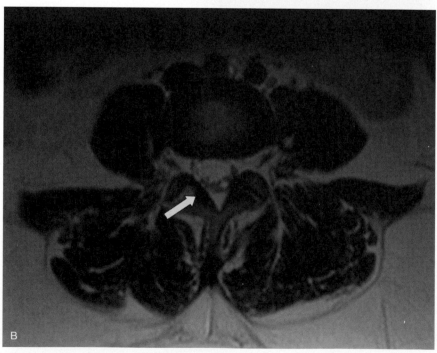

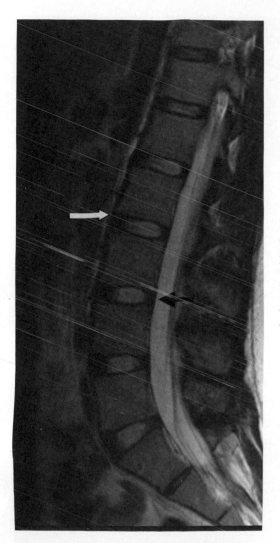

Figure 7. Sagittal MRI demonstrating the anterior (white arrow) and posterior (black arrow) longitudinal ligaments, coursing between the adjacent vertebral bodies. Although the appearance of the two structures is similar on imaging, the anterior longitudinal ligament significantly resists hyperextension of the spinal column, whereas the posterior longitudinal ligament adds little to the structural integrity of the vertebral column.

LUMBAR MUSCLES AND FASCIA

Three muscle groups comprise the lumbar paravertebral muscles. The first group is made up of the psoas major and psoas minor muscles, which course anterolaterally from the vertebral bodies. The second group is comprised of the intertransversarii lateralis and quadratus lumborum muscles, which course ventrolateral to the transverse processes of the vertebra. The third group, the posterior lumbar muscles, is further divided into three subgroups: the short intersegmental muscles, the polysegmental muscles (multifidus, and the lumbar segments of the longissimus and iliocostalis muscles), and the long polysegmental muscles (the thoracic segments of the longissimus and iliocostalis lumborium muscles) (Figure 8). The posterior lumbar muscles are attached to the erector spine aponeurosis and the three layers of the thoracolumbar ˜ia.

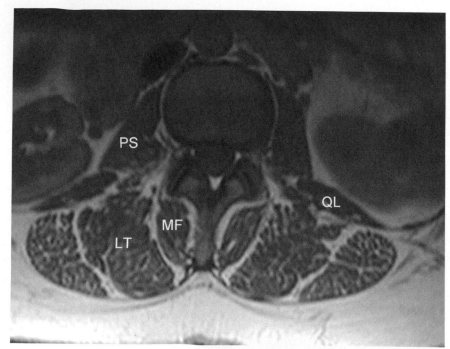

Figure 8. Axial T1W MRI demonstrating the paraspinous muscles; PS – psoas major; QL – quadratus lumborum; LT – longissimus thoracis; MF – mutifidus.

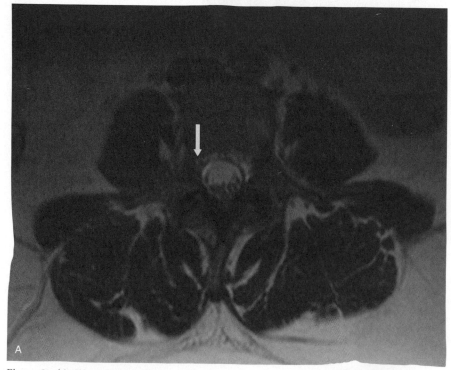

Figure 9. (A–G) Axial MRI sequence demonstratin the course of the nerve root (arrow) as it exits the vertebral column.

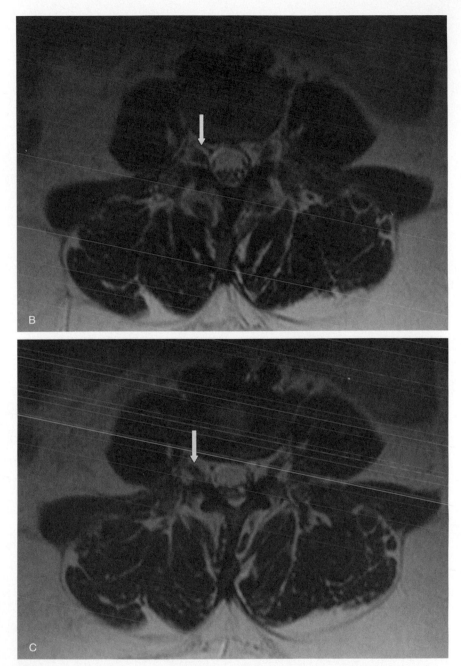

Figure 9. (*continued*)

NERVE SUPPLY OF THE LUMBAR SPINE

The exiting dorsal and ventral nerve roots join to form the spinal nerve, which subsequently divides into the larger ventral and smaller dorsal rami (Figure 9). The ventral ramus receives additional innervation from the sympathetic trunk, located along the anterolateral aspect of the lumbar spine.

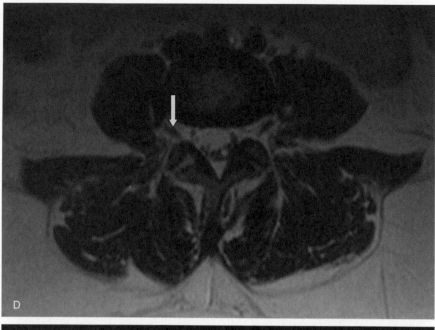

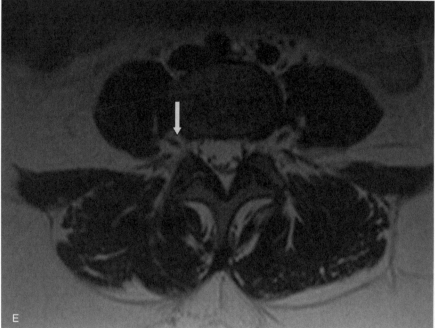

Figure 9. (*continued*)

The nerve supply to the lumbar paravertebral muscles is extensive and occurs in a segmental manner. The ventral ramus of the spinal nerve innervates the psoas major, quadratus lumborum, and intertransversarii muscles. The dorsal ramus of the spinal nerve innervates the posterior lumbar muscles and other structures posterior to the intervertebral foramen. The dorsal ramus subdivides into three major branches: the lateral branches of the dorsal ramus innervate the iliocostalis lumborum muscle, the intermediate branches supply the longissimus

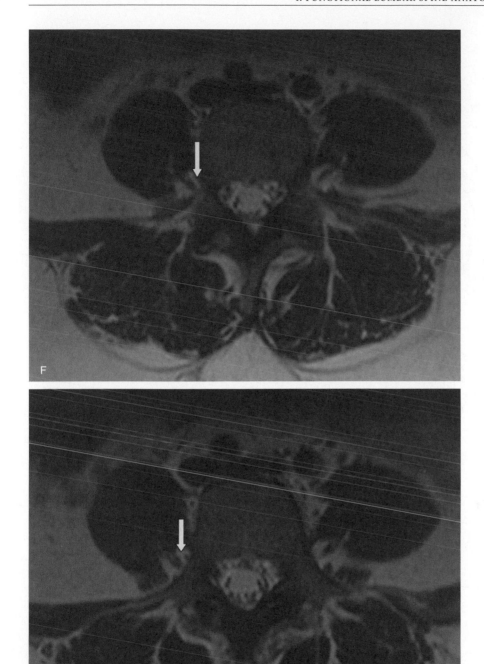

Figure 9. (*continued*)

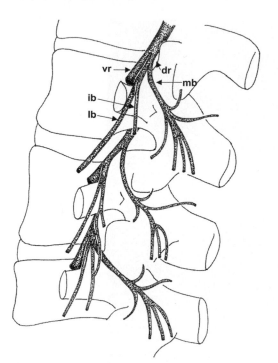

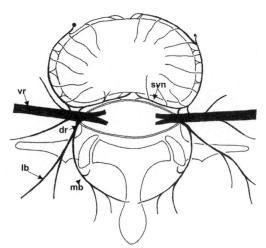

Figure 10. Sagittal drawing of the lumbar spine demonstrating branches of the nerve root after exiting from the neural foramina; vr – ventral nerve root; dr – dorsal nerve root; mb – medial branch of the dorsal nerve root; ib – intermediate branch of the dorsal nerve root; lb – lateral branch of the dorsal nerve root. [Adapted from (1).]

Figure 11. Lumbar spine innervation. The posterior elements, as well as the posterior musculature, derive their innervation from the smaller dorsal ramus (dr). The anterior elements derive their innervation from the larger ventral ramus (vr); svn – sinuvertebral nerves; lb – lateral branch of the dorsal root; mb – medial branch of the dorsal root. [Adapted from (1).]

muscles, and the medial branches innervate the short multifidus muscle, interspinous ligament, and the facet joints (Figures 10 and 11).

The vertebral bodies are innervated by the gray rami communicantes (from the sympathetic trunk) and the ventral ramus forming the anterior longitudinal and posterior longitudinal plexuses. The intervertebral discs are innervated by multiple sources: the gray rami communicantes anterolaterally, the ventral rami posterolaterally, and the sinuvertebral nerves posteriorly. The sinuvertebral nerves are recurrent branches of the ventral ramus and supply the posterior longitudinal ligament, the posterior (dorsal) aspect of the disc, and the anterior (ventral) aspect of the dura mater. The posterior (dorsal) aspect of the dura, however, has no nerve supply.

Innervation of the disc space is limited to the outer third of the annulus, which contains nerve fibers and free nerve endings. In addition, neuropeptides have been identified in the disc space, confirming the nociceptive role of these free nerve endings.

REFERENCE

1. Clinical Anatomy of the Lumbar Spine and Sacrum (4th ed.), Bogduk N (ed.). Elsevier, Churchill Livingstone, 2005.

Percutaneous Vertebroplasty

Mitchell T. Smith and Charles E. Ray, Jr.

INTRODUCTION

The first percutaneous vertebroplasty (PVP) using imaging guidance was performed in France in 1984 (1). The injection of polymethylmethacrylate (PMMA) by Galibert et al. into a painful C2 hemangioma relieved the patient's pain (1). Since that time, the interest and technical efficacy have improved to the point where PVP is used to treat osteoporotic and malignant compression fractures as well as primary and metastatic neoplasms of the vertebral bodies at all levels.

Prior to the development of PVP, painful vertebral compression fractures (VCFs) were treated conservatively. Indeed, current recommendations for PVP include failure of conservative treatment as a procedural prerequisite. The initial treatment of patients with painful VCF is a combination of immobilization, external bracing, and analgesic drugs (2).

Many pharmacological therapies are aimed at preventing the bone demineralization that can lead to compression fracture. The commonly prescribed medications include bisphosphonates, alendronate, and risedronate, which bind to hydroxyapetite and inhibit resorption. These agents are usually well tolerated and available in once weekly preparations (3,4). Calcitonin, administered as a nasal spray, prevents osteoclast-mediated bone resorption and may have analgesic properties. Finally, teriparatide, a truncation product of human parathyroid hormone, stimulates bone formation and is available for subcutaneous injection. The use of these agents can decrease the incidence of VCFs by 60% in one year (5,6).

Surgical intervention is needed in a small percentage of patients with VCFs. This is usually secondary to a neurological deficit resulting from the fracture deformity. The operations are frequently difficult and the osteoporotic bone affords marginal pedicle screw purchase (7,8). Complications include surgical wires cutting through bone and hardware failure, which can lead to a worsening spinal deformity.

A number of techniques can be used to improve results with conventional surgery. Optimization of nutritional status has been shown to be associated with increased healing and decreased mortality (9). Additionally, the use of longer constructs with multiple fixation points, sublaminar wires, and large pedicle screws with or without methylmethacrylate and bone graft can improve outcomes (10–12).

A more recent development for treatment of VCFs involves the injection of cement into the vertebral body. This is thought to splint the internal fracture and thereby decrease pain. There are two techniques that are commonly used: vertebroplasty and kyphoplasty.

Kyphoplasty, which uses a balloon tamp inflated to >200 psi to create a space within the vertebral body prior to injection of cement, was developed in 1998 by Reileyin and described by Lieberman et al. in 2001 (13). It is thought that the balloon expansion may help restore vertebral body height and, therefore, reduce the kyphotic deformity. Dublin et al. demonstrated that PVP improves pretreatment vertebral body height by approximately 47.6%, with only 15% showing no improvement in pretreatment height (14). This compares favorably to Lieberman's data, which demonstrated a restoration of 47% of pretreatment height in 70% of patients (13). Hiwatashi et al. demonstrated a 2.7-mm increase in anterior vertebral body height, 2.8 mm centrally and 1.4 mm posteriorly in 72 of 85 patients treated with PVP for osteoporotic compression fractures ($p < 0.05$ for all levels compared to pretreatment) (15). The overall height increase was more modest, but not statistically different, in patients treated for collapse caused by neoplasm (15).

Another purported benefit of kyhoplasty is a reduction of leakage or embolic events thought to be associated with the tamping procedure and the injection of higher viscosity PMMA under lower pressures. At this time, there are no firm clinical data to support this claim. The relief of pain is similar for both procedures, but kyphoplasty is more expensive due to the added equipment and is occasionally done under general anesthesia with its attendant risks . For a more in-depth discussion about kyphoplasty, please see Chapter 6.

CLINICAL INDICATIONS
Insufficiency Fractures

Compression fractures of vertebral bodies are an increasingly common problem with our aging population, and approximately 700,000 new fractures occur per year (16). The toll of these fractures is high on both the patients and our health care system. Compression fractures result in more than 150,000 hospitalizations, 161,000 physician office visits, and 5,000,000 restricted daily activities in patients 65 years and older (17,18). The lifetime risk of a symptomatic compression fracture is 16% for Caucasian females and 5% for Caucasian males (17). With increasing longevity of our aging population, osteoporosis and its clinical consequences, including vertebral compression fractures, are expected to increase fourfold (16).

Osteoporotic VCFs are associated with increased mortality. Kado et al. (1999) followed 9,575 women for eight years and found that the presence of a VCF increases mortality between 23% and 34% (19). The five-year survival rate for patients with VCF is approximately 61%, which compares unfavorably to a rate of 76% in age-matched peers (20).

Osteoporosis that leads to VCFs can be either primary or secondary. Primary osteoporosis is secondary to the uncoupling of bone remodeling; this starts at age 30 and progresses with 3–5% loss of bone per decade (21). Radiographically identified compression fractures of the thoracolumbar spine are observed in up to 26% of women older than 50 years of age, with a concomitant loss of 15% of the vertebral height (22). Men appear to be affected approximately half as often as women (81 per 100,000 person-years compared to 153 per 100,000 person-years, respectively) (23).

Secondary osteoporosis is common in patients being treated with steroids for asthma, chronic obstructive pulmonary disease, rheumatoid arthritis, and transplantation. Secondary osteoporosis is also seen as a side effect of anti-androgenic therapy for prostate cancer (24). Some estimates indicate that in all patients with osteoporosis, 50% of men and 20% of women have secondary causes (25,26).

The most striking outcome post-PVP is a decrease in the patient's pain. Kobayashi et al. performed 205 PVPs in 175 patients and demonstrated that their pain, as measured on an 11-level visual analog scale (VAS), dropped from 7.22 to 2.07 one day after the procedure ($p < 0.0001$) (27). The pain improved in 96.4% of patients and disappeared in 44% of them (27). McGraw et al. performed 156 PVPs in 100 patients and demonstrated improvement of pain in 97% 12 to 24 hours postprocedure that, as measured by a 0–10 VAS, improved from 8.91 to 2.02 ($p < 0.001$) (28). Additionally, 91 of 99 patients were able to decrease the amount of oral pain medication required (28). Hodler et al. showed that pain was absent or better in 86% of treated patients initially; and at a mean follow-up of 8.8 months, 88.4% had remained pain free or had improvement relative to their preprocedural state (29). Grados et al. demonstrated persistent pain relief at the treated level and no progression of vertebral deformity 12–84 months postprocedure (mean follow-up = 48 months) (30).

Additional benefits include improved quality of life and ambulation. Kobayashi et al. compared a PVP group to a conservatively treated control group and found that the interval to ambulation was decreased by 22 days (1.9 compared to 23.9 days) (27). Evans et al. reported on a patient group where 72% of a pretreatment group displayed impaired ambulation that improved to 28% posttreatment. Activities of daily living, as assessed by a questionnaire, demonstrated a statistically significant improvement ($p < .001$) (31). In addition to showing decreasing pain for a two-year interval, Trout et al. showed that early PVP in fracture patients can reduce hospital stays (32).

Burst Fractures

There is some evidence that, in carefully selected patients, PVP can be used to treat burst fractures. Chen and Lee selected six patients with anterior- and middle-column burst fractures, minimal retropulsion of bony fragments, and persistent pain after conservative therapy for PVP (33). These patients reported a statistically significant decrease in their pain (scored on a 0–100 pain VAS) from 84.3 at baseline to 34.7 on postoperative day 3 and 30.2 at postoperative month 3 (33). There was also the suggestion that PVP in this small sample was associated with an increase in mobility (33). Four of six treated vertebrae in this series had PMMA leakage through the end plate and into the disc space without any clinical symptoms (33). With the amount of leakage, this technique may be most suitable for subacute to chronic fractures that have not improved with conservative treatment.

NEOPLASTIC INDICATIONS

Indications for PVP in neoplasia include treatment of painful hemangiomas or compression fractures secondary to osteolytic metastases or myeloma, and as a method for the treatment of refractory spinal pain in patients with multiple metastases.

Hemangiomas

Hemangiomas of the vertebral bodies are common lesions that have been seen at autopsy in up to 11% of patients (34). In 67% of patients, these are solitary, incidental findings on radiograph, computed tomography (CT), or magnetic resonance imaging (MRI) scans of the thoracic spine (35,36). Hemangiomas come to clinical attention secondary to pain with or without pathological fracture, spinal cord compression with resultant neurological deficit, or expansion of the vertebral body and/or posterior elements (36–38). Traditional methods for the treatment of vertebral hemangiomas have included irradiation, surgery with or without radiation therapy, or preoperative embolization with subsequent surgery (39). PVP in the setting of hemangioma is typically used for an analgesic effect, to retard secondary deformation of the vertebral body, or as a preoperative measure to diminish operative blood loss. The mechanism for the analgesic effect is unknown, but it has been postulated that this effect is likely due to chemical ablation of pain-sensitive nerve endings and/or from the stabilization of microfractures. PVP of hemangiomas has been demonstrated to reduce the risk of hemorrhage with spinal surgery (40).

Neoplastic Compression Fractures with and without Refractory Pain

Pain that can limit activity and lead to associated increases in morbidity and mortality from bedsores, deep venous thrombosis, and pulmonary complications is often seen in patients with metastatic disease to the spine. PVP can help to relieve pain and stabilize fractures in the palliative setting late in life (41–43).

Weill et al. treated 37 cancer patients with 52 vertebroplasties and found that 73% of the procedures performed for analgesia resulted in clear improvement, seven showed moderate improvement, and two demonstrated no improvement (41). The improvement was stable in 73% of patients at six months (41). Cortet et al. treated 40 vertebrae in 37 patients and found that 97.3% reported a decrease in their pain within 48 hours with 13.5% being completely pain free (44). The reduction in pain was not correlated to the extent of cement filling the vertebral body and persisted in 75% of treated cases at 6 months (44).

Timing of Intervention

As a general rule, patients with acute compression fractures who demonstrate bone marrow edema on T2 or STIR MRI sequences will benefit from PVP. Brown et al. compared outcomes of 15 patients with bone marrow edema on MRI to 45 patients without bone marrow edema (45). Although marrow edema was not precisely correlated with fracture age, all patients with edema had elimination or reduction of pain and 67% reported improved mobility; in patients without marrow edema, 80% reported elimination or reduction of pain and 57% reported improved mobility (differences between the groups were not statistically different) (45).

There were initial studies that reported poor outcomes with subacute or chronic fractures at 6 or 12 months (46,47). More recently, a report by Brown et al. found that patients with fractures treated by PVP that were 12–24 months old had mobility improvement (although not significantly different) from a control group of patients with acute fractures treated with PVP (48). Even though mobility was improved, the relief of pain was less robust in the older treated fractures (48). Kaufmann et al. performed 122 PVPs in 75 patients whose mean fracture age was 19 weeks and reported decreased pain and increased mobility for the entire cohort (49).

In summary, the effectiveness of PVP for a given fracture on the basis of age has not been clearly established in the literature, although imaging studies suggest bone marrow edema seems to be associated with positive outcomes.

TECHNIQUE

Physical Exam

A pertinent clinical history should be obtained prior to procedural intervention to exclude causes of back pain not treatable by PVP. These include disc disease with resultant spinal cord or nerve root compression, spinal stenosis, facet disease, and discogenic back pain. Patients with a compression fracture will usually report sudden onset of pain at a specific spinal level that is exacerbated with weight bearing and relieved by the supine position. Physical exam should confirm pain with palpation at a single site that corresponds to a compression deformity on radiograph. If multiple deformities are present, additional imaging should be performed to determine the specific site for intervention.

Preprocedural Imaging

Lateral radiographs of the spine will typically demonstrate diffuse osteopenia with one or more wedge compression deformities. The treatment decision is uncomplicated if the patient has one compression deformity, can recall an exact time of injury, and demonstrates pain with palpation at that specific level. In the absence of these three indicators, serial radiographs may be helpful in determining the acuity of several fractures and the level to be treated.

A thin-slice CT scan with multiplanar reformations may be of use if there is a question of posterior cortex involvement, which would be a relative procedural contraindication.

In the absence of clearly defined fractures, an MRI or bone scan may be useful for determination of treatment level. MRIs looking for edema on T2-sensitive or STIR sequences, or enhancement on fat-saturated gadolinium-enhanced T1 sequences, can help to pinpoint a vertebral body for treatment (Figure 1). MRI also has the advantage of obtaining anatomic information regarding other potential causes for the patient's pain (metastatic or disc disease) and for evaluation of cord compromise (50).

In patients who cannot receive an MRI exam, a bone scan can help to elucidate the treatment level in a patient with multiple compression fractures. Maynard et al. used bone scans as preprocedural planning in 28 PVPs and found subjective pain relief in 93% of cases, with an improvement in mobility seen in half the cases (improvement of one level on a five-point subjective scale) (46). A caveat with bone scans is that patients two years out from fracture may have continued activity on the bone scan and the efficacy of PVP in patients that far removed from injury has not been fully evaluated.

The preprocedural workup in the setting of neoplasm should include CT or MRI to evaluate the extent of tumoral burden and to evaluate for destruction of posterior vertebral body cortex or epidural tumor, both relative contraindications due to risk of cement extravasation.

Contraindications

Absolute contraindications to PVP include local infection (including osteo-myelitis, discitis, and epidural abscess). Patients with generalized signs of infection (fever or infectious leukocytosis) should not be treated until their signs resolve. Anyone with significant coagulopathy should have this corrected prior to the introduction of the large-bore needles used for PVP; the authors use an

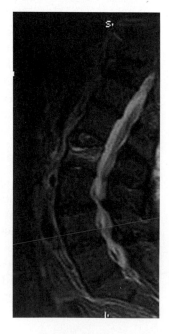

Figure 1. MRI of osteoporotic compression fracture. Sagittal STIR image demonstrates a 20–30% compression deformity of the L2 vertebral body. There are associated moderate marrow edematous changes and a linear transversely oriented fracture compatible with an acute event. Note also the compression deformity of T11, with decreased signal intensity; the patient had a previous kyphoplasty at this level. (Image courtesy of Robert Allen, MD.)

INR >2.0 as a contraindication. Finally, the patient should have no documented allergies to any of the components in the cement mixture (such allergies are exceedingly rare).

Relative contraindications include severe radiculopathy, tumor extension into the epidural space, posterior cortical defects, and retropulsion of osseous fragments with canal compromise (even in asymptomatic patients).

Procedural Imaging

PVP is typically performed using either multiplanar fluoroscopic guidance or, in some institutions, CT guidance. Some authors have used a single-plane C-arm using an oblique projection advancing the needle into the pedicle prior to advancing the needle into the anterior third of the vertebral body on the lateral view and confirming a central location on the posteroanterior view (51).

One area where fluoroscopic guidance is likely superior to CT is intraprocedural evaluation of cement injection. With CT evaluation of cement injection, care must be taken to evaluate a large enough field of view to be certain that leakage is not occurring outside the field of view.

Technique

CERVICAL SPINE

The cervical spine has been amenable to PVP using a direct transoral or anterolateral approach (52–56). The transoral approach is the most straightforward, but it usually requires general anesthesia, excellent visualization, and superb disinfection of oral mucosa. This technique has been used to treat an aneurismal bone cyst with pain relief at 18 months postprocedure and C1/2 instability at six months (54).

The anterolateral approach requires extension of the head to expose the neck and elevate the mandible with palpation and lateral displacement of the carotid space (56). The needle is placed 1 cm below the level of the angle of the mandible and inserted until contact is made with the vertebral body (56). The needle will traverse, in order, the parapharyngeal, retropharyngeal, and prevertebral spaces (56). Once placement is confirmed radiographically, cement injection is performed in the standard fashion.

THORACIC AND LUMBAR SPINE

Treatment of the vertebral bodies in the thoracic and lumbar spine uses a unipedicular, bipedicular, parapedicular, or transcostovertebral approach. The transpedicular route is the most commonly used; it is advantageous as it offers a defined anatomic landmark and places no other structures (lung, nerve root, spinal cord, or vasculature) at significant risk. With small pedicles (i.e., in the upper thoracic spine), a parapedicular or transcostovertebral approach is used to avoid pedicle fracture and to, in theory, allow more uniform filling of the vertebral body as the needle is closer to midline. Kim et al. found that they were able to fill both halves of the vertebral body in 96% of patients using a unipedicular approach that enters the pedicle lateral to the superior articulating facet (57).

An antibiotic is administered prior to the start of the procedure; the authors use 1 g of cefazolin intravenously. Regardless of the approach used, the subcutaneous soft tissues and bony periosteum of the upper lateral pedicle are anesthetized using 5–10 ml of 0.25% bupivicaine or 1% lidocaine. A small incision is made in the skin and the vertebroplasty needle is advanced to the pedicle. To violate the periosoteum and advance the needle, a twisting motion or sterile orthopedic hammer can be used. Lateral and PA fluoroscopy should be used to position the needle in the anterior third of the vertebral body as close to midline as possible.

Intravertebral venography has received much attention as a method to prevent unwanted PMMA leakage. There are multiple arguments in the literature both for and against venography, and multiple contrast agents have been investigated (58–63). McGraw et al. performed 135 intraosseus venograms and demonstrated that bilateral marrow blush was 95% predictive of contralateral hemivertibrae cement deposition (60). Other authors have stated that viscosity differences between contrast and PMMA are not predictive of spread and that venography increases the risk of contrast reaction (64). It is likely that as the operator's experience and skill increase, the need for venography will decrease.

Choice of cement, opacifying agents, and intravertebral antibiotics is operator dependent, and many different combinations have been used successfully. PMMA Simplex P (Stryker-How-Medica-Osteonics, Rutherford, NJ) was the first cement used for PVP and, at the time of preparation of this manuscript, the only FDA-approved cement for pathological fractures of the spine. However, many different cement formulas have been used; patients should be informed that a particular mixture is an "off-label" use and told the physician's reasons for using the particular mixture. More important than the actual cement is the prevention of leaks during the procedure.

The authors use PMMA powder mixed with tobramyacin powder and barium sulfate for opacification (additional opacifying agents include tantalum powder and tungsten powder). The components are combined in a sterile vacuum and mixed until a cake-glaze consistency is obtained. The cement is prepared after the needles are in place. The injection of cement can be accomplished with either 1-ml syringes or a device specifically for cement injection under either high or low pressure (Parallax Medical, Scotts Valley, CA). Other devices and kits are frequently being introduced into the market and are commercially available from a variety of vendors.

Regardless of the device used for injection, the opacification of the vertebral body should be done with continuous fluoroscopic observation or intermittently after the injection of 0.1–0.2 ml. The injection is continued until resistance is met (which may indicate a plug at the end of the needle or tubing that needs clearing), cement reaches the posterior fourth of the vertebral body, or the desired volume is achieved. Absolute contraindication to continuing cement injection is epidural, foraminal, or venous extravasation.

The amount of cement needed to stabilize fractures or produce pain relief has not been empirically determined. A guideline proposed by Mathis and Wong is that the amount of cement should fill between 50% and 70% of the remaining vertebral body (64). This is up to 4 ml in the thoracic spine and up to 8 ml in the lumbar spine (64). *In vitro* testing demonstrates that 2 ml of PMMA will increase strength, but 4–8 ml is needed for restoration of stiffness (65).

At the completion of the procedure, the cannula is removed without the reintroduction of the stylet as this will push the contents of the cannula into the vertebral body. Cement deposition in the needle tract is a complication that may require surgical intervention. This can be avoided by redirecting the needle superiorly and advancing toward the superior end plate prior to the removal of the needle (66). Direct pressure at the end of the procedure is used for homeostasis and to prevent subcutaneous hematoma.

Figure 2 demonstrates the pertinent steps in performing vertebroplasty.

Postprocedural Imaging

Postprocedural imaging may be performed to evaluate for additional compression deformities in a patient with a new history of back pain. The previously described modalities are all appropriate for this indication.

More problematic is to evaluate the vertebroplasty itself. Dansie et al. used MRI to evaluate 51 treated vertebrae in 30 patients to determine the normal postprocedural appearance (67). Moderate to severe marrow edema was observed in 66% of preprocedural vertebrae, in 63% imaged at 0–6 weeks post-PVP, and in 22% of vertebrae more than six months post-PVP (67).

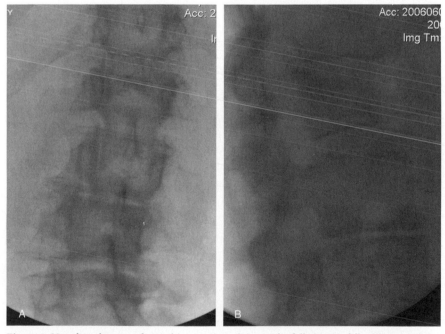

Figure 2. Vertebroplasty performed in a patient three weeks following a fall with acute pain and a compression fracture. (A) Preprocedural spot AP fluoroscopic image demonstrates a moderate compression deformity of the L1 vertebral body. (B) Preprocedural spot lateral fluoroscopic image demonstrates the compression deformity. (C) Spot fluoroscopic image demonstrating needles placed via both pedicles into the vertebral body. (D) Lateral image during early cement injection demonstrating filling of the anterior portion of the vertebral body. (E) Final image demonstrating cement preferentially in the upper portion of the vertebral body. (F) Final image demonstrating cement post-injection. (Images courtesy of Robert Allen, MD.)

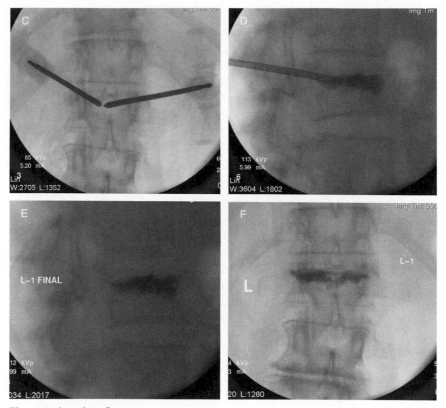

Figure 2. (*continued*)

Additional height loss postprocedure was noted in 18% of treated vertebral levels (67). As suggested by this study, because the patients did not have postprocedural pain at the level treated, edema and height loss should not be used as evidence of persistent pathology at a treated level (67).

Due to the lack of evidence documenting the best postprocedural imaging modality, which modality to use is left largely to the discretion of the operator. The absolute need for imaging is also open to debate, with most operators finding clinical follow-up sufficient.

Complications

CEMENT EXTRAVASATION

The most common complication from PVP is cement extravasation. This complication is usually clinically silent and in some reported series occurs in up to 67% of patients (68). Cement leakage that results in spinal cord compression or radiculopathy is more common in PVP treatment of metastatic disease or myeloma than in treatment of osteoporotic vertebral bodies. In treating osteoporotic compression fractures, Chiras reported complication rates of only 4% and 0.5% for radiculopathy and cord compression, respectively (69).

Schmidt et al. compared radiographs, fluoroscopy, and CT scans for determination of cement extravasation and found that only 34% of leaks were identified with a lateral radiograph from a total of 81% identified by CT scan (70).

Embolism of glue particles into the basivertebral venous system, and ultimately the broader systemic circulation, is a serious complication. Seo et al. described a polymerized 14-cm segment of glue in the IVC with concomitant pulmonary embolus in a 72-year-old treated with PVP (71). Monticelli et al. described a fatal pulmonary embolus from a vertebroplasty (72). The patient became hypoxic 15 minutes postprocedure and died from cement embolism (72). In their report, the authors postulate that insufficient polymerization secondary to unbalanced monomer-to-powder ratio may have been to blame (72). Francois et al. report on a cement embolus that was treated by pulling the embolus with a catheter-based basket into the lobar branch of the right pulmonary artery prior to removal during open heart surgery (73). An even more rare complication was described by Park et al. when an embolized particle of cement eroded through the right ventricular wall and caused ST elevation, hemopericardium, and acute pericarditis (74). The acrylic fragments were removed during open heart surgery (74).

CONTIGUOUS VERTEBRAL BODY COLLAPSE

A second controversy regarding PVP is whether or not it causes contiguous vertebral body collapse. Lindsay et al. demonstrated that 21.9% of Caucasian females who have one compression fracture secondary to osteoporosis will develop a subsequent fracture within one year (75). Uppin et al. found that of an initial study group that contained 177 patients treated with PVP, 22 patients (12.4%) suffered 36 additional compression fractures; 67% of these fractures occurred at levels contiguous to the previous PVP (76). Syed et al. observed 253 patients for one year following PVP and found that 21.7% of the study group developed additional fractures within the year (77). To our knowledge, there are no controlled or cohort studies to determine whether these results represent fractures induced by the initial PVP or represent disease progression.

Ex vivo studies have suggested that both PVP and kyphoplasty will transmit greater pressure to the nucleus pulposus, although neither procedure will increase pressure over the *in vivo* state (78). Grados et al. found that the odds ratio of a subsequent fracture at a level contiguous to previous PVP was 2.27 (79). This was greater than 1.44, which was the odds ratio for a new fracture next to an untreated vertebral body (79).

Although there is some evidence that PVP will increase the risk of contiguous vertebral body fracture, the overall incidence does not appear higher in the small study groups in the literature. Overall, approximately 1/5 of women who have a first osteoporotic vertebral compression fracture can expect to have an additional fracture in one year (75). This appears to be true whether or not PVP has been performed.

CONCLUSIONS

PVP is a minimally invasive technique that reduces pain from osteoporotic and malignant vertebral compression fractures as well as from spinal neoplasms. Long-term results are good and include increased mobility and early discharge from the hospital. There are few contraindications and, in experienced hands, the significant complication rate is low.

REFERENCES

1. Galibert P, Deramond H, Rosat P, Le Gars D. Preliminary note on the treatment of vertebral angioma by percutaneous acrylic vertebroplasty. Neurochirurgie. 1987; 33:166–8.

2. Tamayo-Orozco J, Arzac-Palumbo P, Peon-Vidales H. Vertebral fractures associated with osteoporosis: patient management. Am J Med. 1997;18:S44–50.

3. Simon JA, Lewiecki EM, Smith ME, Petruschke RA, Wang L, Palmisano JJ. Patient preference for once-weekly alendronate 70 mg versus once-daily alendronate 10 mg: a multicenter, randomized, open-label, crossover study. Clin Ther. 2002;24:871–86.

4. Brown JP, Kendler DL, McClung MR, et al. The efficacy and tolerability of risedronate once a week for the treatment of postmenopausal osteoporosis. Calcif Tissue Int. 2002;71:103–11.

5. Harris ST, Watts NB, Genant HK, et al. Effects of risedronate treatment on vertebral and nonvertebral fractures in women with postmenopausal osteoporosis: a random-ized controlled trial. Vertebral Efficacy With Risedronate Therapy (VERT) Study Group. JAMA. 1999;282:1344–52.

6. Neer RM, Arnaud CD, Zanchetta JR, et al. Effect of parathyroid hormone (1–34) on fractures and bone mineral density in postmenopausal women with osteoporosis. N Engl J Med. 2001;344:1434–41.

7. Fujita T, Kostuik JP, Huckell CB, Sieber AN. Complications of spinal fusion in adult patients more than 60 years of age. Orthop Clin North Am. 1998;29:669–78.

8. Linville DA, Bridwell KH, Lenke LG, Vedantam R, Leicht P. Complications in the adult spinal deformity patient having combined surgery. Does revision increase the risk? Spine. 1999;24:355–63.

9. Hu SS, Fontaine F, Kelly B, Bradford DS. Nutritional depletion in staged spinal reconstructive surgery. The effect of total parenteral nutrition. Spine. 1998;23: 1401–5.

10. Hu SS. Internal fixation in the osteoporotic spine. Spine. 1997;22(24 Suppl):43S–8S.

11. Sarzier JS, Evans AJ, Cahill DW. Increased pedicle screw pullout strength with vertebroplasty augmentation in osteoporotic spines. J Neurosurg. 2002;96(3 Suppl): 309–12.

12. Wuisman PI, Van Dijk M, Staal H, Van Royen BJ. Augmentation of (pedicle) screws with calcium apatite cement in patients with severe progressive osteoporotic spinal deformities: an innovative technique. Eur Spine J. 2000;9:528–33.

13. Lieberman IH, Dudeney S, Reinhardt MK, Bell G. Initial outcome and efficacy of "kyphoplasty" in the treatment of painful osteoporotic vertebral compression frac-tures. Spine. 2001;26:1631–8.

14. Dublin AB, Hartman J, Latchaw RE, Hald JK, Reid MH. The vertebral body fracture in osteoporosis: restoration of height using percutaneous vertebroplasty. Am J Neu-roradiol. 2005;26:489–92.

15. Hiwatashi A, Moritani T, Numaguchi Y, Westesson P. Increase in vertebral body height after vertebroplasty. Am J Neuroradiol. 2003;23:185–9.

16. Riggs BL, Melton LJ III. The worldwide problem of osteoporosis: insights afforded by epidemiology. Bone. 1995;17:505S–11S.

17. Melton LJ III. Epidemiology of spinal osteoporosis. Spine. 1997;22(Suppl 24):2S–11S.

18. Jacobsen SJ, Cooper C, Gottlieb MS, et al. Hospitalization with vertebral fracture among the aged: a national population based study, 1986–1989. Epidemiology. 1992;3(6):515–8.

19. Kado DM, Browner WS, Palermo L, Nevitt MC, Genant HK, Cummings SR. Verte-bral fractures and mortality in older women: a prospective study. Study of Osteo-porotic Fractures Research Group. Arch Intern Med. 1999;159:1215–20.

20. Cooper C, Atkinson EJ, Jacobsen SJ, O'Fallon WM, Melton LJ III. Population-based study of survival after osteoporotic fractures. Am J Epidemiol. 1993;137: 1001–5.

21. World Health Organization Study Group. Assessment of fracture risk and its application to screening for postmenopausal osteoporosis. Report no. 843. Geneva; 1994.

22. Melton LF III, Kan SH, Frye MA, Wahner HW, O'Fallon WM, Riggs BL. Epidemiology of vertebral fractures in women. Am J Epidemiol. 1989;129:1000–11.

23. Cooper C, Atkinson EJ, O'Fallon WM, Melton LJ III. Incidence of clinically diagnosed vertebral fractures: a population-based study in Rochester, Minnesota, 1985–1989. J Bone Miner Res. 1992;7:221–7.

24. Ross RW, Small EJ. Osteoporosis in men treated with androgen deprivation therapy for prostate cancer. J Urol. 2002;167:1952–6.

25. Fitzpatrick LA. Secondary causes of osteoporosis. Mayo Clin Proc. 2002;77:453–8.

26. Nolla JM, Gomez-Vaquero C, Romera, M, et al. Osteoporotic vertebral fractures in clinical practice: 669 patients diagnosed over a 10 year period. J Rheumatol. 2001;28:2289–93.

27. Kobayashi K, Shimoyama K, Nakamura K, Murata K. Percutaneous vertebroplasty immediately relieves pain of osteoporotic vertebral compression fractures and prevents prolonged immobilization of patients. Eur Radiol. 2005;15:360–7.

28. McGraw JK, Lippert JA, Minkus KD, Rami PM, Davis TM, Budzik RF. Prospective evaluation of pain relief in 100 patients undergoing percutaneous vertebroplasty: results and follow-up. J Vasc Intervent Radiol. 2002;13:883–6.

29. Hodler J, Peck D, Gilula LA. Midterm outcome after vertebroplasty: predictive value of technical and patient-related factors. Radiology. 2003;227:662–8.

30. Grados F, Depriester C, Cayrolle G, et al. Long-term observations of vertebral osteoporotic fractures treated by percutaneous vertebroplasty. Rheumatology. 2000;39:1410–4.

31. Evans AJ, Jensen ME, Kip KE, et al. Vertebral compression fractures: pain reduction and improvement in functional mobility after percutaneous polymethylmethacrylate vertebroplasty retrospective report of 245 cases. Radiology. 2003;226:366–72.

32. Trout AF, Gray LA, Kallmes DF. Vertebroplasty in the inpatient population. Am J Neuroradiol. 2005;26:1629–33.

33. Chen JF, Lee ST. Percutaneous vertebroplasty for treatment of thoracolumbar spine bursting fracture. Surg Neurol. 2004;62:494–500.

34. Schmorl G, Junghanns H. The Human Spine in Health and Disease. 2nd ed. New York: Grune and Stratton, 1971.

35. Laredo JD, Reizine D, Bard M, Merland JJ. Vertebral hemangiomas: radiographic evaluation. Radiology. 1986;161:183–9.

36. Krueger EG, Sobel GL, Weinstein C. Vertebral hemangioma with compression of the spinal cord. J Neurosurg. 1961;18:331–8.

37. McAllister VL, Kendall BE, Bull JW. Symptomatic vertebral haemangiomas. Brain. 1975;98:71–80.

38. Nguyen JP, Djindjian M, Gaston A, et al. Vertebral hemangiomas presenting with neurologic symptoms. Surg Neurol. 1987;27:391–7.

39. Acosta F, Dowd C, Chin C, Tihan T, Ames C, Weinstein P. Treatment strategies and outcomes in the management of symptomatic vertebral hemangiomas. Neurosurgery. 2006;58:287–95.

40. Ide C, Gangi A, Rimmelin A, et al. Vertebral haemangiomas with spinal cord compression: the place of preoperative percutaneous vertebroplasty with methyl methacrylate. Neuroradiology. 1996;38:585–9.

41. Weill A, Chiras J, Simon JM, et al. Spinal metastases: indications for and results of percutaneous injection of acrylic surgical cement. Radiology. 1996;199:241–7.

42. Cotten A, Dewatre F, Cortet B, et al. Percutaneous vertebroplasty for osteolytic metastases and myeloma: effects of the percentage of lesion filling and the leakage of methyl methacrylate at clinical follow-up. Radiology. 1996;200:525–30.

43. Pilitsis JG, Rengachary SS. The role of vertebroplasty in metastatic spinal disease. Neurosurg Focus. 2001;11:1–4.

44. Cortet B, Cotten A, Boutry N, et al. Percutaneous vertebroplasty in patients with osteolytic metastases or multiple myeloma. Rhum Engl Rev Ed. 1997;64:177–83.

45. Brown DB, Glaiberman CB, Gilula LA, Shimony JS. Correlation between preprocedural MRI findings and clinical outcomes in the treatment of chronic symptomatic vertebral compression fractures with percutaneous vertebroplasty. Am J Roentg. 2005;184:1951–5.

46. Maynard AS, Jensen ME, Schweickert PA, Marx WF, Short JG, Kallmes DF. Value of bone scan imaging in predicting pain relief from percutaneous vertebroplasty in osteoporotic vertebral fractures. Am J Neuroradiol. 2000;21:1807–12.

47. Jensen ME, Dion JE. Percutaneous vertebroplasty in the treatment of osteoporotic compression fractures. Neuroimaging Clin N Am. 2000;10:547–68.

48. Brown DB, Gilula LA, Seghal M, Shimony JS. Treatment of chronic symptomatic vertebral compression fractures with percutaneous vertebroplasty. Am J Roentg. 2004;182:319–22.

49. Kaufmann TJ, Jensen ME, Schweickert PA, Marx WF, Kallmes DF. Age of fracture and clinical outcomes of percutaneous vertebroplasty. Am J Neuroradiol. 2001;22:1860–3.

50. Do HM. Magnetic resonance imaging in the evaluation of patients for percutaneous vertebroplasty. Top Magn Reson Imaging. 2000;(4):235–44.

51. Koyama M, Takizawa K, Kobayashi K, et al. Initial experience of percutaneous vertebroplasty using single-plane C-arm fluoroscopy for guidance. Radiat Med. 2005; 23(4):256–60.

52. Cotten A, Dewatre F, Cortet B, et al. Percutaneous vertebroplasty for osteolytic metastases and myeloma: effects of the percentage of lesion filling and the leakage of methyl methacrylate at clinical follow-up. Radiology. 1996;200:525–30.

53. Martin JB, Gailloud P, Dietrich PY, et al. Direct transoral approach to C2 for percutaneous vertebroplasty. Cardiovasc Intervent Radiol. 2002;25:517–19.

54. Gailloud P, Martin JB, Olivi A, Rufenacht DA, Murphy KJ. Transoral vertebroplasty for a fractured C2 aneurysmal bone cyst. J Vasc Interv Radiol. 2002;13:340–1.

55. Tong FC, Cloft HJ, Joseph GJ, Rodts GR, Dion JE. Transoral approach to cervical vertebroplasty for multiple myeloma. Am J Roentgenol. 2000;175:1322–4.

56. Mont'Alverne F, Vallee JN, Cormier E, et al. Percutaneous vertebroplasty for metastatic involvement of the axis. Am J Neuroradiol. 2005;26(7):1641–5.

57. Kim A, Jensen M, Dion J, Schweickert P, Kaufmann T, Kallmes D. Unilateral transpedicular percutaneous vertebroplasty: initial experience. Radiology. 2002;222: 737–41.

58. Tanigawa N, Komemushi A, Kariya S, Kojima H, Sawada S. Intraosseous venography with carbon dioxide contrast agent in percutaneous vertebroplasty. Am J Roentgenol. 2005;184:567–70.

59. Jansen ME, Evans AJ, Mathis JM, et al. Percutaneous polymethylmethacrylate vertebroplasty in the treatment of osteoporotic vertebral body compression fractures: technical aspect. Am J Neuroradiol. 1997;18:1897–904.

60. McGraw JK, Heatwole EV, Strnad BT, Silber JS, Patzilk SB, Boorstein JM. Predictive value of intraosseous venography before percutaneous vertebroplasty. J Vasc Interv Radiol. 2002;13:149–53.

61. Weill A, Chiras J, Simon JM, et al. Spinal metastases: indications for and results of percutaneous injection of acrylic surgical cement. Radiology. 1996;99:241–7.

62. Gaughen JR, Jensen ME, Schweickert PA, Kaufmann TJ, Marx WF, Kallmes DF. Relevance of antecedent venography in percutaneous vertebroplasty for the treatment of osteoporotic compression fractures. Am J Neuroradiol. 2002;23:594–600.

63. Gaughen JR Jr., Jensen ME, Schweickert PA, Kaufmann TJ, Marx WF, Kallmes DF. Is percutaneous vertebroplasty without pretreatment venography safe? Evaluation of 205 consecutive procedures. Am J Neuroradiol. 2002;23:913–7.

64. Mathis JM, Wong W. Percutaneous vertebroplasty: technical considerations. J Vasc Interv Radiol. 2003;14:953–60.

65. Belkoff SM, Mathis JM, Jasper LE, Deramond H. The biomechanics of vertebroplasty: the effect of cement volume on mechanical behavior. Spine. 2001;26:1537–41.
66. Kaufmann TJ, Wald JT, Kallmes DF. A technique to circumvent subcutaneous cement tracts during percutaneous vertebroplasty. Am J Neuroradiol. 2004;25: 1595–6.
67. Dansie DM, Luetmer PH, Lane JI, Thielen KR, Wald JT, Kallmes DF. MRI findings after successful vertebroplasty. Am J Neuroradiol. 2005;26:1595–600.
68. Cotten A, Dewatre F, Cortet B, et al. Percutaneous vertebroplasty for osteolytic metastases and myeloma: effects of the percentage of lesion filling and the leakage of methyl methacrylate at clinical follow-up. Radiology. 1996;200:525–30.
69. Chiras J. Percutaneous vertebral surgery: techniques and indications. J Neuroradiol.1997;24:45–52.
70. Schmidt R, Cakir B, Mattes T, Wegener M, Puhl W, Richter M. Cement leakage during vertebroplasty: an underestimated problem? Eur Spine J. 2005;14:466–73.
71. Seo JS, Kim YJ, Choi BW, Kim TH, Choe KO. MDCT of pulmonary embolism after percutaneous vertebroplasty. AJR Am J Roentgenol. 2005;184:1364–5.
72. Monticelli F, Meyer HJ, Tutsch-Bauer E. Fatal pulmonary cement embolism following percutaneous vertebroplasty (PVP). Forensic Sci Int. 2005;149(1):35–8.
73. Francois K, Taeymans Y, Poffyn B, Van Nooten G. Successful management of a large pulmonary cement embolus after percutaneous vertebroplasty: a case report. Spine. 2003;28(20):E424–5.
74. Park JH, Choo SJ, Park SW. Images in cardiovascular medicine: acute pericarditis caused by acrylic bone cement after percutaneous vertebroplasty. Circulation. 2005;111(6):e98.
75. Lindsay R, Silverman SL, Cooper C, et al. Risk of new vertebral fracture in the year following a fracture. JAMA. 2001;285:320–3.
76. Uppin AA, Hirsch JA, Centenera LV, Pfiefer BA, Pazianos AG, Choi IS. Occurrence of new vertebral body fracture after percutaneous vertebroplasty in patients with osteoporosis. Radiology. 2003;226(1):119–24.
77. Syed MI, Patel NA, Jan S, Harron MS, Morar K, Shaikh A. New symptomatic vertebral compression fractures within a year following vertebroplasty in osteoporotic women. Am J Neuroradiol. 2005;26:1601–4.
78. Ananthakrishnan D, Berven S, Deviren V, et al. The effect on anterior column loading due to different vertebral augmentation techniques. Clinical Biomechanics. 2005; 20:25–31.
79. Grados F, Depriester C, Cayrolle G, et al. Long-term observations of vertebral osteoporotic fractures treated by percutaneous vertebroplasty. Rheumatology. 2000; 39:1410–4.

6

Kyphoplasty

Frances D. Faro, Anthony P. Dwyer, and Vikas V. Patel

As the world population ages, vertebral fractures have increased in incidence to a staggering 700,000 in the United States annually (1). Vertebral fractures result in a significant burden on the health care system with approximately 150,000 hospital admissions and 161,000 office visits annually (1). Most fractures are due to osteoporotic bone and are managed nonoperatively with analgesic medications, bracing, bed rest, and/or activity modification. In some patients, however, suffering fractures and their sequelae can mean the difference between independent living and institutionalization. In addition, inactivity in an elderly patient has significant risks with respect to pulmonary toilette, deep vein thrombosis, lost bone density, and decreased muscle mass. Narcotic medications carry their own risks including constipation, sedation, and increased fall risk. Although conservative management typically leads to improvement in pain, residual kyphotic deformity has considerable impact on pulmonary function, self-image, and social functioning (2–5). Initially conceived in the mid-1990s, kyphoplasty is a form of percutaneous vertebral augmentation that uses a balloon tamp and injected bone cement to restore lost vertebral height. Because the inflatable balloon tamp was approved by the FDA in 1998, approximately 200,000 vertebral fractures have been treated in this manner. By providing early pain relief and some restoration of vertebral height, kyphoplasty has become a viable alternative to medical therapy, bracing, and vertebroplasty in the treatment of painful vertebral fractures (Figure 1).

PREOPERATIVE CONSIDERATIONS
Indications and Contraindications

Kyphoplasty has been used to treat painful vertebral body compression fractures due to osteoporosis or osteolytic tumors that have failed conservative management. On physical exam, the patient must have pain or tenderness to palpation at the vertebral level that correlates with the vertebral fracture found on imaging. Acute and chronic fractures may be treated by kyphoplasty; however, the restoration of vertebral height achieved with chronic fractures is significantly less (6). Vertebral fractures that involve the posterior cortex, pedicles,

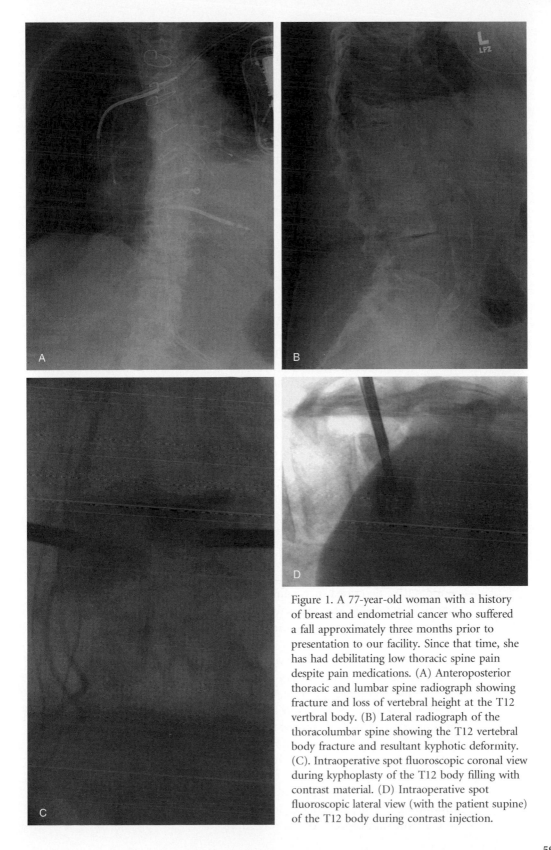

Figure 1. A 77-year-old woman with a history of breast and endometrial cancer who suffered a fall approximately three months prior to presentation to our facility. Since that time, she has had debilitating low thoracic spine pain despite pain medications. (A) Anteroposterior thoracic and lumbar spine radiograph showing fracture and loss of vertebral height at the T12 vertbral body. (B) Lateral radiograph of the thoracolumbar spine showing the T12 vertebral body fracture and resultant kyphotic deformity. (C). Intraoperative spot fluoroscopic coronal view during kyphoplasty of the T12 body filling with contrast material. (D) Intraoperative spot fluoroscopic lateral view (with the patient supine) of the T12 body during contrast injection.

or facets should not be treated by kyphoplasty. Fractures that are caused by solid tumors or osteomyelitis are also contraindications to kyphoplasty. In addition, vertebral fractures that have resulted in compression of neural elements and primarily radicular pain are more appropriately treated with decompressive procedures. There are also several medical considerations prior to surgery; allergies to contrast, coagulopathies, intolerance to being prone, and localized infection at the operative site should all be evaluated prior to the procedure. Ultimately, the patient must clearly understand that the goal of the procedure is alleviation of the pain from the treated fracture, not spinal or radicular pain at other levels or pain from other causes. As the decision to treat has important social ramifications with respect to mobility and independence, in addition to the history and physical exam, the physician must have an understanding of the patient's social situation and work with the patient to meet their functional goals.

Imaging

Plain films should be acquired to confirm the presence of a fracture at the level of the patient's symptoms, and the authors advocate long-standing films to evaluate overall alignment. Magnetic resonance imaging (MRI) with short tau inversion recovery (STIR) images is recommended as this modality of MRI is sensitive in detecting marrow edema consistent with acute fractures (Figure 2) (7). In addition, MRI aids in visualization of the posterior elements and canal contents to rule out burst fractures and posterior compromise that would require decompression and stabilization not provided by kyphoplasty. Few authors advocate the use of bone scan or computed tomography as the primary imaging methods for preoperative planning; however, these modalities can be used if contraindications to MRI exist.

Timing

The early recommendations by Garfin et al. described treating patients within three months of the fracture event (8). However, in subsequent studies, the authors have described successfully treating patients as early as a week and as late as 32 months following fracture (7,9). Crandall et al. conducted a prospective analysis comparing outcomes of kyphoplasty in patients who had acute versus chronic vertebral fractures differentiated as less than or greater than four months, respectively (6). There was no significant difference between the acute and chronic groups with respect to pain relief postoperatively; however, there was significantly more vertebral height restoration in the acute group. In 60% of acute fractures, vertebrae were restored to within 10% of their normal height; in contrast, only 26% of chronic fractures achieved this level of height restoration (7). In our experience, best results are attained when fractures are treated within three months of their occurrence. Although a trial of conservative treatment is appropriate, waiting too long to pursue operative intervention can introduce further morbidity with decreased muscle mass and bone density from inactivity and prolonged dependence on narcotics, as well as a decrease in the reduction capacity of the procedure.

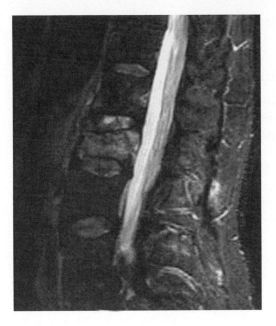

Figure 2. An active man of 64 years with a history of melanoma who sustained an injury to his lower back after falling down a flight of stairs and landing directly on his back. He presented three weeks after the injury with a decrease in his initial pain, but continued narcotic pain requirements and significant limitations in his activities. The patient underwent kyphoplasty at L2 due to the edema noted on the MRI examination. MRI STIR images show increased signal in the L2 vertebral body, indicating edema and acute fracture.

TECHNICAL CONSIDERATIONS

Although some patients undergo kyphoplasty as a same-day procedure, most are admitted overnight for observation. Preoperative antibiotics covering skin flora are used as prophylactics. Anesthesia ranges from monitored anesthesia care with local anesthesia to general anesthesia, depending upon the comfort, compliance, and comorbidities of the patient (10). The patient is placed in the prone position on a fluoroscopic table with chest and pelvis bolsters to place the spine in extension (11,12). Although kyphoplasty can be performed with a single rotating C-arm, two fluoroscopy machines may be useful to acquire simultaneously anteroposterior and lateral images of the spine.

Technique

Using fluoroscopy, the fractured vertebral body is identified. There is some variance in the type of approach. Many studies describe using a transpedicular approach in the thoracolumbar and lumbar spine, and an extrapedicular approach to the upper thoracic spine. Due to the shape of the upper thoracic vertebrae as well as the pedicular orientation, the extrapedicular approach may allow more medial and anterior placement of cement (13). In at least one study, however, this approach was associated with more leakage of cement (14). Most studies describe a simultaneous bilateral technique, although a few authors have described a unilateral approach in the upper thoracic spine (8,13,15). A biomechanical study by Steinmann et al. compared unipedicular kyphoplasty to bipedicular kyphoplasty in thirty cadaveric vertebral bodies. Although the power of the study was limited by the small sample, the data showed no significant difference between the approaches with respect to stiffness, strength, height restoration, or lateral wedging (16). Our experience is to use a bilateral transpedicular approach at all levels; the subsequent description will utilize this approach.

Author's Preferred Technique

Through a 5-mm incision made lateral to the pedicles to accommodate the trajectory of the pedicle and trocar, a working cannula/trocar is advanced through the pedicle past the posterior cortex of the vertebral body. Frequent biplanar fluoroscopy is used to ensure that the medial cortex of the pedicle is not violated. At this point, in patients with a known malignancy, a bone biopsy can be obtained using a biopsy cannula or ENT pituitary rongeur. Through the working cannula, a drill bit is placed and a corridor for the balloon tamp is drilled under the collapsed superior endplate. The drill bit is removed and replaced with a balloon tamp (Kyphon, Sunnyvale, CA). Balloon tamps come in a variety of sizes and directionality for special cases; typically, a 15- or 20-mm round balloon tamp is used. The balloon tamp has a radiopaque marker at each end to ensure correct placement in the bone before inflation. Once the procedure is repeated on the contralateral side, the balloons are inflated simultaneously with contrast material until one of the following criteria is met: the fracture is reduced, the balloon pressure reaches 220 psi, maximum balloon volume is attained, or a balloon contacts one of the cortical margins of the vertebra. After the contrast is withdrawn, the deflated balloon is removed through the cannula. This leaves a cavity in the bone, which is often visible on the lateral view as an "air vertebrogram" (17). The cement is mixed and cured to a viscous consistency and then injected simultaneously by hand with bone-void-filler tubes through the bilateral working cannulae. Cement fill begins at the anterior cortex, filling approximately two-thirds of the way back to the posterior cortex. The cement volume is generally 1–2 ml greater than the balloon-induced void as the cement interdigitates with the bony trabeculae. Estimates of average cement fill per vertebrae vary from 2 to 12 ml, though a typical fill in our hand is 2–4 ml (8,9,17,18).

Most kyphoplasties use polymethylmethacrylate (PMMA). Different formulations of PMMA have been investigated and have shown little difference in postaugmentation stiffness and strength (19). PMMA has some theoretical drawbacks including monomer toxicity and thermonecrosis that occur with the curing of the cement. Togawa et al. histologically evaluated four human vertebrae excised one month to two years following kyphoplasty and, in this limited sampling, did not find extensive necrosis in the region surrounding the PMMA (20). Calcium phosphate and calcium sulfate have been proposed as fillers in kyphoplasty and have the attractive feature of osteoconductivity as opposed to PMMA which, is biologically inert. Biomechanical studies have shown that both calcium phosphate and calcium sulfate provided similar stiffness and strength in fractured cadaveric vertebrae as PMMA (19,21,22). However, *in vivo* studies of calcium sulfate in other applications have revealed it to be quickly resorbed and therefore may be a poor option for kyphoplasty vertebral augmentation. In addition, both calcium phosphate and calcium sulfate have low viscosity and poor handling characteristics that have prevented them from becoming viable alternatives to PMMA. Some bioactive acrylic cements are under investigation but osteoconductivity in human vertebrae has yet to be proven (9). Alternatives to the current standard PMMA will be required to have a short liquid phase and long "doughy" working phase with the ability to be inserted percutaneously and interdigitate with bony trabeculae.

After cement fill of the vertebrae, the working cannulae are withdrawn and the incisions are closed, typically with a single stitch. Patients are returned to the supine position and anesthesia is ceased. Postoperative hospital stay varies among studies – some patients undergo the procedure as outpatients, although the majority requires a 23-hour stay; prolonged hospital stays were usually due to comorbidity factors. After discharge, the patient should be followed as an outpatient to ensure that they are recovering appropriately, not experiencing complications such as fractures of adjacent vertebrae, and are receiving the appropriate level of assistance for their living situation.

OUTCOMES
Overview

The most striking characteristic about the body of available literature is the lack of a single prospective, randomized study with long-term follow-up evaluating the outcomes of kyphoplasty to those of vertebroplasty or conservative treatment. There are approximately two dozen studies on vertebral compression fractures treated with kyphoplasty published from 2001 to 2006. Of the 2,000 patients evaluated by these studies, two-thirds were studied prospectively, but only 4% of patients were compared to controls. The average follow-up is less than two years in all but two studies. Nevertheless, some solid conclusions can be drawn from the available data.

Pain Relief

All studies reported a significant improvement in pain with many patients describing immediate relief of pain. An initial multicenter study of 603 fractures treated by kyphoplasty in 350 patients by Garfin et al. reported that 95% of patients had significant pain relief from the procedure (8). Subsequent studies have reported a high percentage of patients reporting improvement in pain following the procedure, ranging from 84% to 100% (11,23–27). A prospective study of 70 fractures treated in thirty patients by Lieberman et al. quantified pain relief using the Short Form 36 (SF36) bodily pain score, which averaged 11.6 preoperatively and 58.7 postoperatively (9). Other studies using the SF36 scores have shown similar improvements in bodily pain assessment (13,28). Some studies have used the visual analog scale (VAS) to quantify improvements in pain. Rhyne et al. evaluated 52 patients in which 82 kyphoplasty procedures were performed. An average VAS of 9.2 was reduced to 2.9 following surgery (17). Similarly, Grohs et al. evaluated patients preoperatively as well as at three postoperative time points, and found that the reduction in VAS from 7.4 preoperatively to 2.0, four months following surgery was maintained at two-year follow-up (29). Although it is clear that pain is improved in the majority of patients treated with kyphoplasty, there has been no analysis to determine factors predisposing patients to improved postoperative pain level.

Functionality

Reduction in pain is clearly linked to improved functionality, and some studies have quantified this with various disability indices. Studies by both Coumans and Lieberman reported significant improvements in the physical function, vitality, mental health, and social functioning scores of the SF36 (9,13). Ledlie et al. evaluated the ambulatory status of seventy-nine patients and found that by one month, the percentage of fully ambulatory patients had increased from 35% to 83% (23). Some studies have evaluated patient functionality using the Oswestry Disability Index (ODI) and demonstrated significant functional improvements (7,15). Gaitanis et al. reported that a consecutive series of thirty-two patients demonstrated a 53% increase in daily activities by the ODI scoring (18). In comparing forty patients treated with kyphoplasty to twenty patients treated nonoperatively, Grafe et al. reported an average of 5.3 physician office visits over 12 months in the kyphoplasty group, versus 11.6 visits over 12 months in the nonoperative group (30). Although an indirect measurement of pain and functionality, this measurement is an important reflection of improvement in quality of life following kyphoplasty.

Vertebral Height Restoration

With the balloon tamp inflation, some vertebral height can be restored. All studies that evaluated vertebral height before and after kyphoplasty showed improvement in vertebral height; however, the range of improvement was wide, with the procedure restoring from 12% to 71% of the lost vertebral height. Garfin's original study of 603 kyphoplasties showed a posttreatment height restoration averaging 66%, as midline vertebral height improved from 76% to 92% of predicted normal height (8). Ledlie et al. studied 133 procedures and found a similar pattern with a midline vertebral height increasing from 65% to 90% of predicted normal (23). A 2005 study by Gaitanis et al. reported that 88% of treated vertebrae were restored to predicted normal height.

Other studies have reported less impressive height restitution (18). Studies by both Lieberman and Dudeney described height restoration rates of approximately 35% (9,28). Kasperk et al. reported that kyphoplasty only reestablished 12% of lost vertebral height (31). Other investigators have reported their height restoration in terms of reduction of kyphosis. Phillips et al. reported being able to reduce kyphosis by 7.9° for lumbar fractures and 9.7° for thoracic fractures per vertebral level treated (12). Both Garfin and Berlemann reported an approximately 50% improvement in kyphosis (8,24).

Although long-term follow-up in these studies is lacking, some data appear to suggest that this height restoration is a lasting effect. Grafe et al. described an increase in vertebral height from 59% to 68% of predicted height that was still maintained at one year following surgery (30). Ledlie et al. measured preoperative vertebral height as 61% predicted normal height; immediate postoperative films and two-year follow-up films showed 87% and 88% predicted, respectively (27). Kasperk et al. compared kyphoplasty patients to nonoperative controls and found that the former only had a 12% improvement in height that was maintained at a year; in contrast, the control patients lost 8% in that same year (31).

There is some debate about the direct effect of the height restoration attained by kyphoplasty. Citing studies that describe the impact of spinal deformity on disability as partially independent of pain, Yuan et al. have hypothesized that increased kyphosis from vertebral compression fractures impacts the overall spinal alignment, sagittal balance, and body biomechanics. They extrapolate that restoring vertebral height and decreasing kyphosis will restore sagittal balance and improve functionality, improve quality of life, and even decrease subsequent hip fractures (32). This idea is biomechanically logical and attractive; however, *in vivo* restoration of vertebral height does not seem to restore overall sagittal alignment (33). The increase in height is mainly midline, and 7° restored at one vertebra balances with soft tissues and does not translate into a 7° improvement in overall sagittal balance (34). In addition, there has been no relationship identified between restoration of height and improved pain or functionality scores (30).

COMPLICATIONS

Extravasation of Cement

A fairly common phenomenon in vertebroplasty (34,35), extravasation of cement has been closely monitored in kyphoplasty procedures. The rate of cement leakage per treated level has ranged from 0.3% to 33%; however, there are no reports of cement leakage that became symptomatic. Initial studies revealed extravasation rates from 0.3% to 8.6%, with leakage occurring into the epidural, disc, and paraspinal spaces (8,9,28). Phillips et al. evaluated the pattern of contrast material injected before both vertebroplasty and kyphoplasty cementing; invariably, contrast fill of epidural vessels and/or the inferior cava as well as transcortical leakage was seen with vertebroplasty. Contrast injected following balloon inflation in kyphoplasty had some leakage of contrast, which was dramatically less than that witnessed with vertebroplasty. This study likely overestimates the leakage rates of cement as the contrast material is much less viscous than the cement; however, it does appear that using the bone tamp in the vertebral body has an impact on cement extravasation (12). Combining this study with the increased viscosity of cement injected in kyphoplasty explains the higher rates of cement leakage seen clinically in vertebroplasty (34–37).

Subsequent Fractures

A multicenter study of approximately 2,700 women showed that the incidence of a second vertebral fracture in the years following a primary vertebral fracture was 19.2%. Percentages of subsequent fracture in the studies of kyphoplasty range from 5% to 21% (24,29). A study by Fribourg et al. analyzed the postoperative course of 38 patients and concluded that the majority of subsequent fractures present within the first 60 days following kyphoplasty and are adjacent to the treated vertebra (Figure 3). Nonadjacent fractures tend to occur further out from the procedure (38). Steroid-induced osteoporosis is a risk factor for a second fracture. Harrop et al. found that patients with secondary osteoporosis had an incidence of second fractures of 49%, whereas patients with primary osteoporosis had a rate of only 11% (39). A finite-element model by Villaraga et al. showed little change in the stresses placed on the segments of the spine following kyphoplasty and theorized that successive fractures were part of the natural history of osteoporosis (40).

Other Complications

There have been a few reports of pulmonary emboli of cement following kyphoplasty. The FDA register of complications with kyphoplasty from

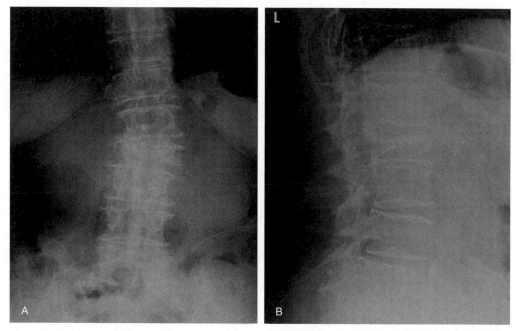

Figure 3. A woman of 79 years who presented to our facility with one month of back pain after bending over to do her laundry. She was diagnosed at that time with an L2 compression fracture and despite narcotic pain medications had a severe decrease in her daily function and debilitating pain that prevented her from living independently. Kyphoplasty was performed at L2, but subsequent fractures with clinical sequelae occurred at L1, L3, L4, and L5. One month following her last procedure, the patient had only mild back pain to palpation and had returned to independent living. (A) Anteroposterior views of the lumbar spine in which the L2 vertebral fracture has resulted in asymmetrical loss of vertebral height. (B) Lateral radiograph of the lumbar spine reveals overall loss of height as well as increased kyphosis at the L2 level. (C) Postkyphoplasty radiograph of the lumbar spine taken two weeks after kyphoplasty reveals an L1 fracture adjacent to the prior kyphoplasty level (compare with A). (D) Lateral radiograph of the lumbar spine confirms adjacent fracture at L1 (compare with B). (E) Lateral radiograph of the lumbar spine following kyphoplasty at L1 and L2 show further adjacent fractures at levels L4 and L5. (F) Postkyphoplasty anteroposterior radiograph of the lumbar spine after kyphoplasties of levels L3 through L5 (and prior kyphoplasties at L1 and L2).

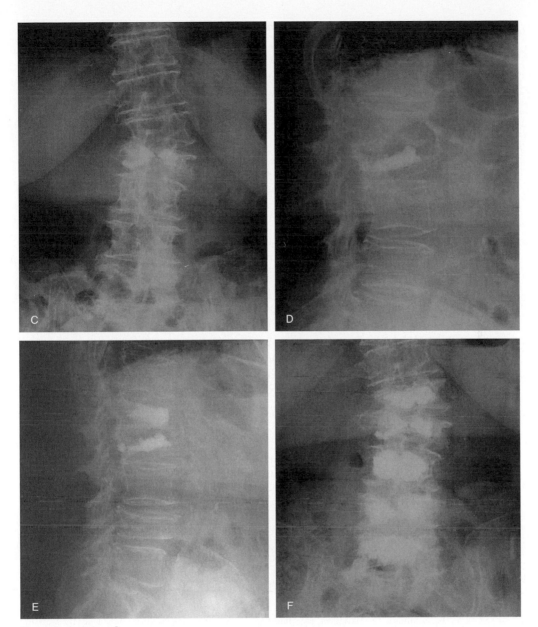

Figure 3. (*continued*)

1999 to 2003 lists one pulmonary embolus that caused an extended hospital stay (41). Choe et al. acquired chest films after kyphoplasties and vertebroplasties and found that cement emboli were present after 4.6% of procedures. The patients with emboli all had multiple myeloma, and the emboli were all asymptomatic and required no intervention (42). Gaitanis et al. reported three instances of spinal stenosis following kyphoplasty that required laminectomy for resolution of symptoms (18). Canal intrusion with damage to neural elements is a definite risk with the transpedicular approach and has been documented as occurring five times for the 50,000 procedures done between 1999 and 2005 (41). In addition, there have been reports of an epidural hematoma that required evacuation, a pneumothorax, fractured ribs, and an anterior cord syndrome (9,41). Though complications are not common, these procedures should only be performed with ready availability of access to posterior spinal decompression. A practitioner should develop a relationship with a spinal surgeon to discuss the early recognition and treatment of complications from kyphoplasty.

CONCLUSIONS

Since it was first described in 2001, kyphoplasty has grown rapidly in its utilization across the country. When used for the right indications, kyphoplasty is a swift and effective procedure that helps to improve the quality of life of already frail vertebral fracture patients. In comparison to vertebroplasty, kyphoplasty is more expensive and usually involves an overnight stay in the hospital; however, the ability to restore vertebral height and the decreased rate of cement extravasation may balance out these drawbacks. This cannot be evaluated thoroughly without a truly randomized and controlled study comparing kyphoplasty to vertebroplasty. As kyphoplasty becomes solidly established as an effective means of pain control for osteoporosis or neoplastic vertebral fractures, other avenues of treatment are opening up. Use of novel bone cements, treatment of traumatic vertebral fractures, and the addition of chemotherapeutic agents are current areas of investigation.

REFERENCES

1. Riggs BL, Melton LJ 3rd. The worldwide problem of osteoporosis: insights afforded by epidemiology. *Bone*. 1995 Nov;17(5 Suppl):505S–11S.
2. Gold DT. The clinical impact of vertebral fractures. Quality of life in women with osteoporosis. *Bone*. 1996;18(Suppl):185S–9S.
3. Leech JA, Dulberg C, Kellie S, Pattee L, Gay J. Relationship of lung function to severity of osteoporosis in women. *Am Rev Respir Dis*. 1990;141:68–71.
4. Lombardi I Jr., Oliveira LM, Mayer AF, Jardim JR, Natour J. Evaluation of pulmonary function and quality of life in women with osteoporosis. *Osteoporos Int*. 2005; 16(10):1247–53. Epub 2005 Apr 2.
5. Schlaich C, Minne HW, Bruckner T, et al. Reduced pulmonary function in patients with spinal osteoporotic fractures. *Osteoporos Int*. 1998;8(3):261–7.
6. Crandall D, Slaughter D, Hankins PJ, Moore C, Jerman J. Acute versus chronic vertebral compression fractures treated with kyphoplasty: early results. *Spine J*. 2004;4(4):418–24.
7. Baur A, Stabler A, Bruning R, et al. Diffusion-weighted MR imaging of bone marrow: differentiation of benign versus pathologic compression fractures. *Radiology*. 1998;207(2):349–56.
8. Garfin SR, Yuan HA, Reiley MA. New technologies in spine: kyphoplasty and vertebroplasty for the treatment of painful osteoporotic compression fractures. *Spine*. 2001;15;26(14):1511–5.
9. Lieberman IH, Dudeney S, Reinhardt MK, Bell G. Initial outcome and efficacy of "kyphoplasty" in the treatment of painful osteoporotic vertebral compression fractures. *Spine*. 2001;15;26(14):1631–8.
10. Schubert A, Deogaonkar A, Lotto M, Niezgoda J, Luciano M. Anesthesia for minimally invasive cranial and spinal surgery. *J Neurosurg Anesthesiol*. 2006;18(1): 47–56.

11. Fourney DR, Schomer DF, Nader R, et al. Percutaneous vertebroplasty and kypho-plasty for painful vertebral body fractures in cancer patients. *J Neurosurg.* 2003;98 (1 Suppl):21–30.

12. Phillips FM, Ho E, Campbell-Hupp M, McNally T, Todd Wetzel F, Gupta P. Early radiographic and clinical results of balloon kyphoplasty for the treatment of osteo-porotic vertebral compression fractures. *Spine.* 2003;28(19):2260–5; discussion 2265–7.

13. Coumans JV, Reinhardt MK, Lieberman IH. Kyphoplasty for vertebral compression fractures: 1-year clinical outcomes from a prospective study. *J Neurosurg.* 2003; 99(1 Suppl):44–50.

14. Majd ME, Farley S, Holt RT. Preliminary outcomes and efficacy of the first 360 consecutive kyphoplasties for the treatment of painful osteoporotic vertebral com-pression fractures. *Spine J.* 2005;5(3):244–55.

15. Lane JM, Hong R, Koob J, et al. Kyphoplasty enhances function and structural align-ment in multiple myeloma. *Clin Orthop Relat Res.* 2004;(426):49–53.

16. Steinmann J, Tingey CT, Cruz G, Dai Q. Biomechanical comparison of unipedicular versus bipedicular kyphoplasty. *Spine.* 2005;30(2):201–5.

17. Rhyne A 3rd, Banit D, Laxer E, Odum S, Nussman D. Kyphoplasty: report of eighty-two thoracolumbar osteoporotic vertebral fractures. *J Orthop Trauma.* 2004; 18(5):294–9.

18. Gaitanis IN, Hadjipavlou AG, Katonis PG, Tzermiadianos MN, Pasku DS, Patward-han AG. Balloon kyphoplasty for the treatment of pathological vertebral compressive fractures. *Eur Spine J.* 2005;14(3):250–60.

19. Tomita S, Molloy S, Jasper LE, Abe M, Belkoff SM. Biomechanical comparison of kyphoplasty with different bone cements. *Spine.* 2004;29(11):1203–7.

20. Togawa D, Bauer TW, Lieberman IH, Takikawa S. Histologic evaluation of human vertebral bodies after vertebral augmentation with polymethyl methacrylate. *Spine.* 2003;28(14):1521–7.

21. Perry A, Mahar A, Massie J, Arrieta N, Garfin S, Kim C. Biomechanical evaluation of kyphoplasty with calcium sulfate cement in a cadaveric osteoporotic vertebral com-pression fracture model. *Spine J.* 2005;5(5):489–93.

22. Tomita S, Kin A, Yazu M, Abe M. Biomechanical evaluation of kyphoplasty and vertebroplasty with calcium phosphate cement in a simulated osteoporotic compres-sion fracture. *J Orthop Sci.* 2003;8(2):192–7.

23. Ledlie JT, Renfro M. Balloon kyphoplasty: one-year outcomes in vertebral body height restoration, chronic pain, and activity levels. *J Neurosurg.* 2003;98(1 Suppl):36–42.

24. Berlemann U, Franz T, Orler R, Heini PF. Kyphoplasty for treatment of osteoporotic vertebral fractures: a prospective non-randomized study. *Eur Spine J.* 2004;13(6): 496–501.

25. Theodorou DJ, Theodorou SJ, Duncan TD, Garfin SR, Wong WH. Percutaneous balloon kyphoplasty for the correction of spinal deformity in painful vertebral body compression fractures. *Clin Imaging.* 2002;26(1):1–5.

26. Bartolozzi B, Nozzoli C, Pandolfo C, Antonioli E, Guizzardi G, Morichi R, Bosi A. Percutaneous vertebroplasty and kyphoplasty in patients with multiple myeloma. *Eur J Haematol.* 2006;76(2):180–1.

27. Ledlie JT, Renfro MB. Kyphoplasty treatment of vertebral fractures: 2-year outcomes show sustained benefits. *Spine.* 2006;31(1):57–64.

28. Dudeney S, Lieberman IH, Reinhardt MK, Hussein M. Kyphoplasty in the treatment of osteolytic vertebral compression fractures as a result of multiple myeloma. *J Clin Oncol.* 2002;20(9):2382–7.

29. Grohs JG, Matzner M, Trieb K, Krepler P. Minimal invasive stabilization of osteo-porotic vertebral fractures: a prospective nonrandomized comparison of vertebro-plasty and balloon kyphoplasty. *J Spinal Disord Tech.* 2005;18(3):238–42.

30. Grafe IA, Da Fonseca K, Hillmeier J, et al. Reduction of pain and fracture incidence after kyphoplasty: 1-year outcomes of a prospective controlled trial of patients with primary osteoporosis. *Osteoporos Int.* 2005;16(12):2005–12.

31. Kasperk C, Hillmeier J, Noldge G, et al. Treatment of painful vertebral fractures by kyphoplasty in patients with primary osteoporosis: a prospective nonrandomized controlled study. *J Bone Miner Res.* 2005;20(4):604–12.

32. Yuan HA, Brown CW, Phillips FM. Osteoporotic spinal deformity: a biomechanical rationale for the clinicalconsequences and treatment of vertebral body compression fractures. *J Spinal Disord Tech.* 2004;17(3):236–42.

33. Pradhan BB, Bae HW, Kropf MA, Patel VV, Delamarter RB. Kyphoplasty reduction of osteoporotic vertebral compression fractures: correction of local kyphosis versus overall sagittal alignment. *Spine.* 2006;31(4):435–41.

34. Schmidt R, Cakir B, Mattes T, Wegener M, Puhl W, Richter M. Cement leakage during vertebroplasty: an underestimated problem? *Eur Spine J.* 2005;14(5):466–73.

35. Cortet B, Cotten A, Boutry N, Flipo RM, Duquesnoy B, Chastanet P, Delcambre B. Percutaneous vertebroplasty in the treatment of osteoporotic vertebral compression fractures: an open prospective study. *J Rheumatol.* 1999;26(10):2222–8.

36. Cotten A, Dewatre F, Cortet B, Assaker R, Leblond D, Duquesnoy B, Chastanet P, Clarisse J. Percutaneous vertebroplasty for osteolytic metastases and myeloma: effects of the percentage of lesion filling and the leakage of methyl methacrylate at clinical follow-up. *Radiology.* 1996;200(2):525–30.

37. Cyteval C, Sarrabere MP, Roux JO, Thomas E, Jorgensen C, Blotman F, Sany J, Taourel P. Acute osteoporotic vertebral collapse: open study on percutaneous injection of acrylic surgical cement in 20 patients. *AJR Am J Roentgenol.* 1999;173(6):1685–90.

38. Fribourg D, Tang C, Sra P, Delamarter R, Bae H. Incidence of subsequent vertebral fracture after kyphoplasty. *Spine.* 2004;29(20):2270–6; discussion 2277.

39. Harrop JS, Prpa B, Reinhardt MK, Lieberman I. Primary and secondary osteoporosis' incidence of subsequent vertebral compression fractures after kyphoplasty. *Spine.* 2004;29(19):2120–5.

40. Villarraga ML, Bellezza AJ, Harrigan TP, Cripton PA, Kurtz SM, Edidin AA. The biomechanical effects of kyphoplasty on treated and adjacent nontreated vertebral bodies. *J Spinal Disord Tech.* 2005;18(1):84–91.

41. Nussbaum DA, Gailloud P, Murphy K. A review of complications associated with vertebroplasty and kyphoplasty as reported to the Food and Drug Administration medical device related web site. *J Vasc Interv Radiol.* 2004;15(11):1185–92. Review.

42. Choe du H, Marom EM, Ahrar K, Truong MT, Madewell JE. Pulmonary embolism of polymethyl methacrylate during percutaneous vertebroplasty and kyphoplasty. *AJR Am J Roentgenol.* 2004;183(4):1097–102.

7

Epidural Steroid Injections

Brian D. Petersen, Kirkland W. Davis, and James Choi

Epidural injections have been used to treat low-back and radicular pain for the past 100 years; these injections have included corticosteroids for the past 50 years. As the technique has evolved and become more widespread, epidural steroid injections have become an important part of the armamentarium in treating low-back pain, sciatica, and, to a lesser degree, neck pain.

The solution to back pain continues to vex physicians and their patients. Most patients with acute disc herniations will improve without surgery (1); however, even those who recover without invasive therapy often suffer pain and disability in the meantime. This may lead to lost wages and diminished productivity. Although epidural steroid injections are not a cure for the root cause of pain, they may reduce or eliminate the pain in the short and intermediate term (2), allowing rehabilitation to proceed and a speedier return to normal activities (3). Even though occasional patients experience permanent, complete relief from epidural steroid injections, one cannot advise patients that they will achieve lasting relief purely from the injection. The goal is to improve symptoms, which will allow a more normal lifestyle and facilitate other modes of therapy (4).

This chapter reviews the relevant anatomy for epidural injections, history of the technique, medications, practical steps, and other relevant information of epidural injections. A variety of routes will be discussed.

ANATOMY

The epidural space exists from the skull base through the sacrum. Within the spinal canal, the epidural space lies between the dura mater and the osseous confines of the spinal canal (5,6). The outer margin of the epidural space is the peridural membrane, denoted by the periosteum of the osseous canal, the posterior borders of the intervertebral discs, the inner edge of the ligamenta flava, and the anterior margin of the interspinous ligament (7,8). The plica mediana dorsalis occasionally is present, dividing the posterior epidural space into halves; this may confine epidural injections to one side of the canal (5,6,9,10). When present, this variant is usually limited to the sacral and lower lumbar spine.

The lumbar epidural space is most prominent in the posterior midline. Here, the epidural space usually is triangular and filled with fat, and readily identifiable on magnetic resonance (MR) and computed tomography (CT) scans by its clear fat signal/attenuation. This site is the target when the "interlaminar" approach is used (Figure 1). The posterior epidural space may be small for many reasons: spinal stenosis or postsurgical scarring often obliterates it and the posterior epidural space is usually only a potential space at L5/S1, with no visible fat to target. Likewise, there is little to no fat visible in the cervical spine. In these locations, placing the needle within the epidural space relies in part on touch.

The sacrum comprises five embryonic vertebrae that fuse *in utero*, with three to five rudimentary vertebrae forming the coccyx, which is attached to the caudal tip of the sacrum. When one chooses a caudal approach to reach the lumbosacral epidural space, the portal is the sacral hiatus (Figure 2), where the posterior elements of the S4 and S5 segments do not fuse in the midline dorsally. The sacral cornua lie along the lateral margins of the hiatus and are often palpable landmarks for entry into the hiatus. The hiatus is covered by the sacrococcygeal ligament and the floor is the posterior aspect of S5. The thecal sac extends into the sacral portion of the spinal canal in normal patients; one should not puncture the thecal sac when performing caudal epidural injections. The thecal sac reportedly typically extends to the lower S1 level in adults and to the S3 level in children, but studies of cadavers suggest that the position of the thecal sac tip is at the middle third of the S2 body in the average patient (11,12).

HISTORY

In 1901, the first reported epidural injections for lumbargo or sciatica included cocaine as a medication. Many substances and combinations were tried as epidural injections evolved. For instance, Viner described using 20 ml of 1% procaine in 50–100 ml of Ringer's solution, normal saline, or petrolatum in

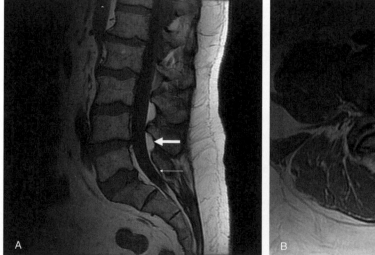
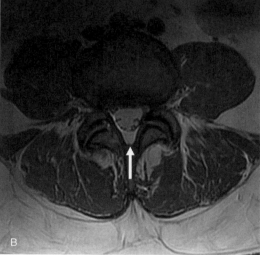

Figure 1. Epidural space. (A) Sagittal T1-weighted sequence showing the target site for the interlaminar epidural steroid injection (ILESI) (thick arrow). The epidural space tends to be largest at the level of the disc space. Note the absence of significant epidural space at L5/S1 (thin arrow). (B) ILESI target on axial image (arrow).

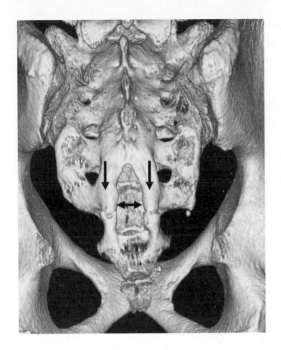

Figure 2. Sacral hiatus: three-dimensional surface rendered reconstruction of a traumatic pelvic CT shows the paired cornua (thin arrows) and the midline sacral hiatus (double-headed arrow).

1925 (13,14). Five years later, Evans reported the use of massive volumes of 1% novocaine or saline (often >100 ml) in 40 patients. He quoted side effects as, "abnormal sensations or paraesthesiae, such as formication. A few [patients] said that they had found it difficult to control a desire to shout or scream." One of his patients, treated with 2% novocaine, was unconscious for one hour and was incontinent for 12 hours, suggesting the need for caution with regard to the anesthetic concentration. Through all this, Evans reported that 22 of the patients were "cured," and another five "improved" over baseline (15).

Differences in volume of injected and number of procedures also evolved. For instance, Kelman in 1944 reported good results using 50–100 ml of saline, 1% novocaine, or 0.75% metycaine in saline injected every other day for four to six procedures (16).

These early practitioners believed that the benefits of epidural injections resulted from breaking up adhesions around incarcerated nerve roots and displacing nerves away from herniated discs, in addition to the effects of the anesthetics. To achieve these purported hydrodynamic effects, a large volume was needed, justifying the common side effects of epidural injections in their hands, including pain, headache, and dizziness (1).

The first report of injecting corticosteroids into the epidural space was in 1952 (17). The following year, Lievre et al. administered hydrocortisone through an S1 foraminal injection in 46 patients with sciatica. They reported that eight patients had a very good response, fifteen good, and eight mediocre (1). The first epidural injection of corticosteroids in the United States was described by Goebert et al., who administered three daily injections of 30 ml procaine and 125 mg hydrocortisone acetate (18). Since those early reports, volumes have diminished, from a maximum of 200 ml (19), and various combinations of steroid preparations, anesthetics, and saline have been tested. Recommendations of the current authors are included in the technique portion of this chapter.

There remain two significant controversies regarding epidural steriod injection (ESI). Efficacy is the first. Because acute radicular pain due to disc herniations often improves without therapy, early support for the technique has been lessened by conflicting results of controlled trials. This subject will be examined in the next section.

Second, some have questioned the safety of administering available steroid preparations into the epidural space. Theoretically, the risk arises if the steroids are inadvertently injected into the thecal sac or if there is transdural transit of the steroids (20). It is known, from prior treatment of patients with spinal multiple sclerosis, that multiple intentional doses of intrathecal steroids can be associated with myelographic signs of arachnoiditis (not necessarily symptomatic), although direct causality is not established (21). However, current belief is that there is essentially no risk that a single inadvertent intrathecal injection of corticosteroids would cause arachnoiditis (6).

One Australian physician has lobbied against the performance of ESIs because of the purported neurotoxicity of the preservative polyethylene glycol, which is contained in two of the steroids used for ESI, triamcinolone diacetate (Aristocort Intralesional; Fujisawa Pharmaceutical, Osaka, Japan) and methylprednisolone acetate (Depo Medrol; Upjohn Pharmaceutical Co., Kalamazoo, MI) (20). Notably, the preservative shown to be potently neurotoxic is propylene glycol, not polyethylene glycol. It turns out that polyethylene glycol is not neurotoxic at commercially available concentrations (4,22). In his recent review, Spaccarelli points out that several studies now refute the risk of neurotoxicity or arachnoiditis of epidural steroids used in current practice (23).

MECHANISMS OF ACTION
Medications

STEROIDS

The original supposition that epidural injections relieve pain by displacing nerve roots and lysing adhesions, proposed by Evans in 1930 (15), is no longer credible. The surgical descriptions of White in 1983, pointed out that such adhesions are notoriously difficult to dissect with a scalpel, thus rendering doubtful any possible mechanical effect of even large fluid injections (24). The theory of fluid displacing and stretching nerve roots (25) has never been proved.

Current belief is that epidural steroids provide relief through anti-inflammatory effects. Spinal nerves are often inflamed during surgery (26) and evidence points to the presence of inflammation in patients with lumbar radiculopathy and disc degeneration. In a canine study, McCarron et al. provoked a strong inflammatory response by injecting autologous disc material into the epidural spaces, with subsequent rapid onset of fibrosis (27). High levels of phospholipase A2 (PLA2) were discovered around symptomatic disc herniations and painful discs by Franson et al. This group then provoked a strong inflammatory response by injecting PLA2 into the paws of mice (28). The inflammatory reaction evoked by PLA2 exerts is due to the liberation of arachidonic acid from cell membranes (4) and corticosteroids are known to inhibit this action of PLA2 (29,30).

There may be additional biochemical effects of corticosteroids when used for epidural injections. Johansson et al. demonstrated that corticosteroids injected into mice diminish transmission of impulses along the unmyelinated C-fibers, which carry pain information, but not in myelinated fibers (31).

For many years, the most common corticosteroids used in ESI were methylprednisolone acetate (Depo Medrol) and triamcinolone diacetate (Aristocort Intralesional). These preparations confer high local tissue levels for two weeks or more (32). Given the concerns about the potential neurotoxicity of polyethylene glycol (since refuted: see History section), Silbergleit et al. advocate the use of either triamcinolone acetonide (Kenalog-40; Bristol-Myers Squibb, Princeton, NJ) or a betamethasone preparation (Celestone Soluspan; Schering, Kenilworth, NJ) (10). Celestone Soluspan comprises betamethasone sodium phosphate and betamethasone acetate. Betamethasone sodium phosphate should have a more rapid onset due to its water solubility, whereas betamethasone acetate, which is not water soluble, is longer lasting (33).

Corticosteroid doses have diminished over the years. Knight and Burnell recommended limiting the dose of methylprednisolone acetate to 3 mg/kg patient weight in 1980; this dose was substantially lower than many reported doses prior to that time (34). Today, most authors suggest the dose equivalent of 80–120 mg methylprednisolone acetate for the typical patient (23,28). In our facility, the first choice for interlaminar epidurals is 80 mg (2 ml) Kenalog-40, due to higher efficacy when compared to Celestone Soluspan in a review of returned patient pain surveys (35). This is postulated to be secondary to the larger particle size and more pronounced depot effect of Kenalog. For transforaminal epidural injections, we prefer the smaller particle size of Celestone Soluspan, largely due to the perceived decreased risk of vascular occlusion should a radicular artery be encountered (36). Standards for number and timing of injections have not yet been established (23). In our institution, patients are limited to three injections over a six-month period, although some referring physicians will not refer their patients more than three times per year.

ANESTHETIC

Many authors believe that including an anesthetic in the injectate may provide several benefits: it may result in muscle relaxation, provide psychological benefit from rapid pain relief, and break the pain-muscle spasm-ischemia-pain cycle (23,25), although this last assertion is particularly difficult to prove. Occasionally, there can be partial anesthesia of the dura with an ESI (5,24); as long as a less concentrated dose of the anesthetic is chosen, a significant motor or sensory block is rare in these instances.

In addition, there are physiological changes in the density and threshold potential of pain fibers in patients with chronic pain. This is the basis for treatment of chronic pain with lidocaine (usually in the form of Lidoderm patches). Lidocaine, as a sodium channel blocker, decreases the activity of chronically activated nerves and can reset the pain stimulus threshold, giving more long-term relief (37).

The authors use preservative-free 0.5% lidocaine for two reasons. First, it is important to note that anesthetics containing preservatives such as methyl paraben or phenol can cause flocculation of depot steroid preparations (33). Second, bupivicaine and other longer acting anesthetics should be eschewed to limit the duration of the occasional case of a significant block from a lumbar

ESI. If bupivicaine is chosen, it should be limited to the 0.25% concentration (24).

Expectations

Typically, patients want to know what results they can expect from an epidural steroid injection. The consent process should address these questions, including the following points: the anesthetic often gives initial pain relief that recedes over the next few hours. The effects of the corticosteroid is not expected for 2–6 days (26). Accordingly, a patient may experience a bimodal relief pattern, with symptoms initially improving, then returning over the first few days, followed by a longer period of relief. Rarely, symptoms can be paradoxically worse during the interval between the effects of the anesthetic and the steroids. Obviously, some patients will not respond and others will respond to only the anesthetic or the steroid, without a bimodal effect. Additionally, patients vary widely in their degree of pain relief.

Finally, the authors ensure that patients understand that initial nonresponders may benefit from a second or even third injection sometimes (19,38); for this reason, some referring doctors will routinely preschedule three monthly injections for their patients.

MIDLINE EPIDURAL STEROID INJECTIONS: LUMBAR (ILESI) AND CAUDAL APPROACHES
Indications: Caudal and Lumbar ILESI

Typically, radiologists do not have control over who is referred for ESI. The current authors are willing to perform the procedure on all our referrals, provided they do not have contraindications, based on the safety of epidural steroid injections and numerous anecdotal successes in patients whose indications are not supported by clinical trials. It is difficult to deny a patient a chance at relief, even if that chance is small, especially if they have exhausted other conservative options. Still, all who perform ESIs need to be familiar with typical indications and be able to discuss the likelihood of success with their patients and referring clinicians.

LUMBAR/CAUDAL

Radicular pain, with or without low-back pain, is the principal indication for lumbar ESI (32,39–41). Although commonly performed, substantial efficacy of ESI in mechanical or nonradiating pain has not been routinely supported (23,32). Some, such as Rivest et al., report diminished success in patients with symptoms from spinal stenosis, rather than from herniated discs (42); however, others have not supported this discrepancy.

Second, most investigators describe higher success rates in patients with short-term pain (less than three or six months) (1,26,39,43,44) than in those with pain lasting more than a year, possibly because inflammation eventually gives way to fibrosis (23). Third, a study by Hopwood and Abram demonstrated a statistically significant increased risk of failure when patients were unemployed, smoked, and had nonradicular and long-term pain (45).

Postoperative patients (26,39,46) and those with neurogenic claudication (47) have been shown to have much lower success with ESI. Fredman et al. point out that surgical adhesions and scar tissue may often prevent the medication from reaching the source of the pain, a concept supported by the pattern of contrast injections on postoperative patients (46). This idea prompted Revel et al. to use forceful injection of 40 cc of saline following injection of caudal steroid to theoretically break up adhesions (48). Although they achieved mediocre results overall, the forceful injection group did statistically better than the steroid-alone injection group. Fukusaki et al. suggested that neurogenic claudication is an ischemic neuropathy, rather than inflammatory, explaining the lack of efficacy of ESI for this population (47). Finally, neoplasm, infection, or spondyloarthropathy is not indication for epidural injection.

Contraindications: Caudal and Lumbar ILESI

As for all invasive procedures, patients with a hemorrhagic diathesis, local infection, or a history of reaction to the medications should not undergo ESI. Even a systemic or distant infection is a contraindication because steroids impair the immune system (5,23,32). Other contraindications in the literature include cauda equina syndrome, pilonidal cysts, and neurological disorders that could be masked by this procedure (5).

Importantly, the safety of aspirin and other antiplatelet medications in ESI has been the subject of two studies. These two reports documented no evidence of epidural hematoma in a total of 637 epidural injections and infusions (38,49). Because the authors employ a 25-gauge needle, patients may continue taking aspirin prior to an ESI.

Interestingly, ESI with a 25-gauge needle may be safe even in anticoagulated patients. Waldman et al. described a series of 336 epidural blocks using morphine sulfate and bupivicaine in cancer patients who were either medically anticoagulated or thrombocytopenic and had intractable pain. In their series, there were only two ecchymoses in the superficial tissues and no evidence of epidural hematoma. Although they do not promote routine use of ESI in anticoagulated patients, they thought it likely to be safe when absolutely necessary (50).

Although diabetes and cardiac disease are not contraindications to ESI, these conditions do require extra caution. Corticosteroids are known to increase the lability of blood glucose levels in patients with diabetes. In patients controlled with oral medications or diet, notifying patients that their blood sugar may transiently elevate is thought to be sufficient by the authors. Insulin-dependent patients can increase the dose of insulin they use at the discretion of their endocrinologist/primary care physician. Extremely brittle diabetics may require a decrease in the dose of steroid administered.

Steroids may also lead to water retention and possibly initiate congestive heart failure in patients with poor cardiac reserve (32,51). As such, the current authors reduce the steroid dose by 25–50% in these patients.

Technique: Caudal and Lumbar ILESI

The following descriptions of these procedures reflect the techniques used in the authors' department. Various details of these procedures can be varied and these techniques may be adjusted according to training, experience, equipment, and preferences.

Neither the lumbar/interlaminar nor the caudal approach has an advantage in efficacy. As such, the choice of route depends on operator preference and equipment. The lumbar/interlaminar method usually allows placement of the needle closer to the lesion and has a lower risk of intravenous positioning. The caudal approach may be easier in postoperative patients, allows better access to the L5/S1 space, and carries a lower risk of intrathecal injection (23,29,52).

Prior to the procedure the patient's images are reviewed and a route is selected. Most practitioners prefer to be within two levels of the pathology (ideally at or below it), Harley demonstrated that 6 ml of contrast injected at the L4/5 level consistently spread up to L1 and down over the sacrum (43). For interlaminar injections, it is important to target a level with a sufficient posterior epidural recess filled with fat. If the patient does not have a cross-sectional study (MR or CT) immediately available, a caudal approach is safer than a blind lumbar interlaminar attempt. MR or CT may also demonstrate findings that may preclude or alter the procedure, including Tarlov cysts or spinal dysraphism.

The procedure is described to the patient and informed consent is obtained. Risks that are quoted include infection, bleeding, intrathecal injection, and allergic reaction. Focused questions regarding history of diabetes, cardiac conditions, and allergies are posed. In the authors' institution, a significant number of calls and questions are avoided with a general warning regarding some of the short-term side effects of systemic absorption of steroids: face flushing, insomnia, diarrhea, mood swings, and itching are the most common side effects encountered. The patient is informed that these side effects are seen in a small fraction of patients, correlate to the peak activity of the steroids (2–7 days following injection) and should be self-limited. We do not routinely use IV sedation for any of our spinal injections, so a detailed discussion of the risks implicit in sedation is not required. Additionally, the patient's cardiovascular status is not monitored during the procedure.

We use a multipurpose C-arm fluoroscopy machine with both transverse and craniocaudal obliquity capability because numerous authors report frequent misplacement of needles when inserted blindly (20,53). White et al. reported malposition in 30% of interlaminar and 25% of caudal approaches performed without fluoroscopy (54). The rate of intrathecal injection ranges from 0.6% to 10% but is usually quoted as 2.5% for injections without fluoroscopy (55,56). Intravascular placement occurs from 0.2% to 11% of the time without fluoroscopy, and up to three-quarters of these will not be demonstrated by aspiration (9,29,54–57). The theoretical risks related to inadvertent intravascular injections include cardiac toxicity, respiratory arrest, and seizure, and there is at least one report of a case of intravascular injection of lignocaine causing convulsions during an attempted ESI (55). Hence, injection of the medication in its intended location demands fluoroscopic guidance and confirmation with contrast.

LUMBAR INTERLAMINAR EPIDURAL STEROID INJECTION

The patient is placed prone on the fluoroscopy table. A pillow or bolster under the abdomen spreads the spinous processes, facilitating passage of the needle. Rotation of the C-arm may be necessary to center the spinous processes. Craniocaudal tilt can be used to assess the interspinous distance and the needle angulation needed to intersect the epidural space at the appropriate level. If the interspinous space is obliterated (Baastrup's sign), a paramedian approach may be the only approach to afford epidural space entry (see following hints). With a direct midline approach, the needle passes between the spinous processes to reach its target. The intended site of entry is marked, typically overlying the upper portion of the more inferior spinous process (Figure 3A).

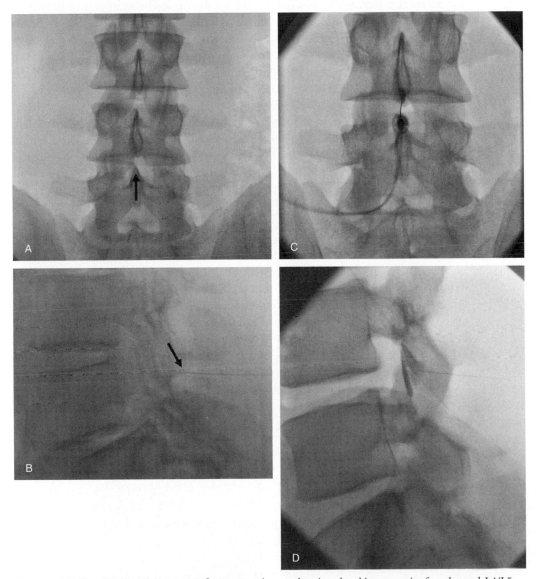

Figure 3. Midline ILESI. (A) Scout AP flouro spot image showing the skin entry site for planned L4/L5 ILESI (arrow). (B) Lateral flouro spot image showing target site for needle tip placement 1–2 mm deep to the dorsal margin of the inferior articulating process. This usually places the needle tip in the ligamentum flavum and where air release technique should start (arrow). (C) AP flouro spot image following air release and injection of a small amount of contrast. The contrast pools around the tip of the needle. (D) Lateral flouro spot image showing contrast pooling along the dorsal epidural space.

Standard preparation and drape procedures are followed by anesthesia of the skin and local tissues with 1% lidocaine buffered with sodium bicarbonate. Under frontal fluoroscopic guidance, a 25-gauge, 3.5-inch spinal needle is advanced, usually employing a slight cranial angulation. Knowing that a spinal needle tracks in a direction opposite of its bevel, the needle can be steered to keep it centered and on line to reach the target. Once the needle lies within the interspinous ligament, it is unusual for it to deflect laterally; from this point, the needle is advanced with lateral fluoroscopic visualization.

One stops advancing the needle when it crosses the posterior margin of the facets (see Figure 3B), positioning the needle tip in the ligamentum flavum. A check of the AP projection ensures continued midline placement. Subsequently, the "air release technique" with AP fluoroscopic guidance is used for further needle advances. The air release technique is accomplished by attaching a glass or low-resistance plastic syringe to the needle (10) and attempting to inject 0.5 ml of air. While the needle tip remains posterior to the epidural space, and within the firm ligamentum flavum, the plunger will bounce back (with the exception of a small space posterior to the ligamentum flavum – see hints). Continue advancing a millimeter at a time, and alternate with an air puff, until there is no bounce back, signaling needle tip entry into the epidural space.

Contrast is then instilled via short, flexible extension tubing, under continuous AP fluoroscopy. When contrast is appropriately within the epidural space, it pools around the needle tip (Figure 3C). However, if the needle tip lies within the thecal sac, the contrast quickly diffuses and does not pool at the needle tip. Check the lateral projection, which should show contrast collecting at the dorsal margin of the thecal sac (Figure 3D) and eventually extending slightly anterior to the thecal sac when there is enough contrast to flow around the sides of the thecal sac. If the needle tip is misplaced into a vein, contrast does not pool but whisks away into branching/tortuous venous structures (Figure 4). Contrast within the thecal sac will layer on the dependent ventral margin of the thecal sac (Figure 5). Luckily, when fluoroscopy is employed, intrathecal injection occurs less than 1% of the time.

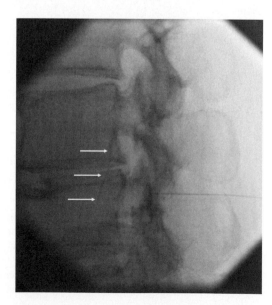

Figure 4. Midline ILESI showing a small vessel filling with contrast. Small-needle manipulations are usually sufficient to ensure a purely extravascular location.

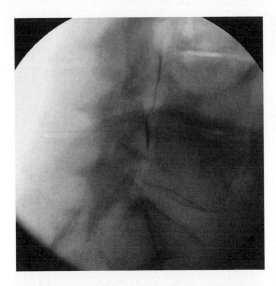

Figure 5. Intrathecal needle placement. The contrast layers in a thin line dependently along the ventral aspect of the thecal sac, forming a fluid-fluid level.

Inadvertent intrathecal placement obviates injection at that level. To proceed would cause a spinal block and the steroids would wash away in the CSF. While Silbergleit et al. terminate the procedure and reschedule if this happens (10), most authors will immediately choose another level; there are no reported mishaps from this practice (8,43,46). The current authors will make a second attempt at a next contiguous level if the spinal needle is a 25-gauge one. If the needle is larger, such as a 22-gauge one, we will reschedule the procedure in 5–7 days, sufficient time for the dural puncture to become healed. This is based on our anecdotal experience (Figure 6A, C).

When the needle position within the epidural space has been documented, a solution containing 2 ml Kenalog-40 and 5 ml preservative-free 0.5% lidocaine is instilled over 1–2 minutes, with initial visualization in the lateral plane. Unless the needle becomes dislodged, the contrast pool will increase initially, from the small residual contrast remaining in the tubing, followed by contrast dilution and dispersal by the radiolucent medication. Some patients experience discomfort or even pain during the injection. This should improve with a reduced injection rate. Spot images should be obtained in the AP and lateral planes, documenting epidural contrast as proof of appropriate needle tip placement. These spot images will aid the next operator if the patient returns for a subsequent injection; additionally, if the patient subsequently develops a headache, the spot images will exclude intrathecal positioning as a cause of spinal headache (corticosteroids may cause headaches as a side effect). The needle is removed, the puncture site is cleansed with alcohol, and a bandage is placed. Some patients experience lightheadedness following the procedure, mandating close assistance while patients slowly rise from the procedure table.

Our practice has been to release ESI patients after the brief time it takes to clean up and have a short discussion regarding change in pain after the procedure. The rare patient who requires conscious sedation or who suffers from a significant motor nerve anesthesia may be detained longer. We caution patients to limit their activities on the day of the procedure and then resume normal activities the next day, including providing work releases for the day of the procedure. All patients must bring a driver.

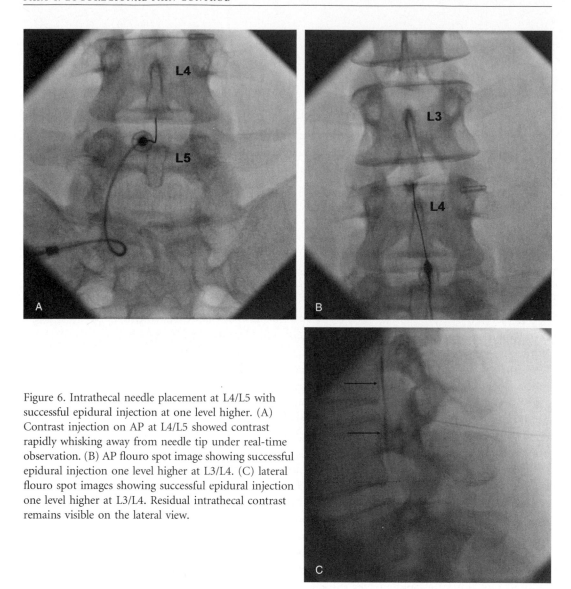

Figure 6. Intrathecal needle placement at L4/L5 with successful epidural injection at one level higher. (A) Contrast injection on AP at L4/L5 showed contrast rapidly whisking away from needle tip under real-time observation. (B) AP flouro spot image showing successful epidural injection one level higher at L3/L4. (C) lateral flouro spot images showing successful epidural injection one level higher at L3/L4. Residual intrathecal contrast remains visible on the lateral view.

HINTS
Optimize the Planned Needle Route

Sometimes, ESI must be tailored to suit the situation. One should evaluate for adequate space between the spinous processes at the selected level. If the space is not sufficient, it will often improve sufficiently with the addition of a second bolster under the abdomen. In these patients, checking one's approach at the beginning in the lateral fluoroscopic position, or with craniocaudal angulation of the tube, will ensure that the selected skin site will allow a direct course to the target.

Paramedian Technique

If bolstering fails to increase the interspinous distance adequately to allow passage of a needle (Figure 7) or there is presence of interspinous ligamentous

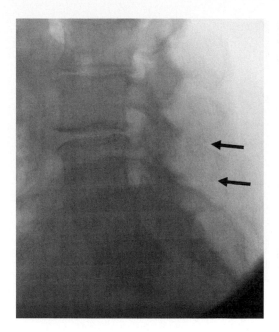

Figure 7. Lateral flouro spot image with bolster in place, showing close approximation of the spinous processes (arrows), precluding the midline interlaminar approach. A paramedian approach is necessary.

calcification or articulation of adjacent spinous processes (Baastrup's sign), a paramedian approach can still allow an interlaminar injection.

Once the level is selected, the laminar notches on either side of the spinous process are localized. The tube is craniocaudally tilted to align the apex of the notch with the upper margin of the disk space. Ten degrees of lateral angulation to one side is sufficient to open the laminar notch and bring the needle tip into the posterior epidural space (Figure 8A). Frequently, we check both sides to choose the laminar notch that is the least impeded by osseous protuberances from the spinous process. The top of the laminar notch is used as the landmark and, using a bull's-eye approach, the needle is advanced, keeping the tip closer to the spinous process (medially) than the lamina (laterally) (Figure 8B). The interspinous ligament is not encountered in this approach and the first significant resistance is felt at the ligamentum flavum.

Medial or lateral deviation of the needle is occasionally necessary to arrive at a midline location at the appropriate depth. The straight AP projection is used to ensure that the needle is coursing toward the midline (Figure 8C). On lateral projection, the same osseous landmarks are used to begin checking air release. If air release is achieved, the position of the needle tip is checked in the AP projection to ensure an appropriate midline position and contrast then injected to confirm needle tip position (Figure 8D, E).

We apply this technique commonly in patients with degenerative disease of the spine, with great success. Many practitioners use this approach exclusively, due to the ease of alignment and the guaranteed unencumbered course to the epidural space.

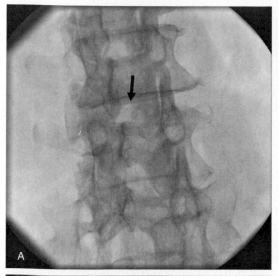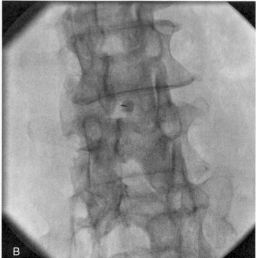

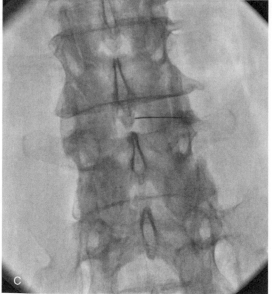

Figure 8. Paramedian technique. (A) Rightward angulation of 10°–15° and appropriate craniocaudal angulation to align the laminar notch (arrow) with the disc space. (B) Bull's-eye approach with 25-gauge, 3.5-inch spinal needle. (C) Confirmation in the AP projection that the needle is coursing toward the midline in order to intersect the epidural space appropriately. (D) Injection of contrast in AP projections following air release, confirming epidural needle tip location. (E) Injection of contrast in lateral projections following air release, confirming epidural needle tip location.

Target the Largest Portion of the Epidural Space

The epidural space is typically the largest at the level of the disc space. This can vary between patients and, however, review of a preprocedural MRI can provide a more specific target level. Typically, the disc space is a convenient landmark on both the AP and lateral views, usually indicating the greatest epidural space at a particular level.

Preview Needle Course in Lateral Plane

Some patients require no needle angulation to reach the epidural space, which can affect skin entry site. When in doubt, previewing in the lateral plane will help.

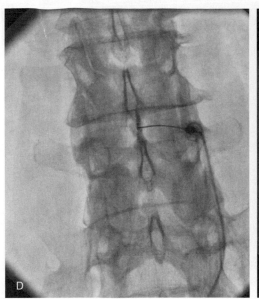
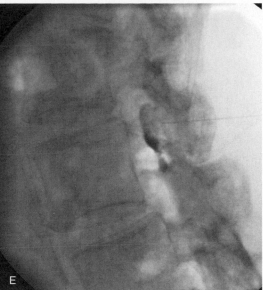

Figure 8. (*continued*)

Tilt the Tube

If the needle contacts the bone and it is uncertain which bone is obstructing the path, tilting the tube (in the AP plane) down the barrel of the needle often will reveal the culprit.

Use a Needle of Adequate Length

Larger patients may require a longer needle to reach the epidural space. Unfortunately, 25-gauge needles longer than 3.5 inches are quite difficult to steer; thus, in large patients we use a 6-inch, 22-gauge spinal needle.

Beware the "Partial" and "Premature" Air Release

While performing the air release technique, a bounce back may be followed by a partial air release after the next advancement. Although this "partial" air release is unsatisfying, it invariably signals initial entry of a portion of the needle lumen into the epidural space, and further needle advancement (just to be sure) may only position the needle within the thecal sac. To confuse matters, though, when a partial or a full air release occurs before expected, the position of the needle tip may be posterior to the ligamentum flavum, a space that can accept air insufflation as easily as the epidural space (Figure 9). If contrast injection shows a retrolaminar collection, the needle must be advanced slowly with intermittent contrast injection to confirm eventual epidural needle placement. After the contrast has been injected initially, the air release technique occasionally works but is not reliable.

Clear the Needle

After each set of three needle advances and air puffs, reinsertion of the stylet is advisable to clear soft tissue that may be clogging the needle tip.

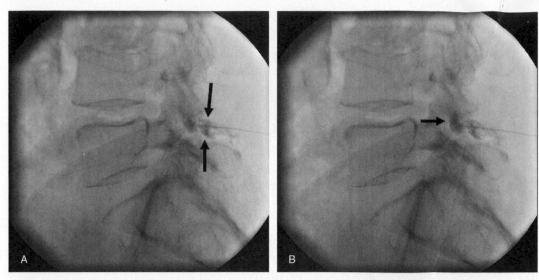

Figure 9. Air release prompted retrolaminar injection of contrast. (A) Contrast is seen extending into the interspinous space (arrows). Air release technique is no longer reliable once contrast has been injected into the needle. (B) Needle advancement in the lateral projection with intermittent contrast injection will confirm epidural needle placement (arrow).

Gadolinium as Alternative

Finally, if the patient is allergic to iodinated contrast, gadolinium is an acceptable alternative. Gadolinium is quite visible with high-quality fluoroscopic equipment, especially if a digital subtraction run is employed.

CAUDAL

Caudal epidural steroid injections are best performed in the prone position; the lateral decubitus position with the hips flexed may be employed if a patient cannot lie prone. Padding may be placed under the pelvis to provide an optimal angle of approach. The sacral hiatus is located by running a finger down the midline sacrum, until the coccyx is reached. The sacral cornua are just above the coccyx, about a centimeter lateral of midline, and often palpable (Figure 2). The location of the hiatus, the target for entry to the sacral epidural space, should be verified with lateral fluoroscopy and marked. Then, gauze is placed within the gluteal crease to protect the sensitive perineum from spillage of sterilizing solution. After standard sterile preparation and drape, local anesthesia of the skin and sacral periosteum is achieved with 1% lidocaine buffered with sodium bicarbonate.

Because caudal ESI patients complain of less pain with a 25-gauge spinal needle (3.5-inches) than a 22-gauge needle, we select the former. Although some practitioners employ a 20-gauge or larger needle, these may cause prolonged pain because of irritation caused by the needle scraping along the periosteum. Additionally, smaller needles are more flexible, allowing one to follow the sacral contour and avoid ventral penetration of the sacrum into the perirectal regional or dorsal penetration through the sacral roof to the skin (Figure 10). Due to the sensitivity of the sacral periosteum, a liberal amount of lidocaine is administered at the level of the cornua. Placing a curve on the end of the needle helps the needle to follow the slope of the sacrum.

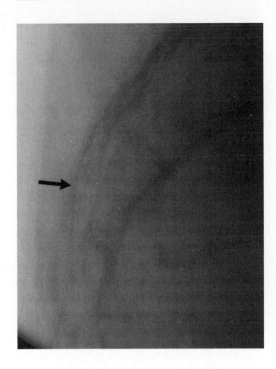

Figure 10. Needle penetration of the dorsal sacral cortex. Placing a gentle curve at the needle tip and advancing while rotating the needle will help to avoid periosteal or cortical penetration.

Entering at a 45° angle with the bevel down, the needle is advanced through the sacrococcygeal ligament and stopped upon encountering the underlying bone. After fluoroscopic verification of appropriate midline position within the sacral canal, the needle is withdrawn slightly from the periosteum and the needle is laid almost horizontal, until it parallels the sacral canal. The needle is advanced cephalad through the canal. Appropriate orientation of the bevel and a gentle rotating motion may help the needle to follow the curved contour of the sacral canal. Midline position of the needle within the canal must be intermittently confirmed with fluoroscopy. The final target is the middle or upper half of the S3 segment, certainly below the S2/3 junction (Figure 11A).

Following needle placement, extradural position of the needle tip is confirmed by injection of 1–2 cc of contrast (Omnipque-300) with fluoroscopic monitoring. If the needle is appropriately placed, the epidurogram resembles a Christmas tree and the contrast does not disperse rapidly (Figure 11B). If the needle tip is in an epidural vein, the contrast will flow into serpentine structures. To extricate the needle from the vessel, slight advancement should be attempted first. If this is unsuccessful, the needle may have to be completely withdrawn and replaced. Theoretically, it may help to direct the needle dorsally, because the epidural veins are more prominent ventrally within the sacral epidural space. If the patient has a plica mediana dorsalis, the contrast will fill only one side of the epidural space; in this event, redirecting the needle or repuncture may be required to achieve satisfactory medication delivery.

If the needle is intrathecal, the procedure must be terminated. Readjusting of the needle is not recommended after piercing the sacral thecal sac and the procedure should be rescheduled in 5–7 days.

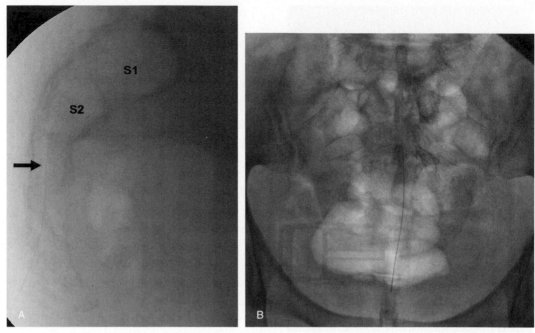

Figure 11. (A) Lateral projection showing proper needle tip position at the mid to superior portion of the S3 vertebral body. (B) "Christmas tree" appearance of contrast distribution in a caudal injection.

After confirming epidural needle tip position and documenting it with AP and lateral spot radiographs, the medication may be injected. Our solution consists of 2 ml of Kenalog-40 with 5–8 ml of preservative-free 0.5% lidocaine. Recommendations for volume of injectate vary. More recent reports (58,59) have demonstrated that 10 ml of injectate consistently reaches the low- to mid-lumbar spine. This amount of lidocaine will not overdilute the steroids. Some practitioners choose to inject the steroids first with the preservative-free lidocaine as a "chaser." In our experience, the majority of patients can tolerate 10 ml of injectate. In the occasional patient who does not tolerate this volume, the chaser method ensures that the patient has received the entire steroid dose.

The injection should not encounter any resistance; if so, needle malposition should be considered. If the patient complains of pressure or dull or shooting pain down the legs, a decreased injection rate should allow symptoms to resolve. After the procedure, the needle is removed, the puncture site is cleansed with alcohol, and a bandage is applied. The patient is assisted while rising slowly. The postprocedure routine is the same as for lumbar injections.

Complications: Caudal and Lumbar ILESI

Complications from epidural injections are uncommon, but they vary from minor to severe. Watts and Silagy compiled a list of adverse effects in their meta-analysis of controlled trials of ESI; those adverse effects included subarachnoid tap (2.5%), transient headache (2%), and transient increase in low-back or radicular pain (2%). There was one report of irregular menses (41).

Other authors have reported side effects including transient vasovagal response, angina, and respiratory difficulty with an inadvertent spinal block (39). In a report on 5,489 consecutive fluoroscopy-guided ESIs, Johnson et al. noted only four complications that necessitated hospitalization or an emergency department visit. These complications included one vasovagal reaction and an episode of "significant hypotension," both of which resolved uneventfully; a self-limited cervical epidural hematoma in which symptoms resolved after 18 hours; and a patient who was admitted for 3 days of observation for tachycardia and hypertension, thought to be due to an unusual steroid effect (60).

Epidural injection of steroids is known to cause occasional insomnia, facial flushing, or nausea; despite the epidural placement, a small amount may enter the systemic circulation (51). Other possible systemic effects are Cushingoid effects, which were much more common in the past, when higher doses were typical (34,61); and suppression of the hypothalamic-pituitary axis for about 3 weeks, which has been documented in canine (62) and human (63) studies. This latter effect becomes important if the patient has subsequent surgery (62,63) and may preclude the epidural injection or require steroid supplementation at the time of surgery.

We have not found a study that documents the risk of osteonecrosis from an ESI; although this is one of the known risks of systemic steroid exposure, most practitioners do not believe osteonecrosis is a substantial risk of ESI as it is currently practiced. Risk of inducing osteopenia/osteoporosis has been assuaged by a study by Dubois et al. measuring bone mineral density in 28 patients receiving chronic injections of epidural methyl prednisilone and correlating to cumulative steroid dose (64).

Acute and chronic local effects are also a concern. Abram reviewed the published complications of ESI; his list included five epidural abscesses; one case of aseptic meningitis following an inadvertent intrathecal injection; two cases of bacterial meningitis, one following an intrathecal injection and the other not documented; and no reports of arachnoiditis. Arachnoiditis has only been documented in the setting of multiple intrathecal steroid injections, a former therapy for multiple sclerosis no longer practiced (32). Slucky et al. found no significant alterations/weakening of the dura after ESI in dogs. Interestingly, this group noted a reduction of posterior epidural fat in 17 of 24 specimens (65), arguing against the common notion that local deposit of steroids may cause epidural lipomatosis.

In their study, Botwin et al. reported a 15.6% rate of minor complications from epidural steroid injections (51). The incidence of major complications is uncertain but undoubtedly rare (66).

Efficacy: Caudal and Lumbar ILESI

Neither caudal nor interlaminar epidural injection has been shown to have an advantage in efficacy for patients with symptoms emanating from the lumbar spine (41,67). Although numerous uncontrolled studies have touted the results of ESI, most demonstrate a much higher benefit over the short term (a few months) than the long term (a year or more) (26,32,43,54,68–71). Critics of these studies cite their lack of control patients; however, many provided relief for patients who had already failed other nonsurgical treatments. Spaccarelli reviewed 26 uncontrolled studies and calculated an overall efficacy of 65% (23).

As ESI has become the subject of more rigorous studies, controlled investigations have not uniformly supported the benefits of ESI. Some controlled studies demonstrate a benefit from ESI (3,19,67,72–74), whereas others have not (75–79). Notably, the two studies commonly used to criticize ESI (77,78) were not designed in a way that should produce a successful result given today's understanding of the effects of ESI (68,80). Both studies assessed patients less than two days after the injection, when depot steroids have not taken full effect; and then not again for at least 8 (78) or 13 (77) months, when then natural history of disc herniations would lead one to expect many patients' pain to have resolved anyway. After this long period, one would also expect the depot steroids to have lost any residual effects.

Several authors have made systematic attempts to analyze all of the controlled studies (23,40,68,80,81), a task made quite difficult given the wide range of indications, injection techniques, outcome measures, and length of follow-up periods across the various studies they collected (2,80). Even these authors have not agreed, with some concluding that ESI has at least a short-term benefit (23,40) and others neither documenting nor refuting efficacy of ESI (80,81). The reviewing authors bemoaned the methodological flaws of each controlled study. For instance, a major flaw in all of the studies they reviewed was that none used fluoroscopy to guide and document successful placement of the needle within the epidural space (46,80) despite the fact that several investigators have demonstrated that blind placement of needles into the epidural space is often inaccurate (53,54,57).

In one analysis of 11 randomized controlled trials of ESI, the procedure increased the odds ratio of short-term pain relief (defined as greater than 75% reduction in pain for up to 60 days) to 2.61, versus placebo. The odds ratio for the long term fell to 1.87. Hence, this review supported the short-term success of ESI and also suggested that some, but not as many, patients may experience relief over longer periods (41).

The three most recent studies, not included in the above meta-analyses, showed mixed results as well (73,74,79). In a profoundly flawed randomized, double-blind, controlled clinical trial, Valat et al. (79) showed no difference between epidural saline injection and ESI. Despite compelling evidence for the inaccuracy of blind injections, all injections in the study were performed without image guidance. Only clinical criteria were used to select patients with "presumed sciatica," without imaging support. No long-term follow-up was performed.

Wilson-MacDonald et al. showed significant short-term improvement in the epidural steroid group when compared to saline group, but no long-term ability to avoid surgery. Most patients only received a single injection, also performed blindly. Butterman et al. used fluoroscopically guided injections in 38 of their 50 patients (76%), and permitted multiple injections. Their data showed that 50% of patients who received ESI were able to avoid discectomy. These patients had comparable results measured by visual analog scale (VAS) and Oswestry scores to those patients who underwent successful discectomy.

LUMBAR TRANSFORAMINAL EPIDURAL STEROID INJECTIONS

Indications: Lumbar Transforaminal Epidural Steroid Injection

The transforaminal epidural steroid injection (TFESI) has the benefit of placing the medication closer to the affected nerve root. This allows a more selective treatment of a particular radicular pattern. As such, the patient selection criteria differ slightly from the interlaminar or caudal injection.

Interlaminar and caudal approaches are a "shotgun approach" to the treatment of low-back pain and radiculopathy and are intended to bathe both sides of the epidural space with a steroid mixture. In addition, the interlaminar approach has been shown to predominantly deposit the mixture dorsally in contradistinction to the transforaminal approach, which has been shown to preferentially deposit the steroid mixture in the foramen and anterior epidural space, where discogenic radiculopathy most commonly originates (82).

Controlled studies have shown efficacy of TFSEI predominantly in patients with more lower extremity pain than back pain (83–91). However, further patient selection criteria are broad, with efficacy shown in patients from relatively acute (less than six months) onset of radiculopathy (84,87–89,91) to chronic pain (83). Surgical candidates have been shown to benefit (88,91) as well as those with history of prior surgery (90). Patients with discogenic radiculopathy are probably most likely to benefit (84,87,89,91), although studies have shown benefit in spinal stenosis (88,90,92), degenerative spondylosis (83,90), lateral recess narrowing (83,88,90), and epidural lipomatosis (93).

In general, demographic breakdown of those benefiting from TFESI parallels that of epidural injections. Notable demographic subsets that are statistically less likely to do well are those with worker's compensation settlements pending and those going back to significantly physical labor (90). Some pain management physicians will refuse to treat patients with ongoing workman's compensation claims for this reason.

In our practice, the transforaminal injection is viewed as the injection of choice for those patients with unilateral radiculopathy in a discrete nerve root distribution. With concerted effort put forth to produce epidural reflux, the transforaminal approach may affect nerve root distributions at adjacent levels through epidural spread (usually cephalad) of the steroid injectate. If strictly diagnostic information regarding the affected level is needed, a selective nerve root block (SNRB) would be more useful. If a particular nerve root distribution is affected unilaterally, and therapeutic benefit is of chief concern, the transforaminal approach combines selectivity with a steroid dose equal to that administered through an interlaminar or caudal injection.

Contraindications: Lumbar TFESI

Typical contraindications to interventional procedures apply: hemorrhagic diathesis, local or systemic infection, and allergic reaction to the medications. Coumadin should be stopped three days prior to injection with no international normalized ratio (INR) check required at our institution. Aspirin and antiplatelet medications are acceptable for procedures in the lumbar spine. The special considerations of diabetes and cardiac failure have been addressed previously.

Technique: Lumbar TFESI

The descriptions of these procedures in the following paragraphs reflect the methods and techniques employed in our department. Multiple aspects of these procedures can be varied, and these techniques should be adjusted according to training, experience, facilities, and preferences.

Preprocedural imaging is requisite at our institution, with particular attention paid to the presence of a nerve root sheath cyst or any other anatomic anomaly that may preclude safe injection. The procedure is described to the patient and informed consent is obtained. The risks are similar to that of ILESI, with the risk of nerve damage added to the list. A focused medical history is necessary to exclude significant allergies or medical conditions. The possibilities of minor side effects to the steroids (listed in the ILESI section) are broached, in order to allay the patient's concerns. Patient comfort in a prone position should be explored, as this can be a significant hurdle in those with radicular pain. No IV sedation is necessary in the vast majority of cases.

The patient is placed prone on the fluoroscopy table. No abdominal bolster is routinely necessary, but at times it makes patients more comfortable and may decrease tension on an inflamed nerve root. It is a matter of personal preference as to whether to work on the ipsilateral or contralateral side of intended injection. Most feel that placing the patient on the table and working from the contralateral side affords more freedom from the image intensifier in the oblique orientation. Prior to proceeding with target localization a time-out should be performed to confirm the side of the patient's radiculopathy.

The goal of needle placement in TFESI is the "safe triangle" described by Bogduk et al. (94), in a subpediculate, supraneural, intraforaminal location (Figure 12). To most effectively profile the safe triangle, a direct AP projection is initially attained with obliquities as necessary to line up the spinous processes centered between the pedicles. The disc space is then profiled at the intended

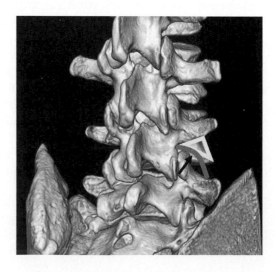

Figure 12. Target for right L4/L5 TFESI. Surface-rendered lumbar CT with right posterior oblique (RPO) angulation and craniocaudal tilt to profile the L4/L5 disc space. The "safe triangle" described by Bodguk and colleagues.

level of intervention. An ipsilateral obliquity of 25°–30° is usually sufficient to attain the "Scotty dog" appearance of the on-end pedicle, transverse process, and superior articular process with the target at the 6 o'clock position of the on-end pedicle (Figure 13). The needle entry site is slightly below the inferior border of the pedicle cortex, and not directly underneath. This is because fluoroscopy summates the various portions of the pedicle cortex with the most prominent visible area being the central, tapered section, thereby underestimating the caliber of the most superficial margin. Therefore, placing the needle directly under the inferior cortex will either block or inferiorly displace the needle during its positioning, preventing ideal position and increasing the risk of nerve injury.

The skin entry site (Figure 14A) is marked with indelible ink and the skin is sterilely prepared and draped. Depending on patient size and the obliquity of the planned needle course a 3.5 or 6-inch 22-gauge needle is selected. The skin and subcutaneous tissues are anesthetized with 1% lidocaine buffered with sodium bicarbonate. The initial needle advancement is made in the oblique projection using a bull's-eye technique just below the 6 o'clock position on the pedicle (Figure 14B). Once the bull's-eye route has gained significant purchase, the needle can be advanced in the true AP and lateral projections. Checking the bull's-eye projection periodically may be necessary to confirm the needle is within the safe triangle. The goal of needle tip placement is intraforaminal on the lateral view and no further medial than 6:30 position on the left and 5:30 position on the right in the direct AP view (Figure 14C, D). Commonly, there is a palpable pop as the foramen is pierced.

After attaining the intended location, the stylet is removed and iodinated contrast (gadolinium in the presence of contrast allergy) is connected to the needle with short flexible tubing. The use of flexible tubing is a recurring theme in our practice, and limits needle tip manipulation when transferring different injection syringes. The ideal injection produces a neurogram of the exiting nerve root and refluxes under the pedicle into the adjacent epidural space (Figure 14C, F). In the event that there is a predominant flow pattern – either epidural or perineural – minimal needle tip manipulations can be attempted

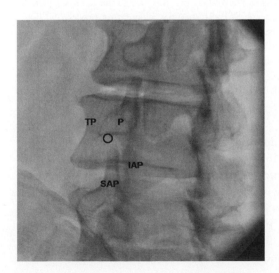

Figure 13. LPO fluoroscopic spot image of 25°–30° showing the target site for left L4/L5 transforaminal epidural. The 6 o'clock position of the on-end pedicle should be targeted. Obliquity needs to be sufficient to move the superior articulating process medial to the course of the needle: P–L4 pedicle; TP–L4 transverse process; IAP–L4 inferior articulating process; SAP–L5 superior articulating process.

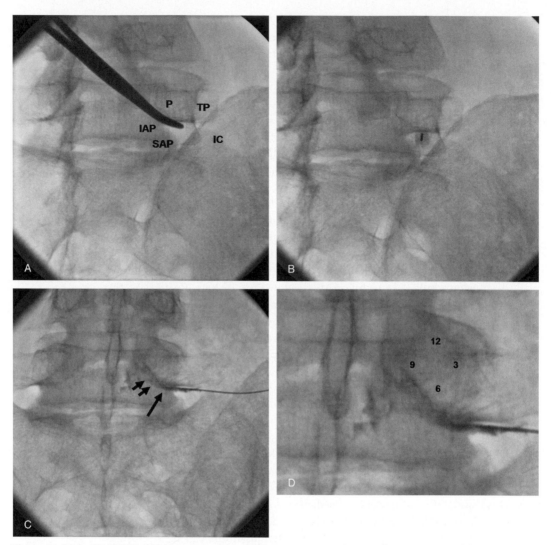

Figure 14. Right L5 TFESI. (A) Target marked with hemostat. Note the significant craniocaudal angulation necessary to profile the L5/S1 disc space and the small window allowed by the presence of the IC: P–L5 pedicle; TP–L5 transverse process; IAP–L5 inferior articulating process; SAP–S1 superior articulating process; IC iliac crest. (B) Bull's-eye needle placement at the 6 o'clock position of the pedicle. (C,D) AP fluoroscopic image showing proper needle tip position (long arrow). The needle tip should not be advanced more medially than the 5:30 clock position on the right pedicle (6:30 position on the left). Contrast should flow under the pedicle into the epidural space (short arrows). (E) Lateral fluoroscopic image showing needle tip placement within the superior aspect of the neural foramen. (F) Right L4/L5 TFESI AP flouroscopic image in a different patient with proper 50/50 contrast flow pattern.

with care to achieve a 50/50 flow pattern. A lateral view after injection of contrast is necessary to exclude inadvertent intrathecal placement (Figure 14E).

Careful consideration of intravascular placement is needed – particularly on the left – prior to proceeding with the steroid injection. Although aspiration has been reported as a means to assess intravascular needle tip placement, this method should be considered inaccurate, with 74% of intravascular needle placements demonstrating no flashback in a large study by Sullivan et al. (95). Meticulous observation under active fluoroscopy is necessary to evaluate

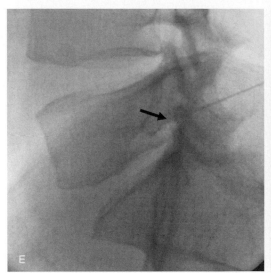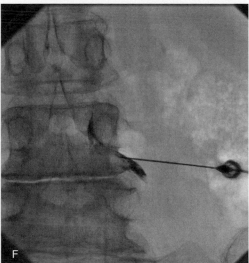

Figure 14. (*continued*)

for any visible arterial flow or rapid contrast clearance indicating vascular clearout. Digital subtraction angiography can be used for equivocal cases. If the needle tip is found to be intravascular, it is usually venous and indicated by larger caliber and slow flow, and advancement or retraction is usually sufficient to find a safe extravascular injection location. If the artery of Adamkiewicz or other radicular artery is identified, the needle should be removed and needle placement pursued at another level (see following paragraphs for further discussion).

The steroid/anesthetic mixture of choice is then infused slowly over approximately one minute. The steroid mixture we use for TFESI is 2 cc Celestone Soluspan (betamethasone sodium phosphate and betamethasone sodium acetate) with 2-cc 1% preservative-free lidocaine. We use Celestone due to the success seen in early work by Botwin et al. (83) and significantly smaller particle size, theoretically decreasing the chance of vascular occlusion compared with Kenalog-40 (triamcinolone acetonide) (95), if inadvertent intravascular injection is performed.

The needle is removed and the field is cleansed with a small bandage placed on the puncture site. The patient is assisted while rising slowly. Patients rarely experience motor block but may need wheelchair assistance following TFESI due to dense paresthesia, particularly if multiple or bilateral injections are performed. The patient is not detained longer than it takes for clean up and a short postprocedure discussion. We require all patients to be accompanied by a driver.

SPECIAL CONSIDERATION – S1 TFESI

The S1 TFESI is a common injection and can be separated from an S1 nerve root block with careful attention. The cross-sectional anatomy of the S1 nerve root (Figure 15) allows a better understanding of the necessary needle placement to allow both perineural and epidural spread of injectate.

The fluoroscopic localization for a S1 TFESI and S1 NRB are the same with no cranial caudal angulation necessary and approx 15° of ipsilateral obliquity

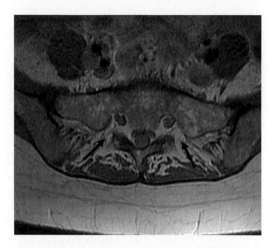

Figure 15. Axial proton density MRI image through the dorsal S1 neural foramen. Note the direct AP orientation of the dorsal S1 foramen, precluding the need for any craniocaudal angulation when performing S1-directed procedures.

(Figure 16A). With this simple obliquity, the S1 foramen becomes apparent and the superomedial portion is localized for a bull's-eye approach. The fibro-osseous tunnel of the S1 foramen is often palpably pierced, and once the direction of the needle is satisfactory, the needle should be advanced in the lateral view, with the goal being needle tip placement 1 mm short of the posterior cortex of the sacral bodies (Figure 16B). This usually allows both perineural and epidural spread of injectate, with small manipulations made after injection of contrast to attempt to maximize the 50/50 flow pattern (Figure 16C, D). This needle position is in contradistinction to the slightly more anterior location necessary for a S1 SNRB (slightly anterior to the posterior sacral cortex) to target the anteriorly exiting S1 nerve root (Figure 17).

Complications: Lumbar TFESI

Complications of TFESI are rare. General risks of infection and bleeding are commonly quoted in the consent but are extremely rare in the lumbar spine in the absence of a profound immunocompromised state or bleeding diastheses (see contraindications).

Nerve laceration from needle placement is a theoretical complication and is increased with a more inferiorly displaced needle route. Usually, a radicular pain occurs prior to intraneural needle placement and can be avoided with slow advancement and careful attention to patient feedback. Intrathecal injection remains a possibility if the needle is advanced medial to the 6 o'clock position or in the presence of a previously unknown nerve root sheath cyst. Rare intradiscal injection during TFESI has been reported (96).

Complications with respect to the iodinated contrast or the steroid depot mixture are similar to midline epidural.

Deserving special consideration are multiple recent reports of catastrophic spinal cord injury related to TFESI (36,97). The transforaminal approach is the most likely of lumbar approaches to demonstrate endovascular needle placement (95). Typically, endovascular contrast is due to a radicular vein and is of little clinical significance – minimal needle manipulation results in a normal extravascular injection. Arterial injection, however, can be catastrophic. There are multiple radicular arteries extending from lumbar arteries

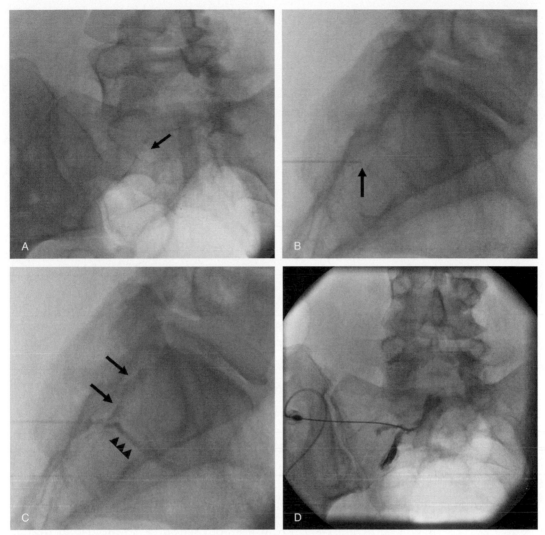

Figure 16. Left S1 TFESI. (A) Obliquity of 15° shows the dorsal S1 foramen to greatest advantage (arrow). (B) Lateral fluoroscopic image shows the needle tip placed 1–2 mm short of the dorsal cortex of the sacral vertebral bodies (arrow). (C) Injection of contrast shows proper 50/50 flow pattern, extending out the ventral S1 neural sheath (arrowheads) and cephalad into the epidural space (arrows). (D) AP fluoroscopic image confirming good epidural and perineural spread of contrast.

to feed either the anterior or posterior spinal cord. The largest of radicular arteries is the artery of Adamkiewicz, which in 80% of the people, enters the spinal canal from the left between the levels of T5 and L1 (98). This course is variable and spinal cord entry of the artery of Adamkiewicz has been reported as low as L4 (98).

Injection of a steroid mixture into a spinal cord radicular artery can cause catastrophic embolic injury to the cord. It has been suggested that an injectate using a steroid of smaller particle size (Celestone Soluspan) confers less embolic risk than the typical depot mixtures containing triamcinolone (Kenalog-40) (36). The benefit of the strong depot effect of Kenalog-40 suspensions has been shown to afford therapeutic advantage over betamethasone (Celestone) in the short term follow-up of interlaminar epidurals (35). However, no such

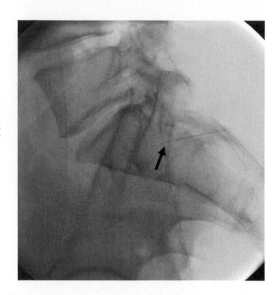

Figure 17. Needle tip position for S1 SNRB for comparison to S1 TFESI. The deeper needle tip position places the needle in the sheath of the ventral ramus of the S1 nerve root and avoids epidural spread that can confound the diagnostic power of the SNRB.

advantage has been shown in transforaminal epidural steroid injections or selective nerve root blocks (99). For these reasons we use betamethasone for TFESI for the theoretical decrease in embolic risk.

Efficacy: Lumbar TFESI

Although TFESI is not immune to the controversy surrounding the efficacy of ILESI, the results of multiple prospective studies seem to favor TFESI in treating unilateral radicular pain (83–85,87–91).

In relieving symptoms, several prospective outcome studies show efficacy for TFESI. Weiner and Fraser showed 80% improvement in 30 patients with a mean follow-up of 3.4 years (100). Lutz et al. studied 69 patients following a series of TFESIs and showed 78% patient satisfaction at an average follow-up time of 80 months (87). TFESI has been shown to be effective in treating chronic unilateral radiculopathy, as well. Botwin et al. prospectively followed 34 patients with unilateral radiculopathy from degenerative stenosis with a mean duration of pain of over two years. 75% of patients showed greater than 50% pain reduction after one year, with 64% and 57% showing improvements in walking and standing tolerance, respectively (83). In a separate case report Botwin et al. showed 80–85% pain relief in two patients with unilateral radiculopathy caused by epidural lipomatosis (93).

In a randomized, prospective, controlled trial, Vad et al. showed 84% of patients with pain reduction of 50% or more compared to patients receiving trigger point saline injections after 1.4 years (91). Karppinen et al. found that TFESI hastened recovery at two weeks compared to saline injection, but those patients who received steroid had greater pain scores at three and six months (84). To explain the paradoxical outcome they proposed a "rebound phenomenon." This rebound phenomenon has not been noted in other studies. Additionally, Karpinnen et al. only allowed a single injection. The prospective studies that showed significant benefit to TFESI uniformly allowed multiple injections, ranging from 1 to 4 (83,87,88,90,91).

TFESI has been shown to decrease the need for surgery. Through a prospective randomized trial, Riew et al. demonstrated that, compared with injection of bupivicaine alone, patients receiving TFESI were less likely to proceed to surgery. Twenty of 28 patients who received TFESI avoided surgery compared to 9 of 27 in the bupivicaine control group (88).

In reviewing the literature, including several of the studies cited above (84–86,88,89,91), DePalma et al. cited moderate (level III) evidence in support of TFESI (101).

Many of these studies have exclusion criteria that are not pertinent in a day-to-day clinical practice. Patients with prior surgery, previous epidural injections, chronic radiculopathy, multilevel pathology, and patients with pending worker's compensation claims are frequently excluded as confounders in the prospective studies highlighted earlier. However, in an interesting study, Tong et al., focused on these demographic factors in prospectively assessing clinical outcomes in 76 patients following a series of TFESIs. This study found that only patients with pending worker's compensation claims and patients who return to physical labor were predictors of poor outcome (90).

CERVICAL INTERLAMINAR EPIDURAL STEROID INJECTION

Indications: Cervical ILESI

Cervical epidural steroid injections are much less often performed than lumbar ESIs. Given this limited utilization, there are few scientific studies of cervical ESI and there is no consensus regarding indications for the procedure. Various studies support a variety of indications, including radicular pain, cervical spondylosis, subacute cervical strain, cervicogenic headache, chronic neck pain (102–106), and a "variety of indications" (106). Some studies suggest reduced efficacy for patients with axial neck pain, although most do not (104).

Contraindications: Cervical ILESI

Similar contraindications exist in the cervical spine as in the lumbar spine. However, given the smaller epidural space and the catastrophic sequelae of a cervical hematoma, bleeding tendencies need to be more carefully considered. In addition to routine cessation of Coumadin for three days prior to any spinal injection with confirmation of normalized INR, aspirin and other platelet inhibitors need to be stopped for seven days. We ask that the patient take no nonsteroidal anti-inflammatory drugs for two days prior to the procedure.

Technique: Cervical ILESI

The patient is placed prone, and comfort is ensured, with the head neutral and facing straight down at the table. To keep the face from being pressed against the table, proper support is necessary. Occasionally, patients experience claustrophobia in this position. This may be avoided if extra time is spent positioning the head to eliminate discomfort and minimize patient anxiety. Firm support pads or towels should be placed under the patient's chest and forehead, in order to elevate the face off the table. The towels should be placed in a fashion that leaves an opening for the patient's face, minimizing the closed-in feeling. Conscious sedation is not routinely required, but it should be considered for patients who are anxious and less cooperative.

Based on the target level selected from the patient's MRI, a mark is made on the patient's neck utilizing AP fluoroscopy. The skin entry site is at the mid-portion of the lower of the two targeted vertebral bodies and halfway between the spinous process and pedicle (Figure 18A). Following standard sterile preparation and drape, local anesthesia of the skin and subcutaneous tissues is achieved with 1% lidocaine buffered with sodium bicarbonate. Many types of needles have been suggested for cervical ESI; we find a 22-guage Tuohy needle is ideal because its blunt tip pushes firm objects away, diminishing the likelihood of inadvertently puncturing the dura. After initial skin entry with the Tuohy needle, the needle is advanced, under active fluoroscopy, toward the interlaminar space with slight medial angulation, while visualizing its advance using a contralateral oblique projection. To obtain this projection, rotate the tube about 45° contralateral to the side of needle entry; when the angle is correct, the laminae resemble the shingle on a roof. This obliquity allows the needle to be viewed in tangent as it is advanced. The needle is stopped just posterior to reaching the spinal canal (Figure 18B). As the needle is advanced, its position should be checked in the AP projection periodically, to verify that it remains directed toward the midline.

Confirmation of epidural needle tip location can be performed in two different ways. In our institution, we prefer to stop the needle advancement at the margin of the spinal canal and connect to a syringe of contrast with flexible tubing. The needle is then advanced in tiny increments with a small amount of contrast administered, following each needle manipulation. Epidural placement of the needle is demonstrated with a longitudinal pattern of contrast flow craniocaudally within the spinal canal (Figure 18C). Epidural contrast should circumscribe the outline of the dura. Instead, if the injection is intrathecal, the contrast will have a diluted appearance and wrap around the spinal cord, simulating a myelogram. In this case, the procedure should be aborted and reattempted in a week. Rarely, the contrast will demonstrate the needle tip within an epidural vein; in such cases, the contrast tracks away from the needle in a tubular structure and washes out with blood flow. Intravenous placement of the needle does not terminate the procedure; moving the needle slightly often solves the dilemma. Sometimes, a different level must be attempted to avoid the vein (Figure 19).

Alternatively, the "hanging drop" technique may be used to ensure correct advancement of the needle into the epidural space after reaching the margin of the spinal canal and returning to the oblique projection. For this technique, contrast is used to overfill the needle hub ("hanging" there), resulting in a convex dome of contrast with surface tension. The needle is slowly advanced. When it is correctly located within the epidural space, the contrast dome will drop down into the needle hub, signaling epidural location. After this initial confirmation of reaching the epidural space, further confirmation of the appropriate needle tip position is achieved by injecting an additional 2 ml of contrast, monitoring in real time with both oblique and AP projections.

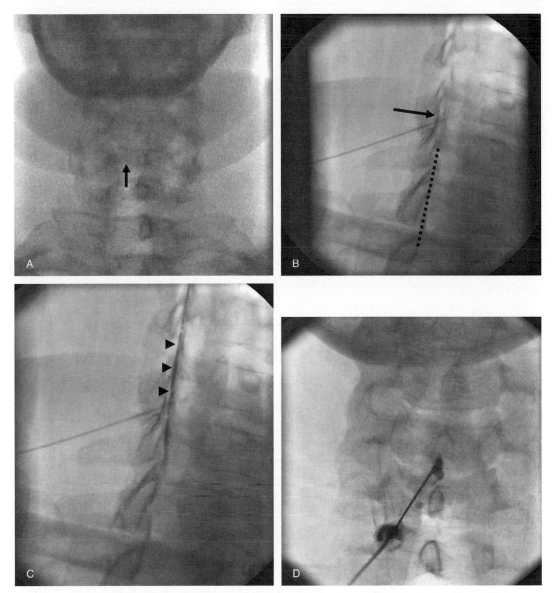

Figure 18. Cervical ILESI. (A) PA fluoroscopic image showing the proper skin entry point for a C5/C6 midline cervical epidural (arrow). (B) Forty-five degree contralateral oblique showing the shingled appearance to the lamina and the needle tip position near the spinal canal (arrow). The dotted line marks the inner cortex of the lamina, indicating the margin of the cervical spinal canal. (C) Contrast injection confirms the epidural location (arrow heads). (D) PA fluoroscopic image shows the needle to be directed toward midline where the diminutive cervical epidural space is the largest.

Once epidural positioning is confirmed, 80 mg (2 ml) of Kenalog-40 is instilled for an average-sized adult, followed by 2 ml of 0.25% preservative-free lidocaine for immediate pain relief. Higher concentrations of anesthetic would risk motor block; because of the devastating results that could accompany motor block in the cervical spine, one should not use a higher concentration of lidocaine. Any resistance to injection should raise suspicion of needle malposition. If the patient experiences pressure at the site of the injection or dull or shooting pain, reducing the rate of injection should improve these symptoms.

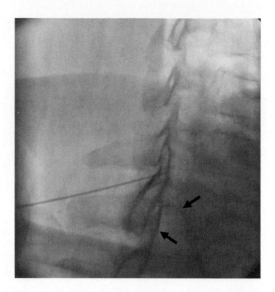

Figure 19. Vascular filling in attempted C6/C7 cervical ILESI. In the same patient as in Figure 18, vascular filling at the initially selected level necessitated needle removal and replacement at the previous level.

After the needle is removed, the skin is cleansed with alcohol and a bandage is applied. The patient is assisted while rising slowly and the remainder of the routine is the same as for lumbar ESI.

Complications: Cervical Ilesi

The same list of adverse effects from corticosteroids that occur in lumbar ESI may also accompany cervical ESI. Logically, there should be a risk of spinal cord injury in cervical ESI, but this has not been well documented. Some side effects, including dyspnea, hypotension, nausea, and neck stiffness, are reportedly more common in cervical injections (107). Finally, reflex sympathetic dystrophy (108) and an epidural hematoma requiring surgical decompression (109,110) have both been reported after cervical ESI.

Efficacy: Cervical Ilesi

Cervical epidural steroid injections are performed much less commonly than lumbar ESI. As such, controlled studies are not available, likely in part due to the reluctance of practitioners to inject a placebo as part of a technically demanding procedure such as cervical ESI. However, cervical ILESI is supported by several uncontrolled studies (103,105,106,111,112). In their retrospective analysis of 25 patients who received a total of 45 cervical ESIs for cervical radiculopathy recalcitrant to conservative measures, Rowlingson and Kirschenbaum reported 64% of patients had a good (75% pain relief) or excellent response to the injections (111). Likewise, a study of 58 cervical ESI patients by Cicala et al. demonstrated 41% excellent and 21% good results at six months (102). Although epidural injections in the cervical spine are considered riskier due to the proximity of the cervical spinal cord, many practitioners consider it an effective method of treatment; moreover, many of these patients have few options (106). However, some surgeons and physiatrists who employ lumbar ESI for their patients with low-back pain will not refer patients with neck pain and radiculopathy for cervical ESI.

CERVICAL TRANSFORAMINAL EPIDURAL STEROID INJECTION

Indications: Cervical Transforaminal Steroid Injection

Cervical transforaminal steroid injections (CTFESIs) are used commonly for unilateral cervical radiculopathy, much like their analogous lumbar counterparts. The use of CTFESI is far less common than lumbar injections, in large part to the historical failure of conservative management in treating cervical pain. Surgery remains the mainstay. In situations where conservative management is indicated or surgery is contraindicated, CTFESI has shown promise in treating cervical radicular pain.

Contraindications: CTFESI

The same contraindications exist for CTFESI as for the cervical interlaminar approach. Anticoagulants of all types are held for the prescribed time period, as discussed in the cervical ILESI section. The ability to hold still in a supine, lateral, or obliqued position (depending on operator preference) should be explored prior to the procedure. If the necessary position is too uncomfortable for the patient, sedation may be required to assure a safe procedure. Small patient movements in cervical procedures can cause significant complications.

Technique: CTFESI

Preprocedural imaging, and a detailed understanding of the anatomy it depicts, is a prerequisite prior to undertaking the procedure. The location and position of the vertebral artery and the exiting nerve should be noted. Significant facet overgrowth can divert the needle anterior, resulting in vascular or nerve injury. The course of the carotid arteries should be evaluated. The presence or absence of nerve root sheath cysts should also be assessed. A nerve root sheath cyst within the target foramen would necessitate selecting an adjacent level for entry.

CTFESI can be performed in several different positions. At our institution, we perform them in a supine position with the patient's head turned away to afford optimal visualization of the ipsilateral cervical neural foramen. An obliquity should be chosen that maximizes the AP dimension of the foramen.

A spot is chosen in line with the anterior cortex of the superior articulating process of the facet, in the midportion of the foramen, where it has maximal AP diameter (Figure 20A). The skin is marked with indelible ink. Prior to local anesthetic placement, gentle palpation of the planned tract can give valuable information regarding the location of the carotid artery and manual manipulation of the carotid may be necessary to clear it from the path. This is usually unnecessary as the structures of the carotid sheath are typically displaced anterior to the needle approach tract when the patient assumes our required position of contralateral head rotation. After sterile preparation has been

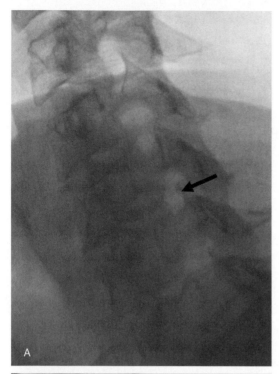

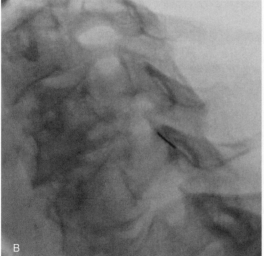

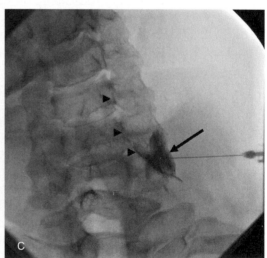

Figure 20. Left C5/C6 TFESI. (A) Ipsilateral oblique fluoroscopic image demonstrates the target site for the TFESI in the posterior portion of the neural foramen (arrow). (B) Twenty-five-gauge needle directed toward the posterior margin of the targeted foramen, coursing toward the waist of the foramen. (C) Straight AP flouroscopic image following contrast injection confirms both foraminal filling (arrow) and reflux into the epidural space (arrowheads). Note the needle tip location in the AP view, approximately halfway across the lateral mass.

performed, the skin and shallow subcutaneous soft tissues are anesthetized with careful consideration of the short distance between the skin and critical vascular and neural elements within the neck.

We typically use a 25-gauge needle 1.5–2.5 inches in length. Under fluoroscopic guidance, the needle is advanced in a bull's-eye fashion to the posterior neural foramen just anterior to the superior articulating process (Figure 20B). Frequent triangulation is necessary with the AP view to assure that the needle tip does not extend medial to the lateral masses or drift anteriorly. A needle position lateral to this will not result in the desired epidural reflux and a position too far medial risks thecal penetration. A needle position that drifts anteriorly risks injury to the vertebral artery with potential catastrophic neurological sequelae.

Once the needle tip is in position, a small amount of iodinated contrast is injected to confirm appropriate location. Meticulous scrutiny is necessary to exclude needle penetration of one of several radicular arteries that provide blood flow to the cervical cord or penetration of the vertebral artery. In the presence of a normal contrast flow pattern (Figure 20C), the contrast syringe can be removed from the flexible tubing and the steroid mixture of choice can be administered under direct visualization. The use of flexible tubing minimizes the chance of inadvertent needle tip motion during syringe exchange.

It can be argued that betamethasone (Celestone Soulspan) should be used when intravascular injection is a possibility but no controlled studies have shown that the difference in particle size between steroid preparations (36,95) has any effect to decrease embolic injury should intra-arterial injection occur. It should be noted that the published complications of either spinal cord or cerebellar infarcts all reported using triamcinolone, although that may be a function of the more widespread use of triamcinolone (113–116).

If intraarterial injection is identified, the procedure should be terminated at that level and either pursued at another level or rescheduled for the future. A nerve root block of the selected nerve root may be a more prudent course for a future injection if a radicular artery is known to reside within the foramen.

Catheter-directed transforaminal cervical epidural steroid has been described, where access is gained to the epidural space through a midline approach at C6/C7 or C7/T1 and a catheter is advanced under fluoroscopic guidance to the desired level and the steroid mixture injected. This is beyond the scope of this chapter.

Complications: CTFESI

A relatively new procedure, CTFESI has not been extensively studied. The genesis of the push-toward cervical transforaminal was born with complications of midline cervical epidural injections from needle trauma to the cervical cord (117,118). Initially thought to be a safe procedure, there have been multiple reported cases of cervical cord and cerebellar injury from cervical transforaminal steroid injections (113–115). Even more concerning is the multiple complications that go unreported, either due to lack of effort or ongoing litigation (116). The safety of cervical transforaminal steroid injection is in question and should only be performed by experienced operators confident in fluoroscopic needle placement, well-versed in the crucial cervical anatomy, and aware of the significant risk.

Efficacy: CTFESI

Due to the sensitive nature of the cervical anatomy, there are no double-blind studies in the literature to compare CTFESI to a sham procedure, so the true efficacy of the procedure continues to be uncertain. Several studies have looked at the prospective and retrospective success of CTFESI in treating upper extremity radicular pain (119–121).

The retrospective review by Slipman et al. showed a 60% satisfaction rate after an average of 21.7 months time and 2.2 injections in 20 patients (120). In a prospective study by Bush, 68 patients received a transforaminal injection; if they failed to improve, they received an interlaminar cervical epidural. Seventy-five percent of patients achieved complete relief of arm pain from a combination of these two treatments (119). Vallee et al. prospectively performed transforaminal cervical epidural injections in 30 patients with upper extremity radicular pain. They demonstrated 53% clinical success at six months, with 29% reporting complete resolution of pain (121).

Overall, there is evidence to suggest that CTFESI is moderately effective in treating patients with cervicogenic upper extremity radiculopathy. Currently, no study has been performed yet to compare interlaminar and transforaminal approach or comparing transforaminal epidural injection to cervical nerve root block.

SUMMARY

ESIs are helpful tools in the treatment of patients with low-back, neck, and radicular pain. Although ESI may not cure the causative lesion, it frequently shortens the clinical course of the disease process, reduces or eliminates hospitalization (54), and provides pain palliation and invaluable lifestyle improvements. ESI is most appropriately performed with fluoroscopic guidance and major complications are rare. Although cervical ESI is less uniformly endorsed, a growing body of evidence and experience is beginning to support its usefulness and safety.

REFERENCES

1. Benzon, H.T., Epidural steroid injections for low back pain and lumbosacral radiculopathy. Pain, 1986. **24**(3): p. 277–95.
2. Rydevik, B.L., D.B. Cohen, and J.P. Kostuik, Spine epidural steroids for patients with lumbar spinal stenosis. Spine, 1997. **22**(19): p. 2313–7.
3. Bush, K. and S. Hillier, A controlled study of caudal epidural injections of triamcinolone plus procaine for the management of intractable sciatica. Spine, 1991. **16**(5): p. 572–5.
4. Rowlingson, J., Epidural steroids: do they have a place in pain management? Am Pain Soc J, 1994. **3**(1): p. 20–27.
5. el-Khoury, G.Y., et al., Epidural steroid injection: a procedure ideally performed with fluoroscopic control. Radiology, 1988. **168**(2): p. 554–7.
6. Link, S.C., G.Y. el-Khoury, and W.B. Guilford, Percutaneous epidural and nerve root block and percutaneous lumbar sympatholysis. Radiol Clin North Am, 1998. **36**(3): p. 509–21.
7. Harrison, G., Topographical anatomy of the lumbar epidural region: an in vivo study using computerized axial tomography. Br J Anaesth, 1999. **83**(2): p. 229–234.
8. Johnson, B.A., Image-guided epidural injections. Neuroimaging Clin N Am, 2000. **10**(3): p. 479–91.

9. Bryan, B., C. Lutz, and G.E. Lutz, Flouroscopic assessment of epidural contrast spread after caudal injection. J Orth Med, 2000. **22**(2): p. 38–41.

10. Silbergleit, R., et al., Imaging-guided injection techniques with fluoroscopy and CT for spinal pain management. Radiographics, 2001. **21**(4): p. 927–39; discussion 940–2.

11. Lanier, V., H. McKnight, and M. Trotter, Caudal analgesia: an experimental and anatomic study. Am J Obstet Gynecol, 1944. **47**: p. 633–641.

12. Ogoke, B., Caudal epidural steroid injections. Pain Physician, 2000. **3**(3): p. 305–12.

13. Hayashi, N., et al., The effect of epidural injection of betamethasone or bupivacaine in a rat model of lumbar radiculopathy. Spine, 1998. **23**(8): p. 877–85.

14. Viner, N., Intractable sciatica – the sacral epidural injection – an effective method of giving pain relief. Canadian Med Assoc J, 1925. **15**: p. 630–4.

15. Evans, W., Intrasacral epidural injection therapy in treatment of sciatica. Lancet, 1930. **2**: p. 1225–9.

16. Kelman, H., Epidural injection therapy for sciatic pain. Am J Surg, 1944. **64**(2): p. 183–90.

17. Robechhi, A. and R. Capra, L'idrocortisone (composto F). Prime esperienze cliniche in campon reumatologico. Minerva Medica, 1952. **98**: p. 1259–63.

18. Goebert, H.W. Jr., et al., Painful radiculopathy treated with epidural injections of procaine and hydrocortisone acetate: results in 113 patients. Anesth Analg, 1961. **40**: p. 130–4.

19. Dilke, T.F., H.C. Burry, and R. Grahame, Extradural corticosteroid injection in management of lumbar nerve root compression. Br Med J, 1973. **2**(5867): p. 635–7.

20. Nelson, D.A., Dangers from methylprednisolone acetate therapy by intraspinal injection. Arch Neurol, 1988. **45**(7): p. 804–6.

21. Roche, J., Steroid-induced arachnoiditis. Med J Aust, 1984. **140**(5): p. 281–4.

22. Delaney, T.J., et al., Epidural steroid effects on nerves and meninges. Anesth Analg, 1980. **59**(8): p. 610–14.

23. Spaccarelli, K.C., Lumbar and caudal epidural corticosteroid injections. Mayo Clin Proc, 1996. **71**(2): p. 169–78.

24. White, A.H., Injection techniques for the diagnosis and treatment of low back pain. Orthop Clin North Am, 1983. **14**(3): p. 553–67.

25. Warr, A.C., et al., Chronic lumbosciatic syndrome treated by epidural injection and manipulation. Practitioner, 1972. **209**(249): p. 53–9.

26. Green, P.W., et al., The role of epidural cortisone injection in the treatment of diskogenic low back pain. Clin Orthop Relat Res, 1980. **153**: p. 121–5.

27. McCarron, R.F., et al., The inflammatory effect of nucleus pulposus. A possible element in the pathogenesis of low-back pain. Spine, 1987. **12**(8): p. 760–4.

28. Franson, R.C., J.S. Saal, and J.A. Saal, Human disc phospholipase A2 is inflammatory. Spine, 1992. 17(6 Suppl): p. S129–32.

29. Cannon, D.T. and C.N. Aprill, Lumbosacral epidural steroid injections. Arch Phys Med Rehabil, 2000. **81**(3 Suppl 1): p. S87–98; quiz S99–100.

30. Derby, R., et al., Response to steroid and duration of radicular pain as predictors of surgical outcome. Spine, 1992. 17(6 Suppl): p. S176–83.

31. Johansson, A., J. Hao, and B. Sjolund, Local corticosteroid application blocks transmission in normal nociceptive C-fibres. Acta Anaesthesiol Scand, 1990. **34**(5): p. 335–8.

32. Abram, S.E., Epidural steroid injections for the treatment of lumbosacral radiculopathy. J Back Musculoskeletal Rehabil, 1997. **8**: p. 135–49.

33. Maldjian, C., M. Mesgarzadeh, and J. Tehranzadeh, Diagnostic and therapeutic features of facet and sacroiliac joint injection. Anatomy, pathophysiology, and technique. Radiol Clin North Am, 1998. **36**(3): p. 497–508.

34. Knight, C.L. and J.C. Burnell, Systemic side-effects of extradural steroids. Anaesthesia, 1980. **35**(6): p. 593–4.

35. Stanczak, J., et al., Efficacy of epidural injections of Kenalog and Celestone in the treatment of lower back pain. AJR Am J Roentgenol, 2003. **181**(5): p. 1255–8.

36. Tiso, R.L., et al., Adverse central nervous system sequelae after selective transforaminal block: the role of corticosteroids. Spine J, 2004. **4**(4): p. 468–74.

37. Yaksh, T. and S.R. Chaplan, Physiology and pharmacology of neuropathic pain. Anesthesiol Clin North Am, 1997. **15**(2): p. 335–52.

38. Benzon, H.T., E.A. Brunner, and N. Vaisrub, Bleeding time and nerve blocks after aspirin. Reg Anaesth, 1984. **9**(2): p. 86–9.

39. Berman, A.T., et al., The effects of epidural injection of local anesthetics and corticosteroids on patients with lumbosciatic pain. Clin Orthop Relat Res, 1984. **188**: p. 144–51.

40. Vroomen, P.C., et al., Conservative treatment of sciatica: a systematic review. J Spinal Disord, 2000. **13**(6): p. 463–9.

41. Watts, R.W. and C.A. Silagy, A meta-analysis on the efficacy of epidural corticosteroids in the treatment of sciatica. Anaesth Intensive Care, 1995. **23**(5): p. 564–9.

42. Rivest, C., et al., Effects of epidural steroid injection on pain due to lumbar spinal stenosis or herniated disks: a prospective study. Arthritis Care Res, 1998. **11**(4): p. 291–7.

43. Harley, C., Extradural corticosteroid infiltration. A follow-up study of 50 cases. Ann Phys Med, 1967. **9**(1): p. 22–8.

44. Heyse-Moore, G.H., A rational approach to the use of epidural medication in the treatment of sciatic pain. Acta Orthop Scand, 1978. **49**(4): p. 366–70.

45. Hopwood, M.B. and S.E. Abram, Factors associated with failure of lumbar epidural steroids. Reg Anesth, 1993. **18**(4): p. 238–43.

46. Fredman, B., et al., Epidural steroids for treating "failed back surgery syndrome": is fluoroscopy really necessary? Anesth Analg, 1999. **88**(2): p. 367–72.

47. Fukusaki, M., et al., Symptoms of spinal stenosis do not improve after epidural steroid injection. Clin J Pain, 1998. **14**(2): p. 148–51.

48. Revel, M., et al., Forceful epidural injections for the treatment of lumbosciatic pain with post-operative lumbar spinal fibrosis. Rev Rhum Engl Ed, 1996. **63**(4): p. 270–7.

49. Horlocker, T.T., D.J. Wedel, and K.P. Offord, Does preoperative antiplatelet therapy increase the risk of hemorrhagic complications associated with regional anesthesia? Anesth Analg, 1990. **70**(6): p. 631–4.

50. Waldman, S.D., et al., Caudal administration of morphine sulfate in anticoagulated and thrombocytopenic patients. Anesth Analg, 1987. **66**(3): p. 267–8.

51. Botwin, K.P., et al., Complications of fluoroscopically guided caudal epidural injections. Am J Phys Med Rehabil, 2001. **80**(6): p. 416–24.

52. Burn, J.M., Treatment of chronic lumbosciatic pain. Proc R Soc Med, 1973. **66**(6): p. 544.

53. Renfrew, D.L., et al., Correct placement of epidural steroid injections: fluoroscopic guidance and contrast administration. AJNR Am J Neuroradiol, 1991. **12**(5): p. 1003–7.

54. White, A.H., R. Derby, and G. Wynne, Epidural injections for the diagnosis and treatment of low-back pain. Spine, 1980. **5**(1): p. 78–86.

55. Dawkins, C.J., An analysis of the complications of extradural and caudal block. Anaesthesia, 1969. **24**(4): p. 554–63.

56. Mulroy, M.F., M.C. Norris, and S.S. Liu, Safety steps for epidural injection of local anesthetics: review of the literature and recommendations. Anesth Analg, 1997. **85**(6): p. 1346–56.

57. Price, C.M., et al., Comparison of the caudal and lumbar approaches to the epidural space. Ann Rheum Dis, 2000. **59**(11): p. 879–82.

58. Kim, K.M., et al., Cephalic spreading levels after volumetric caudal epidural injections in chronic low back pain. J Korean Med Sci, 2001. **16**(2): p. 193–7.

59. Manchikanti, L., et al., Fluoroscopy is medically necessary for the performance of epidural steroids. Anesth Analg, 1999. **89**(5): p. 1330–1.

60. Johnson, B.A., K.P. Schellhas, and S.R. Pollei, Epidurography and therapeutic epidural injections: technical considerations and experience with 5334 cases. AJNR Am J Neuroradiol, 1999. **20**(4): p. 697–705.

61. Stambough, J.L., R.E. Booth, Jr., and R.H. Rothman, Transient hypercorticism after epidural steroid injection. A case report. J Bone Joint Surg Am, 1984. **66**(7): p. 1115–6.

62. Gorski, D.W., et al., Epidural triamcinolone and adrenal response to hypoglycemic stress in dogs. Anesthesiology, 1982. **57**(5): p. 364–6.

63. Kay, J., J.W. Findling, and H. Raff, Epidural triamcinolone suppresses the pituitary-adrenal axis in human subjects. Anesth Analg, 1994. **79**(3): p. 501–5.

64. Dubois, E.F., et al., Lack of relationships between cumulative methylprednisolone dose and bone mineral density in healthy men and postmenopausal women with chronic low back pain. Clin Rheumatol, 2003. **22**(1): p. 12–17.

65. Slucky, A.V., et al., Effects of epidural steroids on lumbar dura material properties. J Spinal Disord, 1999. **12**(4): p. 331–40.

66. Tripathi, M., S.S. Nath, and R.K. Gupta, Paraplegia after intracord injection during attempted epidural steroid injection in an awake-patient. Anesth Analg, 2005. **101**(4): p. 1209–11, table of contents.

67. Swerdlow, M. and W.S. Sayle-Creer, A study of extradural medication in the relief of the lumbosciatic syndrome. Anaesthesia, 1970. **25**(3): p. 341–5.

68. Bowman, S.J., et al., Outcome assessment after epidural corticosteroid injection for low back pain and sciatica. Spine, 1993. **18**(10): p. 1345–50.

69. Hickey, R.F., Outpatient epidural steroid injections for low back pain and lumbo-sacral radiculopathy. N Z Med J, 1987. **100**(832): p. 594–6.

70. Parisien, V.M., Conservative treatment of low back pain with epidural steroids. J Maine Med Assoc, 1980. **71**(3): p. 83–4, 92.

71. Rosen, C.D., et al., A retrospective analysis of the efficacy of epidural steroid injections. Clin Orthop Relat Res, 1988. **228**: p. 270–2.

72. Ridley, M.G., et al., Outpatient lumbar epidural corticosteroid injection in the management of sciatica. Br J Rheumatol, 1988. **27**(4): p. 295–9.

73. Buttermann, G.R., Treatment of lumbar disc herniation: epidural steroid injection compared with discectomy. A prospective, randomized study. J Bone Joint Surg Am, 2004. **86-A**(4): p. 670–9.

74. Wilson-MacDonald, J., et al., Epidural steroid injection for nerve root compression. A randomised, controlled trial. J Bone Joint Surg Br, 2005. **87**(3): p. 352–5.

75. Beliveau, P., A comparison between epidural anaesthesia with and without corticosteroid in the treatment of sciatica. Rheumatol Phys Med, 1971. **11**(1): p. 40–3.

76. Carette, S., et al., Epidural corticosteroid injections for sciatica due to herniated nucleus pulposus. N Engl J Med, 1997. **336**(23): p. 1634–40.

77. Cuckler, J.M., et al., The use of epidural steroids in the treatment of lumbar radicular pain. A prospective, randomized, double-blind study. J Bone Joint Surg Am, 1985. **67**(1): p. 63–6.

78. Snoek, W., H. Weber, and B. Jorgensen, Double blind evaluation of extradural methyl prednisolone for herniated lumbar discs. Acta Orthop Scand, 1977. **48**(6): p. 635–41.

79. Valat, J.P., et al., Epidural corticosteroid injections for sciatica: a randomised, double blind, controlled clinical trial. Ann Rheum Dis, 2003. **62**(7): p. 639–43.

80. Koes, B.W., et al., Efficacy of epidural steroid injections for low-back pain and sciatica: a systematic review of randomized clinical trials. Pain, 1995. **63**(3): p. 279–88.

81. Rosenberg, J.M., T.J. Quint, and A.M. de Rosayro, Computerized tomographic localization of clinically-guided sacroiliac joint injections. Clin J Pain, 2000. **16**(1): p. 18–21.

82. Andrade, A. and E. Eckman. The distribution of radiologic contrast media by lumbar translaminar and selective neural canals in normal human volunteers. In International Spine Intervention Society Meeting. 1992. Keystone, Colorado.

83. Botwin, K.P., et al., Fluoroscopically guided lumbar transformational epidural steroid injections in degenerative lumbar stenosis: an outcome study. Am J Phys Med Rehabil, 2002. **81**(12): p. 898–905.

84. Karppinen, J., et al., Periradicular infiltration for sciatica: a randomized controlled trial. Spine, 2001. **26**(9): p. 1059–67.

85. Kolsi, I., et al., Efficacy of nerve root versus interspinous injections of glucocorticoids in the treatment of disk-related sciatica. A pilot, prospective, randomized, double-blind study. Joint Bone Spine, 2000. **67**(2): p. 113–8.

86. Kraemer, J., et al., Lumbar epidural perineural injection: a new technique. Eur Spine J, 1997. **6**(5): p. 357–61.

87. Lutz, G.E., V.B. Vad, and R.J. Wisneski, Fluoroscopic transforaminal lumbar epidural steroids: an outcome study. Arch Phys Med Rehabil, 1998. **79**(11): p. 1362–6.

88. Riew, K.D., et al., The effect of nerve-root injections on the need for operative treatment of lumbar radicular pain. A prospective, randomized, controlled, double-blind study. J Bone Joint Surg Am, 2000. **82-A**(11): p. 1589–93.

89. Thomas, E., et al., Efficacy of transforaminal versus interspinous corticosteroid injectionin discal radiculalgia – a prospective, randomised, double-blind study. Clin Rheumatol, 2003. **22**(4–5): p. 299–304.

90. Tong, H.C., et al., Predicting outcomes of transforaminal epidural injections for sciatica. Spine J, 2003. **3**(6): p. 430–4.

91. Vad, V.B., et al., Transforaminal epidural steroid injections in lumbosacral radiculopathy: a prospective randomized study. Spine, 2002. **27**(1): p. 11–6.

92. Botwin, K.P., et al., Radiation exposure of the spinal interventionalist performing fluoroscopically guided lumbar transforaminal epidural steroid injections. Arch Phys Med Rehabil, 2002. **83**(5): p. 697–701.

93. Botwin, K.P. and D.P. Sakalkale, Epidural steroid injections in the treatment of symptomatic lumbar spinal stenosis associated with epidural lipomatosis. Am J Phys Med Rehabil, 2004. **83**(12): p. 926–30.

94. Bogduk, N., C. Aprill, and R. Derby, Epidural steroid injections. Spinal Care Diagnosis and Treatment, ed. White A.H. and J. Schofferman. 1995, St. Louis: Mosby. 322–344.

95. Sullivan, W.J., et al., Incidence of intravascular uptake in lumbar spinal injection procedures. Spine, 2000. **25**(4): p. 481–6.

96. Finn, K.P. and J.L. Case, Disk entry: a complication of transforaminal epidural injection – a case report. Arch Phys Med Rehabil, 2005. **86**(7): p. 1489–91.

97. Houten, J.K. and T.J. Errico, Paraplegia after lumbosacral nerve root block: report of three cases. Spine J, 2002. **2**(1): p. 70–5.

98. Alleyne, C.H., Jr., et al., Microsurgical anatomy of the artery of Adamkiewicz and its segmental artery. J Neurosurg, 1998. **89**(5): p. 791–5.

99. Blankenbaker, D.G., et al., Lumbar radiculopathy: treatment with selective lumbar nerve blocks – comparison of effectiveness of triamcinolone and betamethasone injectable suspensions. Radiology, 2005. **237**(2): p. 738–41.

100. Weiner, B.K. and R.D. Fraser, Foraminal injection for lateral lumbar disc herniation. J Bone Joint Surg Br, 1997. **79**(5): p. 804–7.

101. DePalma, M.J., A. Bhargava, and C.W. Slipman, A critical appraisal of the evidence for selective nerve root injection in the treatment of lumbosacral radiculopathy. Arch Phys Med Rehabil, 2005. **86**(7): p. 1477–83.

102. Cicala, R.S., K. Thoni, and J.J. Angel, Long-term results of cervical epidural steroid injections. Clin J Pain, 1989. **5**(2): p. 143–5.

103. Cicala, R.S., L. Westbrook, and J.J. Angel, Side effects and complications of cervical epidural steroid injections. J Pain Symptom Manage, 1989. **4**(2): p. 64–6.

104. Ferrante, F.M., et al., Clinical classification as a predictor of therapeutic outcome after cervical epidural steroid injection. Spine, 1993. **18**(6): p. 730–6.

105. Martelletti, P., et al., Epidural steroid-based technique for cervicogenic headache diagnosis. Funct Neurol, 1998. **13**(1): p. 84–7.

106. Shulman, M., Treatment of neck pain with cervical epidural steroid injection. Reg Anaesth, 1986. **11**: p. 92–4.

107. Bogduk, N., Epidural steroids. Spine, 1995. **20**(7): p. 845–8.

108. Siegfried, R.N., Development of complex regional pain syndrome after a cervical epidural steroid injection. Anesthesiology, 1997. **86**(6): p. 1394–6.

109. Williams, J.W. and T. Powell, Epidural abscess of the cervical spine: case report and literature review. Br J Radiol, 1990. **63**(751): p. 576–8.

110. Williams, K.N., A. Jackowski, and P.J. Evans, Epidural haematoma requiring surgical decompression following repeated cervical epidural steroid injections for chronic pain. Pain, 1990. **42**(2): p. 197–9.

111. Rowlingson, J.C. and L.P. Kirschenbaum, Epidural analgesic techniques in the management of cervical pain. Anesth Analg, 1986. **65**(9): p. 938–42.

112. Shulman, M., U. Nimmagadda, and A. Valenta, Cervical epidural steroid injection for pain of cervical spine origin. Anesthesiology, 1984. **61**(3A): p. A223.

113. Baker, R., et al., Cervical transforaminal injection of corticosteroids into a radicular artery: a possible mechanism for spinal cord injury. Pain, 2003. **103**(1–2): p. 211–5.

114. Brouwers, P.J., et al., A cervical anterior spinal artery syndrome after diagnostic blockade of the right C6-nerve root. Pain, 2001. **91**(3): p. 397–9.

115. Ludwig, M.A. and S.P. Burns, Spinal cord infarction following cervical transforaminal epidural injection: a case report. Spine, 2005. **30**(10): p. E266–8.

116. Rathmell, J.P., C. Aprill, and N. Bogduk, Cervical transforaminal injection of steroids. Anesthesiology, 2004. **100**(6): p. 1595–600.

117. Abram, S.E. and T.C. O'Connor, Complications associated with epidural steroid injections. Reg Anesth, 1996. **21**(2): p. 149–62.

118. Botwin, K.P., et al., Complications of fluoroscopically guided interlaminar cervical epidural injections. Arch Phys Med Rehabil, 2003. **84**(5): p. 627–33.

119. Bush, K. and S. Hillier, Outcome of cervical radiculopathy treated with periradicular/epidural corticosteroid injections: a prospective study with independent clinical review. Eur Spine J, 1996. **5**(5): p. 319–25.

120. Slipman, C.W., et al., Therapeutic selective nerve root block in the nonsurgical treatment of atraumatic cervical spondylotic radicular pain: a retrospective analysis with independent clinical review. Arch Phys Med Rehabil, 2000. **81**(6): p. 741–6.

121. Vallee, J.N., et al., Chronic cervical radiculopathy: lateral-approach periradicular corticosteroid injection. Radiology, 2001. **218**(3): p. 886–92.

Selective Nerve Root Blocks

Brian D. Petersen, Kirkland W. Davis, and James Choi

INTRODUCTION

Flouroscopically directed selective nerve root blocks (SNRBs) were initially described by Macnab in patients with "negative disc exploration" (1). Macnab described needle tip position, reproduction of radicular pain, confirmation of placement with injection of contrast to produce a neurogram, and anesthetization of the affected nerve with lidocaine. The technique has not changed significantly since 1971.

The utility of an SNRB is reflected in the name. It should be selective and, as such, tends to have significant diagnostic and prognostic power in evaluating patients with unclear radicular etiologies. The injection, when combined with a steroid, can be therapeutic as well. In the lumbar spine, if therapeutic benefit is the goal, a transforaminal epidural steroid injection is of more utility with more volume able to be delivered to the affected level with reflux into the epidural space.

In our clinical practice, lumbar SNRBs are performed in order to pinpoint the affected levels in patients with unclear clinical symptoms or discordant symptoms that are discordant with the magnetic resonance images (MRI). It has also been shown to have significant prognostic importance in identifying the level for surgical intervention and in identifying those patients who will benefit from surgery (2,3). Cervical selective nerve root blocks (CNRB) are performed under similar clinical circumstances. Thoracic SNRBs are rarely performed but can have important diagnostic and therapeutic utility in uncommon clinical settings.

ANATOMY

In the absence of significant anatomic abnormality, exiting nerve roots in the cervical, thoracic, and lumbar spine are located in a predictable anatomic location. With knowledge of pertinent spinal anatomy, and using fluoroscopically visible bony landmarks, a needle can be placed percutaneously in the epiradicular space with accuracy.

Nerve roots throughout the spine are covered in a thin membrane of perineurum and epineurum (2). The perineurum is a continuation of the dura to cover the proximal 6–8 mm of the spinal nerve. The perineurum can dilate, resulting in the common appearance of a nerve root sheath cyst. Care must be taken in order to avoid an intrathecal injection when performing transforaminal injections; however, perineural cysts are usually not problematic when performing an SNRB due to the more lateral needle position. The epineurum is a continuation of the epidural membrane and surrounds the nerve to form the epiradicular space. The goal of SNRB is the placement of the injectate within this epiradicular space.

Within the lumbar spine, dorsal and ventral roots coalesce to form the spinal nerve just prior to exiting the neural foramen. The focal thickening of the dorsal root medial to this coalescence is the dorsal root ganglion (DRG), which contains the cell bodies of the sensory fibers of the dorsal root. The dorsal root/DRG complex predominantly carries sensory fibers from the spinal nerve to the spinal cord. The ventral root predominantly carries motor nerves.

The spinal nerve has two divisions. The ventral rami extend anterolaterally to form the lumbar or lumbosacral plexuses. Within the neural foramen, the sinuvertebral nerve is given off from the proximal aspect of the ventral root, which courses medially back through the neural foramen to innervate the lumbar disc annulus and posterior longitudinal ligament. Autonomic nerve fibers communicate with the sympathetic trunk through gray rami communicans extending from the ventral ramus of the spinal nerve (Figure 1) (4).

The dorsal ramus courses posteriorly following bifurcation of the spinal nerve within the neural foramen. The dorsal ramus has three divisions. The lateral and intermediate branches contain predominantly motor fibers with inconsistent cutaneous innervation. The medial branch, however, is of utmost importance as it innervates the facet joints above and below. For example, the L4 spinal nerve gives rise to the L4 dorsal ramus. The medial branch of the L4 dorsal ramus gives off fibers that extend superiorly to innervate the L4/L5 facet and inferiorly to innervate the L5/S1 facet.

Anatomic abnormalities of the lumbar nerve roots should be broached briefly, simply for acknowledgement of their existence. There are three types of anomalies, which can be seen in isolation or in combination (5). Type 1 anomalies are defined as aberrant courses, but with a single nerve root in the appropriate neural foramen. This can manifest as a particularly low exit within the neural foramen or as two nerve roots originating aberrantly from the same dural sleeve but exiting singly. Type 2 anomalies have an abnormal number of roots within the foramen – either two nerve roots exiting in the same foramen with an empty adjacent foramen or supernumerary nerve roots within a single foramen. Type 3 anomalies are those with extradural anastomoses between roots. Fortunately, these anomalies are fairly rare with an estimated total incidence of 8.5% (5). These anomalies can be confounding in a diagnostic workup due to discordant anatomic and symptomatic findings.

Pertinent vascular anatomy in the lumbar spine is centered on the artery of Adamkiewicz. Although this topic has been addressed in the epidural steroid chapter (Chapter 7), a brief review of the normal anatomy should alert the reader to use necessary caution when performing SNRBs. The artery of Adamkiewicz is the largest of the spinal radicular arteries and originates from the aorta. The course of the artery of Adamkiewicz varies significantly but occurs on the left in 70–80% of patients (6,7) and most commonly occurs between the T9 and L1 levels. A study of computed tomography (CT) angiograms in 70 patients detected an artery of Adamkiewicz in 90%, with 92% entering the spinal canal between T8 and L1 (7). In this study, only 71% originated on the left (7). Injection of particulate steroid into this radicular artery can cause infarction of the anterior spinal artery and subsequent devastating neurological complications (8). Care must therefore be taken when performing SNRBs to scrutinize active fluoroscopic contrast injection for filling of this artery.

The cervical spine has similar neural anatomy to the lumbar spine. A distinguishing feature, however, is the presence of eight cervical nerve roots, with the spinal nerve exiting above the pedicle of its associated vertebral body. For example, if the C6 nerve root is the target, the C5/C6 foramen is localized. The ventral rami of C1-C4 form the cervical plexus with those from C5-T1 forming the brachial plexus.

Cervical vascular anatomy deserves special mention, as it is the source of rare catastrophic complications associated with CNRBs. The posterior aspect of the foramen is selected as the target zone in order to steer far clear of the vertebral artery, which is located within the anterior portion of the cervical foramen. It should be noted that the ascending cervical and deep cervical arteries can contribute branches that anastamose with the anterior spinal artery. This is a cause for special concern because these anastamotic radicular arteries have been shown in cadaver dissections to occasionally enter the foramen posteriorly, at the target zone for cervical SNRBs (9). Huntoon's cadaveric dissections found this concerning variant in 1 of 10 cadavers (9), although the true incidence remains a matter of debate.

Neural anatomy in the thoracic spine is similar to the cervical and lumbar spines. Pertinent thoracic anatomy centers around the close approximation of the posteromedial pleura and rib articulation to the target site. Because the posterolateral vertebral body corner is blocked by the costovertebral articulation and the posteromedial pleura, a slightly more superior and medial target is selected. Care must be taken to identify the posteromedial pleura in order to avoid causing a pneumothorax.

As in cervical and lumbar SNRBs, radicular arterial filling must be excluded prior to injection of particulate steroid to avoid devastating complications.

MEDICATIONS

As in interlaminar epidural steroid injections (ILESIs) and transforaminal epidural steroid injections (TFESIs), an anesthetic is typically combined with a steroid for a longer therapeutic benefit. In some clinical settings, sequential anesthetic nerve root blocks can be performed with anesthetic only in order to pinpoint the nerve root causing the chief radicular pain. Once identified, the culprit nerve root can be treated with steroid infiltration as well.

In our institution, we use a 50:50 mixture of triamcinolone acetonide (Kenalog-40; Bristol-Myers Squibb, Princeton, NJ) and 0.5% bupivicaine (Abbot Laboratories, North Chicago, IL) for lumbar SNRBs. Kenalog-40 has been selected over betamethasone sodium phosphate/betamethasone acetate suspension (Celestone Soluspan; Schering, Kenilworth, NJ) at our institution because of the decreased cost of Kenalog-40 for our pharmacy. In a study done at University of Wisconsin by Blankenbaker et al., there was no statistical difference in pain relief when comparing the two medications (10). This is in contradistinction to a similar study from our institution where epidural steroid injections with Kenelog-40 was found to be more efficacious (11). Only 1–2 cc of the solution is injected in the epiradicular space. A small volume is all that is necessary to come to a diagnostic conclusion, and more volume can lead to excessive pain during injection, rupture of the epiradicular membrane, and reflux of injectate into the epidural space, diminishing the diagnostic power of the SNRB.

As in the performance of all fluoroscopically guided spinal procedures, confirmation of the needle tip position with injection of a small amount of iodinated contrast is necessary. In the presence of an iodinated contrast allergy, gadolinium can be substituted. Contrast injection volumes are never sufficient to make gadolinium toxicity a risk.

Sedation for SNRBs is never necessary and would be counterproductive to the diagnostic efficacy of the injection.

LUMBAR SELECTIVE NERVE ROOT BLOCK

Indications

Lumbar SNRBs are performed in patients with lumbar radicular pain and are most commonly used to direct possible surgical intervention in unclear clinical cases. It is used as a preoperative diagnostic procedure in patients with equivocal or multilevel imaging findings prior to operative management, in postoperative patients with persistent radicular signs, and in patients with normal imaging findings but persistent radicular pain.

Contraindications

Contraindications to lumbar SNRB are similar to those of other percutaneous invasive procedures. These would include bleeding diatheses, allergy, overlying infection, or serious systemic infection. Care should be taken in elucidating a history of contrast allergy before the procedure. Diabetics can experience blood glucose lability following steroid injection, and this should be emphasized. We require warfarin to be halted for three days prior to the procedure, whereas the coagulation status of our lumbar SNRB patients are not routinely checked.

Technique

Informed consent is obtained in all patients with attention paid to the theoretical risks of infection and bleeding, as well as the possibility of allergic reaction, side effects to the steroids, and inadvertent nerve damage from the needle. Prior to the injection, the patient is asked to describe the distribution and severity of the pain. We routinely use an 11-point pain scale and, following the procedure, send the patient home with a two-week pain diary to follow the pain level over time.

The patient is placed prone on the fluoroscopy table. The endplates at the desired level are profiled and the tube rotated to the ipsilateral oblique until the posteriorly oriented facets are medially displaced enough for unencumbered access to the target site. At our institution, we target the inferolateral corner of the vertebral body (Figure 1A), 2 mm cephalad and 2 mm medial to the infero-lateral vertebral body cortical margin. If present, osteophytes should be ignored and the skin mark made over the "native" inferolateral vertebral body corner. This inferolateral target allows a selective injection of the nerve root in question without involving the dorsal ramus, sinuvertebral nerve, or adjacent nerve roots within the epidural space. Inclusion of the more proximal spinal nerve or adjacent nerve roots in the injection field can yield a false-positive result by alleviating pain referable to the facet, disc annulus, or adjoining level.

The skin is marked and the patient prepped and draped. The superficial and deep soft tissues are anesthetized with 1% lidocaine buffered with sodium bicarbonate. A bull's-eye approach is made on the target with an appropriately long 22-gauge spinal needle. Deeper soft tissues can be anesthetized if necessary through the spinal needle; however, care must be taken not to administer anesthetic in the vicinity of the spinal nerve prior to eliciting radicular pain. We use the facets as a guide on the lateral view, with lidocaine administration superficial to the facet joints. Administration of lidocaine deep into the facet joints risks anesthesia of the ventral ramus and may not allow the patient to perceive the radicular signs necessary to confirm accurate needle placement. This can also increase the risk of nerve laceration.

The needle is advanced with periodic confirmation of appropriate course and depth in orthogonal planes. Once the level of the foramen is reached on the lateral projection, slow advancement is necessary until radicular signs are pro-duced. The needle advancement is stopped and the pain should resolve, indi-cating that the needle is near, but not within, the nerve. If pain persists, intraneural needle placement is possible and the needle should be withdrawn 1–2 mm. Concordance or discordance with the patient's typical pain pattern should be recorded. If the nerve is not encountered (e.g., lack of reproduction of radicular pain) on the first pass, the vertebral body will act as a backstop. The needle is retracted and a slightly more cephalad course is usually all that is necessary to encounter the nerve.

Once adequate needle position is acheived, a small amount of contrast is injected through flexible tubing with confirmation of a selective neurogram (Figure 1B). Reflux of contrast into the neural foramen and epidural space should be avoided in SNRB in order to prevent false-positive alleviation of pain. The contrast injection should be scrutinized under active fluoroscopic visual-ization in order to avoid intraarterial injection of steroid. This is of particular theoretical importance in high left-sided lumbar SNRBs with the understanding

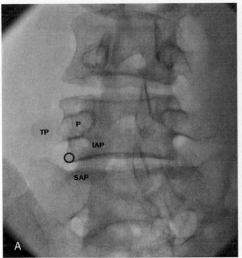
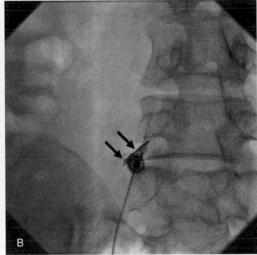
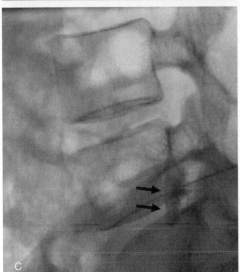

Figure 1. Left L4 SNRB. (A) Left posterior oblique flouroscopic image showing target site for SNRB, 2 mm cephalad and 2 mm medial to the inferolateral corner of the vertebral body. P – pedicle of L4; TP – transverse process of L4; IAP – inferior articulating process of L4; SAP – superior articulating process of L5. (B) Injection of a small amount of contrast confirms the needle tip within the epineural space of the L4 nerve root (arrows), without reflux into the epidural space. (C) Lateral flouroscopic image confirming neurogram (arrows).

that radicular arteries have significant anatomic variability and vigilance must be high regardless of the injection level. We have occasionally justified use of beta-methasone with high lumbar SNRBs because of its lesser viscosity and perceived less risk of arterial occlusion if inadvertent intraarterial injection is performed (12). This concern is probably unfounded given the far peripheral target site we prefer for SNRBs but should be foremost in concern for TFESIs at these levels.

If the desired flow of contrast is achieved anteroposterior (AP) and lateral (Figure 1C) fluoroscopic spot images are obtained to document needle position. A 1:1 mixture (0.5% bupivicaine and 40 mg/ml Kenalog-40) of 1–1.5 cc is slowly injected. The needle tip should not be manipulated. The use of flexible tubing during syringe exchange ensures that the needle tip is not inadvertently displaced. The patient should be questioned as to the nature and location of any discomfort during injection.

The needle is removed and the skin cleansed and the small puncture site dressed with a small bandage. Due to the common parasthesias produced by this procedure, we require all patients to be accompanied by a driver. The patient is aided in slowly coming to a seated position. The patient is kept in the department for only enough time to evaluate for adverse reactions, such as vasovagal reactions or significant motor block, and a short postprocedure interview is performed prior to discharge.

L5 SNRB

L5 SNRB deserves special note due to the significant craniocaudal angulation usually needed to profile the L5/S1 disc space and line up the target site for the L5 nerve root (Figure 2).

Aside from the smaller target tract, the L5 SNRB differs little from other lumbar levels (Figure 3A–C). Rarely, the iliac crest can block the normal route, and a coaxial technique we routinely use for L5/S1 discography is usually successful. In these cases, a 20-gauge guide needle is placed past the iliac crest and lateral to the facets. A 7-inch 25-gauge needle is then coaxially introduced with an appropriate curve placed at its end, such that the needle tip traverses lateral to medial upon exiting the 20-gauge needle. This can also be performed with an 18-gauge guide/22-gauge coaxial combination.

S1 SNRB

The same technique and approach is used for the S1 SNRB as for the S1 TFESI (described previously; see Chapter 7) with the exception of the final needle tip position. In order to favor the epidural spread described for S1 TFESI, the needle tip is located just dorsal to the posterior sacral cortex within the spinal canal. In contrast, in order to ensure more selective infiltration of the S1 periradicular space during S1 SNRB, the needle is advanced antegrade through the ventral S1 neural foramen (Figure 4A, B) until the needle tip is 5–10 mm past the posterior sacral cortex, or until radicular symptoms are encountered. In our experience radicular symptoms of S1 are uncommon, so we rely heavily on the anatomic location of the needle tip and the contrast neurogram to confirm the selective nature of the S1 SNRB. Despite our best efforts, epidural spread with this particular injection is sometimes unavoidable.

CT-guided SNRBs

The authors do not routinely use CT guidance for spinal procedures, although there are many practitioners who use CT nearly exclusively. We believe that fluoroscopy best affords active visualization of contrast injection when the ability to evaluate for vascular filling is of paramount importance given the devastating complications of intraarterial steroid injection.

Complications

Lumbar SNRBs are safe procedures. Complications such as infection and bleeding are raised due to skin puncture, but the actual risk of these is diminishingly

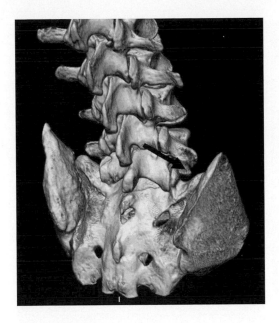

Figure 2. Surface-rendered CT image of the lumbar spine, rotated with craniocaudal and right posterior oblique angulation to adequately visualize the proper target zone for a right L5 SNRB (arrow).

small given the caliber of the needle and the relative paucity of significant vascularity along the needle course. Allergic reaction is a possibility and the use of nonionic contrast is always used to attempt to minimize this possibility. Gadolinium is routinely substituted as contrast in those patients with a documented iodine allergy. Systemic side effects of the steroid (diarrhea, face flushing, insomnia, mood swings) are usually discussed prior to the procedure, as they are self-limited and benign. Intrathecal needle placement is not a risk given the far inferolateral target site. If a more subpediculate target site is used, then the presence of a nerve root sheath cyst can contribute to intrathecal needle placement. Disc entry has been reported (13, personal experience) (Figure 5) but this is rare and benign if recognized and corrected prior to medication administration.

Nerve laceration is a potential risk but can be avoided in most cases by slow advancement of the needle at the appropriate depth and avoiding the use of anesthetic at a depth that may cause premature parasthesia of the spinal nerve. The most catastrophic complication would be infarction of a radicular artery serving the spinal cord. Although the operator needs to be aware of this serious risk, it is exceedingly uncommon and is the subject of case reports at this time.

CERVICAL SELECTIVE NERVE ROOT BLOCK

Indications

Similar to lumbar SNRBs, cervical SNRBs are used in patients with radicular pain and can help to guide surgical intervention in patients with equivocal or confounding imaging studies, atypical pain patterns, or postoperative patients with persistent pain.

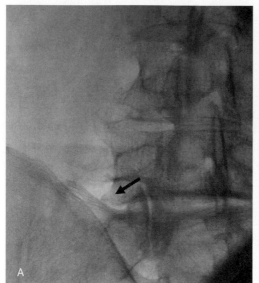

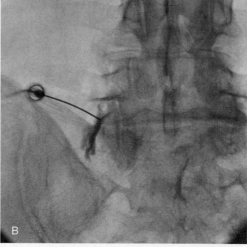

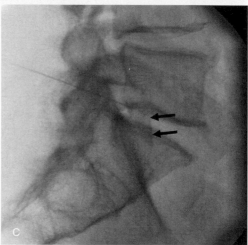

Figure 3. Left L5 SNRB. (A) Left posterior oblique flouroscopic image shows target site (arrow). (B) AP flouroscopic image shows selective left L5 neurogram. (C) L5 neurogram confirmed on lateral flouroscopic projection (arrows).

Contraindications

Similar absolute and relative contraindications exist for cervical SNRBs when compared to other minimally invasive percutaneous spinal procedures. Local and systemic infection, allergies, and uncorrectable bleeding diatheses are all contraindications to percutaneous spinal steroid injections. As in lumbar SNRBs, warfarin should be halted for three days. Due to the smaller area and the more critical consequences of bleeding into the epidural or perineural tissues in the cervical spine, we require an international normalized ratio level be drawn in patients taking warfarin prior to the procedure. This practice is institution specific. We also expand our list of anticoagulative medications that should be halted prior to cervical injection procedures to include platelet inhibitors (clopidogrel, etc.) or aspirin. With the agreement and cooperation of the referring clinician, we require patients to have ceased platelet inhibitors for five days and aspirin for seven days prior to the procedure.

A recent MRI should be available to evaluate for aberrant vasculature and the presence of dural sleeve cysts that could complicate the procedure.

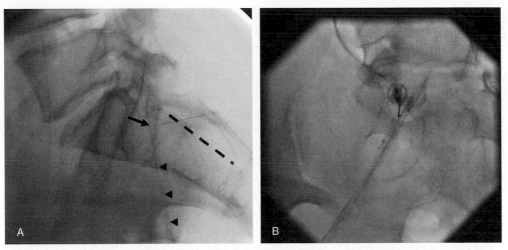

Figure 4. Left S1 SNRB. (A) Lateral flouroscopic image demonstrating the target site (arrow) for needle tip placement in S1 SNRB is more ventral than for a TFESI of the same level: 5–10 mm past the dorsal sacral cortex (dashed line). This allows a selective injection with contrast confined to the S1 epineural space. Contrast is noted surrounding the S1 nerve root (arrowheads). (B) AP flouroscopic image showing a selective S1 neurogram.

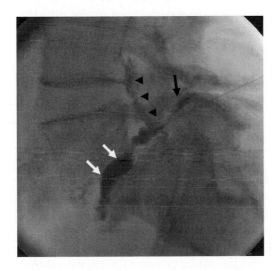

Figure 5. The inadvertant triumvurate. Attempted L5 SNRB resulted in initial filling of the L5/S1 disc (white arrows). Along the retracted needle course, with further injection of contrast, there was filling of the epidural space (arrowheads) and the patient's pars interarticularis defect (black arrow).

Technique

The MRI is scrutinized prior to the procedure with particular attention paid to any anomalous course of the vertebral artery or nerve root sheath cyst that may preclude safely performing the procedure. The selected level is confirmed, taking care to evaluate the proper neural foramen for the targeted nerve root.

The patient is consented in a typical fashion but the risk of stroke, associated with either vertebral artery injury or injection of steroid into a small radicular artery, is broached routinely in our preprocedural consents for cervical injections. The patient's preprocedural pain level is recorded, and a pain survey is given to the patient to record pain response over the next 14 days.

In absence of any anatomic contraindications, the patient is placed supine on the fluoroscopy table with the head turned toward the contralateral shoulder. This moves the carotid artery and jugular vein anteriorly and affords a clear path to the posteroinferior portion of the targeted neural foramen. The fluoroscopy tube is rotated to the ipsilateral side, approximately 45°–55°, until the targeted foramen is profiled optimally. The posteroinferior margin of the foramen, adjacent to the superior articulating process of the facet, is targeted and an indelible mark is placed on the patient's skin (Figure 6A). Targeting the inferior margin of the foramen increases the chances of a more selective injection, usually avoiding encountering the nerve from the cervical level above in the selected level. Targeting the posterior margin of the foramen is of utmost importance as the vertebral artery occupies the anterior portion of the foramen.

Utilizing sterile technique and following conventional prepping and draping of the planned skin entry site, the superficial soft tissues are anesthetized with 1% lidocaine buffered with sodium bicarbonate. Deep soft tissue anesthesia should be performed with extreme care, if at all, given the short distance between the skin entry site and the targeted nerve.

A 25-gauge needle is usually used, but the choice of length and the presence of a stylet or the use of a blunt-tipped needle are all left to operator preference. The argument for a blunt-tipped needle is compelling with the chance of perforating a small radicular artery being decreased; however, the difficulty in traversing the soft tissues and placing the needle accurately within the posteroinferior foramen with a blunt-tipped needle can overwhelm the safety advantages. Opinion varies within our department, with the majority favoring a 1.5-inch 25-gauge needle without stylet, if the distance to the target allows the choice, or a 2.5-inch 25-gauge needle with stylet. We do not find the need to use a 3.5-inch needle in the typical patient, regardless of the level being injected. The shortest needle possible affords the greatest control in this delicate procedure.

The needle is advanced in a bull's-eye fashion (Figure 6B) and the depth of the needle tip is frequently checked in the true AP projection. The needle is slowly advanced until the patient experiences parasthesias or the needle tip extends 1–2 mm medial to the lateral cortical margin of the lateral mass at the desired level. Contrast is injected through short flexible tubing in the AP dimension, and the active fluoroscopic image is scrutinized for selective nerve root contrast extension and intravascular filling (Figure 6C). Digital subtraction angiography, if available, can be used to eliminate any doubt of intravascular filling. If venous filling is noted, the needle can be advanced or retracted into an extravascular location prior to injecting the steroid mixture. In the event, a radicular artery is demonstrated, the procedure should be terminated and the needle removed. The patient should be monitored for neurological symptoms because vasospasm is a risk and possible cause of reported complications (14–19).

The quality of the neurogram is evaluated, and if needle placement is deemed appropriate syringe exchange is performed, leaving the flexible tubing in place. This ensures that no needle tip manipulation will occur between injection of contrast and injection of the steroid mixture. A 1:1 mixture of betamethasone and 0.5% bupivicaine (1–1.5 cc) is then instilled slowly to minimize retrograde flow into the epidural space. We use betamethasone in

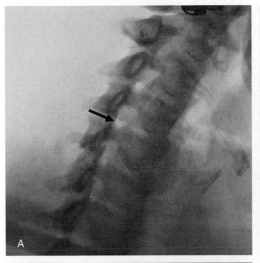
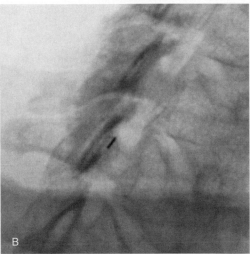
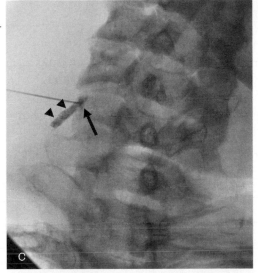

Figure 6. Right C5 SNRB. (A) Fifty-degree ipsilateral oblique projection optimizing the target neural foramen (C4/C5) for a C5 SNRB. Target site is the inferior posterior foramen (arrow). (B) Bull's-eye view of the needle. (C) Direct AP flouroscopic image demonstrating the proper needle tip position just inside the lateral masses (arrow) and a selective right C5 selective neurogram (arrowheads).

cervical SNRBs due to the smaller particle size (when compared to Kenalog-40) and theoretical safety advantages should intravascular injection inadvertently occur (20).

The needle is removed, the skin cleansed, and the puncture site bandaged. The patients are monitored for adverse side effects for the short amount of time it takes for them to comfortably and safely come to a standing position and change their clothes. Postprocedural pain level is recorded and the patient escorted from the department. We require the patient be accompanied by a driver.

We perform cervical SNRBs under fluoroscopy, to maximize the chance of identifying intravascular needle placement. Many operators perform these procedures under CT with good results and low complication rates.

Complications

Cervical injections, both SNRBs and TFESI, have come under scrutiny recently for catastrophic complications including stroke and death (14–19). These procedures should only be undertaken by clinicians with experience in their performance, well versed in the cross-sectional and three-dimensional anatomy of the cervical spine and adjacent soft tissues, and familiar with the possible complications. Prompted by the multiple severe complications reported in the literature, Ma et al. retrospectively evaluated cervical nerve root blocks performed at Washington University between 1999 and 2003 (21). They found 14 complications in a retrospective review of 1,036 cases that included five cases of headache/dizziness, six cases of transient neurological deficits (pain or weakness), one case of hypersensitivity, one case of vasovagal reaction, and one curious case of transient global amnesia. No severe complications were noted (21). They performed their injections in a similar way, as described earlier, with a slightly deeper needle position on average, than we typically advocate. With this large series it would seem that the risk of these procedures is low, even after taking into account the limitations with a retrospective review.

THORACIC SELECTIVE NERVE ROOT BLOCK
Indications

Thoracic SNRBs are rarely indicated in routine practice. We have found them useful for patients with acute thoracic radicular symptoms following trauma or, more commonly in our practice, following vertebroplasty. We have had excellent results in providing the occasional patient with short-term relief of dermotomal thoracic nerve root pain following vertebroplasty (Figure 7A, B).

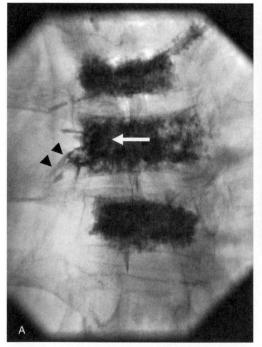
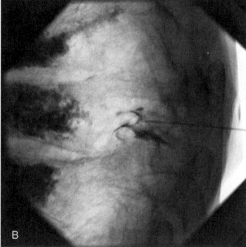

Figure 7. Left T8 thoracic SNRB following vertebroplasty. (A) On the AP flouroscopic spot image, the hub (white arrow) is difficult to see on the background of PMMA cement. A neurogram is demonstrated (black arrowheads). (B) Same patient, lateral flouroscopic image.

Contraindications

Thoracic SNRBs share similar absolute and relative contraindications with all percutaneous spinal injection procedures.

Technique

The technique for thoracic SNRB deserves brief special consideration. Patient consent includes pneumothorax as a risk. The patient is placed prone and the target level is localized. Ipsilateral obliquity is necessary to target inferior to the pedicle, while avoiding the adjacent rib and posteromedial pleura. The target site (Figure 8A) for thoracic SNRB is necessarily more cephalad and medial than for the lumbar SNRB technique described earlier. The posteromedial pleural line needs to be indentified and avoided. Once the needle tip is in an adequate position and radicular signs have been provoked, the contrast injection is performed through flexible tubing. Again, the confirmation of extravascular needle placement is of utmost importance, particularly on the left side. If necessary, digital subtraction angiography can be used to make absolutely sure there is no radicular arterial filling. We use the same steroid injection mixture that we use in the cervical spine (1:1 mixture of betamethasone and 0.5% bupivicaine).

Due to the more superomedial target site necessitated by the presence of the rib and the posteromedial pleura, these injections have a target site more typical of a TFESI. As such, epidural extent is common (Figure 8B). Thankfully, the clinical instances necessitating a truly selective thoracic nerve root block for diagnostic purposes are diminishingly rare.

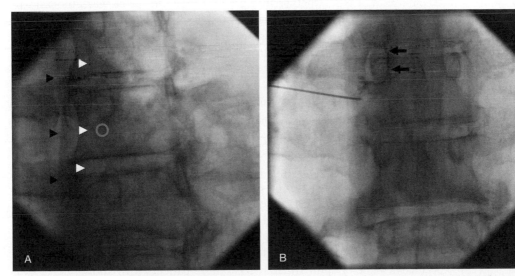

Figure 8. Left T6 nerve root block in a patient with unexplained thoracic dermatomal pain. (A) Left posterior oblique projection demonstrates the target for thoracic nerve root block (circle) with the anteromedial pleural line (black arrowheads) and posterior medial pleural line (white arrowheads) demonstrated. A more superomedial target is necessary in the thoracic level compared to the lumbar level (resembling a transforaminal target site). (B) Straight AP image shows a contrast pattern more typical of a transforaminal epidural injection (arrows). Thoracic NRBs rarely impact surgical planning so a strict selective nerve root block, confined to the epineural space, is rarely necessary.

Complications

Complications are rare with thoracic SNRB but pneumothorax deserves special note. If the posteromedial pleural line is not well visualized during the procedure, or the needle tip is inadvertently deviated laterally, a postprocedural upright chest radiograph should be performed.

SNRB Efficacy

There are many studies that have been published touting the therapeutic benefits of epiradicular steroid injection (22–25). However, all of these describe a technique for TFESI instead of SNRB. The terminology is confusing in the literature with the term "selective nerve root block" being used interchangeably with "transforaminal epidural," "therapeutic selective nerve root block," "therapeutic nerve root block," and "epiradicular steroid injection."

It should be stressed that the authors clearly separate TFESIs from SNRBs. SNRBs should be reserved for diagnostic purposes because, although there is some therapeutic benefit, the amount of steroid–anesthetic mixture is purposefully limited in order to decrease the risk of intraforaminal, epidural, or adjacent nerve root spread. Also, the goal in the above technique is to encounter the nerve peripherally, and to induce and record radicular symptoms experienced by the patient. If therapeutic benefit is the goal, the larger volume steroid–anesthetic injection used with TFESI should be used, and the pain typically associated with the epineural injection in SNRBs can usually be avoided as well.

For diagnostic purposes, the SNRBs, when performed meticulously, demonstrate great diagnostic accuracy in defining the affected level. The greatest advantage in SNRBs, whether they are performed in the cervical, thoracic, or lumbar spine, is to preoperatively assess the affected level in patients with normal imaging, discordant imaging, or multilevel disease.

There are a few studies that show that SNRBs lack the specificity to be used as a predictor of positive postoperative outcomes in the diagnostic pathway of patients with radicular pain (26–29). Common factors of these studies, however, are the use of dorsal ganglionectomy or dorsal rhizotomy as the treatment method. Failure to alleviate the patient's pain after SNRB-directed rhizotomy is cited as evidence for the lack of specificity of the SNRB. It has since been shown that dorsal rhizotomy is unpredictable at best (30–32), and its use has continued to decrease in frequency.

More compelling evidence exists for the support of the sensitivity and specificity of carefully performed SNRBs. Much of the literature predates MRI, where SNRBs were viewed as a dependable and diagnostic adjuvant to clinical exam, myelography, and plain radiography (33–40). van Akkerveeken demonstrated a sensitivity of SNRB of 100%, specificity of 90%, and a positive predictive value of approximately 85% in 46 patients with known nerve root compression (41). Dooley et al. performed a retrospective review of 73 consecutive patients who underwent SNRB and found that all the 44 patients (100%) who had concordant pain with injection and immediate relief (classified as group 1 response) had nerve root pathology at surgery. If patients with postoperative arachnoiditis were excluded, 27 of 32 patients had complete response to single-level decompression giving SNRB an 85% accuracy in predicting which patients will respond to surgery (42). In a prospective study of 105 patients who underwent SNRB, Haueisen et al. found a good positive predictive value for SNRB (40). Of 41 surgically treated patients who had a diagnostic SNRB, surgery confirmed a lesion in 38 (93%). All these patients had a previous myelogram with abnormalities noted on only 24%, and EMG correctly diagnosed the affected level in only 38% (40).

A more recent retrospective review by Sasso et al. of 101 patients who underwent preoperative SNRB is more illustrative of the applicability of SNRBs in the current imaging milieu. All the patients underwent preoperative MRI, with SNRB reserved for the subset of patients with discrepancies between presenting examination and radiological imaging. Ninety-one patients had strongly positive SNRB (greater than 95% pain relief), and 83 of those 91 patients (91%) had a good surgical outcome with clinical follow-up of greater than 12 months. Most interestingly, there were seven patients with an initial negative SNRB at the level requested by the surgeon but with a positive SNRB performed at an adjacent level. All seven patients had surgery at the SNRB-positive level, and all had good outcomes at more than 12 months follow-up. The SNRB was the decisive factor in determining the level to be operated upon. Of four patients with poor surgical outcomes, three (75%) had surgeries performed at the level of a negative SNRB. MRI findings were positive at the operated level in good outcomes 85% of the time, but 13 patients with negative MRI had positive SNRB, findings of nerve entrapment at surgery, and a good surgical outcome (3).

Aspinall et al. presented an abstract evaluating 40 patients prospectively with normal MRI who underwent SNRB. Surgery was performed in all patients with positive SNRBs (11 patients). All 11 patients had nerve root compression found at surgical exploration, with ligamentum flavum compression found in nine, and two with foraminal stenosis. Following surgical correction, 9 of 11 (82%) had complete relief of symptoms (43).

SNRBs can also be useful in patients with atypical pain patterns. It has been shown that the dermatomal maps we have come to rely on may not accurately depict the somatic distribution of nerves in a large percentage of people (44). The term *dynotome* has gained popularity as the intrinsic radicular pattern of pain that an individual experiences when a nerve root is compressed. The discrepancy between the dynatomal and dermatomal distribution can be hypothesized with normal variant lumbar/lumbosacral plexus collaterals (nervus furcalis), anatomic aberrancies, and neural plasticity in patients with chronic pain. SNRBs can elicit this dynotomal pattern with reliability and can confirm single-level disease in patients with confounding clinical presentation.

Specific evidence for the use of cervical SNRBs is less voluminous but supporting nonetheless. Anderberg et al. showed concordance between nerve root compression on MRI and relief of pain following cervical SNRBs in 20 consecutive patients, and concluded that "the SNRB procedure seemed relevant for confirming a relationship between radiological pathology and clinical symptoms and signs"(45). For therapeutic cervical radicular pain benefit, Slipman et al. assessed patients with degenerative cervical spondylosis (46) as well as traumatic cervical radicular pain (47). He found benefit for degenerative spondylosis but no benefit for traumatic cervical radicular pain.

Given the relative paucity of thoracic SNRB indications, there are no studies demonstrating efficacy of thoracic SNRB.

SUMMARY

Although therapeutic benefit is seen in some patients, the term SNRB should be reserved for injections performed peripheral to the foramen to avoid the potential of false-positive findings associated with affecting the sinuvertebral branch of the ventral ramus and the medial branch of the dorsal ramus. If therapeutic benefit is the chief aim, fluoroscopically guided injection can be made transforaminal to allow a higher dose and volume of steroid to be used. SNRBs, when performed with meticulous care in the right clinical setting, are powerful diagnostic tools to confirm pathological levels prior to surgical intervention. SNRBs have been shown to have high sensitivity and specificity in defining pathological levels, as well as good positive and negative predictive values for identifying patients who will benefit from surgery.

REFERENCES

1. Macnab, I., Negative disc exploration. An analysis of the causes of nerve-root involvement in sixty-eight patients. J Bone Joint Surg Am, 1971. **53**(5): p. 891–903.
2. Murtagh, R., The art and science of nerve root and facet blocks. Neuroimaging Clin N Am, 2000. **10**(3): p. 465–77.
3. Sasso, R.C., et al., Selective nerve root injections can predict surgical outcome for lumbar and cervical radiculopathy: comparison to magnetic resonance imaging. J Spinal Disord Tech, 2005. **18**(6): p. 471–8.
4. Bogduk, N. and L.T. Twomey, Lumbar Spine Pain. Clinical Anatomy of the Lumbar Spine, ed. N. Bogduk and L.T. Twomey. 1991, New York: Churchill Livingstone. 151–9.
5. Hasner, E., M. Schalintzek, and E. Snorrason, Roentgenological examinations of the function of the lumbar spine. Acta Radiol, 1952(37): p. 141–9.
6. Alleyne, C.H., Jr., et al., Microsurgical anatomy of the artery of Adamkiewicz and its segmental artery. J Neurosurg, 1998. **89**(5): p. 791–5.
7. Takase, K., et al., Demonstration of the artery of Adamkiewicz at multi-detector row helical CT. Radiology, 2002. **223**(1): p. 39–45.
8. Houten, J.K. and T.J. Errico, Paraplegia after lumbosacral nerve root block: report of three cases. Spine J, 2002. **2**(1): p. 70–5.
9. Huntoon, M.A., Anatomy of the cervical intervertebral foramina: vulnerable arteries and ischemic neurologic injuries after transforaminal epidural injections. Pain, 2005. **117**(1–2): p. 104–11.
10. Blankenbaker, D.G., et al., Lumbar radiculopathy: treatment with selective lumbar nerve blocks – comparison of effectiveness of triamcinolone and betamethasone injectable suspensions. Radiology, 2005. **237**(2): p. 738–41.
11. Stanczak, J., et al., Efficacy of epidural injections of Kenalog and Celestone in the treatment of lower back pain. AJR Am J Roentgenol, 2003. **181**(5): p. 1255–8.
12. Tiso, R.L., et al., Adverse central nervous system sequelae after selective transforaminal block: the role of corticosteroids. Spine J, 2004. **4**(4): p. 468–74.
13. Finn, K.P. and J.L. Case, Disk entry: a complication of transforaminal epidural injection – a case report. Arch Phys Med Rehabil, 2005. **86**(7): p. 1489–91.

14. Baker, R., et al., Cervical transforaminal injection of corticosteroids into a radicular artery: a possible mechanism for spinal cord injury. Pain, 2003. **103**(1–2): p. 211–5.

15. Brouwers, P.J., et al., A cervical anterior spinal artery syndrome after diagnostic blockade of the right C6-nerve root. Pain, 2001. **91**(3): p. 397–9.

16. Karasek, M. and N. Bogduk, Temporary neurologic deficit after cervical transforaminal injection of local anesthetic. Pain Med, 2004. **5**(2): p. 202–5.

17. Ludwig, M.A. and S.P. Burns, Spinal cord infarction following cervical transforaminal epidural injection: a case report. Spine, 2005. **30**(10): p. E266–8.

18. Rathmell, J.P. and H.T. Benzon, Transforaminal injection of steroids: should we continue? Reg Anesth Pain Med, 2004. **29**(5): p. 397–9.

19. Rozin, L., et al., Death during transforaminal epidural steroid nerve root block (C7) due to perforation of the left vertebral artery. Am J Forensic Med Pathol, 2003. **24**(4): p. 351–5.

20. Sullivan, W.J., et al., Incidence of intravascular uptake in lumbar spinal injection procedures. Spine, 2000. **25**(4): p. 481–6.

21. Ma, D.J., L.A. Gilula, and K.D. Riew, Complications of fluoroscopically guided extraforaminal cervical nerve blocks. An analysis of 1036 injections. J Bone Joint Surg Am, 2005. **87**(5): p. 1025–30.

22. Lutz, G.E., V.B. Vad, and R.J. Wisneski, Fluoroscopic transforaminal lumbar epidural steroids: an outcome study. Arch Phys Med Rehabil, 1998. **79**(11): p. 1362–6.

23. Narozny, M., M. Zanetti, and N. Boos, Therapeutic efficacy of selective nerve root blocks in the treatment of lumbar radicular leg pain. Swiss Med Wkly, 2001. **131** (5–6): p. 75–80.

24. Riew, K.D., et al., The effect of nerve-root injections on the need for operative treatment of lumbar radicular pain. A prospective, randomized, controlled, double-blind study. J Bone Joint Surg Am, 2000. **82-A**(11): p. 1589–93.

25. Vad, V.B., et al., Transforaminal epidural steroid injections in lumbosacral radiculopathy: a prospective randomized study. Spine, 2002. **27**(1): p. 11–6.

26. Loeser, J.D., Dorsal rhizotomy for the relief of chronic pain. J Neurosurg, 1972. **36**(6): p. 745–50.

27. North, R.B., et al., Dorsal root ganglionectomy for failed back surgery syndrome: a 5-year follow-up study. J Neurosurg, 1991. **74**(2): p. 236–42.

28. North, R.B., et al., Specificity of diagnostic nerve blocks: a prospective, randomized study of sciatica due to lumbosacral spine disease. Pain, 1996. **65**(1): p. 77–85.

29. Wetzel, F.T., et al., Extradural sensory rhizotomy in the management of chronic lumbar radiculopathy: a minimum 2-year follow-up study. Spine, 1997. **22**(19): p. 2283–91; discussion 2291–2.

30. Geurts, J.W., et al., Efficacy of radiofrequency procedures for the treatment of spinal pain: a systematic review of randomized clinical trials. Reg Anesth Pain Med, 2001. **26**(5): p. 394–400.

31. Geurts, J.W., et al., Radiofrequency lesioning of dorsal root ganglia for chronic lumbosacral radicular pain: a randomised, double-blind, controlled trial. Lancet, 2003. **361**(9351): p. 21–6.

32. van Wijk, R.M., J.W. Geurts, and H.J. Wynne, Long-lasting analgesic effect of radiofrequency treatment of the lumbosacral dorsal root ganglion. J Neurosurg, 2001. **94** (2 Suppl): p. 227–31.

33. Kikuchi, S., Anatomical and experimental studies of nerve root infiltration. Nippon Seikeigeka Gakkai Zasshi, 1982. **56**(7): p. 605–14.

34. Kikuchi, S., et al., Anatomic and clinical studies of radicular symptoms. Spine, 1984. **9**(1): p. 23–30.

35. Kikuchi, S., et al., Anatomic features of the furcal nerve and its clinical significance. Spine, 1986. **11**(10): p. 1002–7.

36. Krempen, J.F. and B.S. Smith, Nerve-root injection: a method for evaluating the etiology of sciatica. J Bone Joint Surg Am, 1974. **56**(7): p. 1435–44.

37. Krempen, J.F., B.S. Smith, and L.J. DeFreest, Selective nerve root infiltration for the evaluation of sciatica. Orthop Clin North Am, 1975. **6**(1): p. 311–5.

38. Tajima, T., K. Furukawa, and E. Kuramochi, Selective lumbosacral radiculography and block. Spine, 1980. **5**(1): p. 68–77.

39. White, A.H., Injection techniques for the diagnosis and treatment of low back pain. Orthop Clin North Am, 1983. **14**(3): p. 553–67.

40. Haueisen, D.C., et al., The diagnostic accuracy of spinal nerve injection studies. Their role in the evaluation of recurrent sciatica. Clin Orthop Relat Res, 1985.198: p. 179–83.

41. van Akkerveeken, P.F., The diagnostic value of nerve root sheath infiltration. Acta Orthop Scand Suppl, 1993. 251: p. 61–3.

42. Dooley, J.F., et al., Nerve root infiltration in the diagnosis of radicular pain. Spine, 1988. **13**(1): p. 79–83.

43. Aspinall, S., S. Mohammed, and P.L. Sanderson. The value of nerve root injections in the evaluation of sciatica in paitents with normal MRI scans. In Spine Society of Australia. 2000. Adelaide, Australia.

44. Wolff, A.P., et al., Do diagnostic segmental nerve root blocks in chronic low back pain patients with radiation to the leg lack distinct sensory effects? A preliminary study. Br J Anaesth, 2006. **96**(2): p. 253–8.

45. Anderberg, L., et al., Selective diagnostic cervical nerve root block – correlation with clinical symptoms and MRI-pathology. Acta Neurochir (Wien), 2004. **146**(6): p. 559–65; discussion 565.

46. Slipman, C.W., et al., Therapeutic selective nerve root block in the nonsurgical treatment of atraumatic cervical spondylotic radicular pain: a retrospective analysis with independent clinical review. Arch Phys Med Rehabil, 2000. **81**(6): p. 741–6.

47. Slipman, C.W., et al., Therapeutic selective nerve root block in the nonsurgical treatment of traumatically induced cervical spondylotic radicular pain. Am J Phys Med Rehabil, 2004. **83**(6): p. 446–54.

Discography

Charles E. Ray, Jr., and Leo J. Rothbarth

First described in 1948 (1), discography consists of the placement of a needle into a disc space using radiologic guidance. Once the needle is in position, provocative procedures are performed in an attempt to mimic a pain response similar to the patient's underlying symptoms. Additionally, images [either computed tomographic (CT), fluoroscopic, or both] are obtained and interpreted. Discography remains a controversial area, with many individuals on both sides of the debate. Proponents believe that discography remains the least invasive way to settle discordance between imaging findings and clinical symptoms; skeptics claim that the high false-positive rate and lack of evidence suggesting better surgical outcomes following discography make the procedure useless. Whether or not discography is performed in any given institution is largely a function of personal belief in the procedure by both the surgical and radiological consultants rather than firm data documenting its utility.

Discography was first described as a method to confirm the diagnosis of herniated nucleus pulposus (HNP) (1). With the advent of cross-sectional imaging modalities and their high accuracy in diagnosing HNP, the indication for discography has changed. It is now largely used to document discogenic pain in the absence of imaging findings that correlate well with the patient's symptomatology, and to determine the symptomatic level in patients with multilevel disease. Although pain may be associated with an HNP, disc fragmentation and herniation is not the only way by which discs can cause pain. Whereas it was long believed that the disc complex itself was devoid of any innervation, it is now recognized that discs possess a nerve supply that may account for pain sensation even in the absence of herniation.

The intervertebral disc complex is composed of three components. The vertebral endplates make up the superior and inferior margins, the ligamentous annulus fibrosis forms the outer (peripheral) margin, and the toothpaste-like nucleus pulposus occupies the inner portion bounded by annulus fibrosis and endplates. In the normal adult disc, the outer third of the annulus is innervated by nerve fibers. Following disc degeneration, however, the innervation grows deeper into the disc complex, with some nerve fibers penetrating into the nucleus pulposus itself (2). These nerve fibers are believed to be at least in part responsible for the pain sensations felt in the presence of disc degeneration, with or without concomitant herniation.

Two theories exist to explain discogenic pain: the mechanical and chemical theories. In the mechanical theory, a progressive breakdown of the normal load-bearing capacity of the disc complex occurs, oftentimes in a stepwise fashion. Unlike the normal disc, where a compressive load is spread uniformly across the disc space, a disc that demonstrates degenerative changes loses its capacity to evenly spread loads that in turn causes significant stress on the annulus fibrosis (2). This uneven distribution results in either vertebral end-plate microfractures or annulus tears. In either case, the integrity of the disc complex is compromised, further degenerative changes occur, leading to worsening of the underlying mechanical stresses, and a downward spiral commences. The initial event causing the initial degenerative change is usually occult.

In the chemical theory, an initial insult to the disc (e.g., vertebral endplate fracture) produces a chemical response with the introduction of inflammatory mediators into the nucleus pulposus itself (2). These mediators change the underlying composition of the nucleus, which can irritate the nerve fibers on the outer third of the annulus (provided an annular tear is present). The changes, and accompanying pain response, may be more marked in patients with preexisting degenerative disc disease due to the irritation of pain fibers that have already grown into the inner annulus or the nucleus pulposus.

It is likely that discogenic pain in any individual patient results from a combination of chemical and mechanical issues. During discography, injections with different pressure may cause variable pain responses. Exquisite pain at low pressures is likely due to a chemical-mediated response and is more typically seen with acute or subacute injuries to the disc. Pain caused only with higher pressure injections is more typically observed after chronic changes in the disc and is more likely caused by mechanical disruptions to the disc. These "chemically sensitized" and "mechanically sensitized" discs are distinguished during discography (discussed later), and provide important information for the spine surgeon to plan interventions.

The indications for discography vary from institution to institution. Guyer and Ohnmeiss published a position paper from the North American Spine Society, which outlined indications for lumbar discography (3). These suggestions are presented in Table 1.

TECHNIQUE

In its simplest form, discography can be performed at one level with a single needle, minimal contrast material, a syringe, and C-arm fluoroscopy. Discography can, however, be a much more elegant procedure that can potentially provide the spine surgeon with vital information necessary to make a surgical intervention more likely to succeed. We describe here the technique used at our institution; however, the reader is cautioned that the number of variations on the technique described is nearly endless. More important than following any described technique is developing a technique with which the operator is familiar and comfortable (Figure 1).

Table 1. Indications for Discography
Determine whether or not an abnormal disc noted on an imaging study is responsible for the patient's pain.
Evaluate the disc as a cause of patient's symptoms in the setting or normal cross-sectional imaging studies.
Evaluate a specific disc where there is discordance between the clinical and radiological findings.
Evaluation of postoperative pain, particularly whether the pain is arising from the disc that was operated upon versus another level.
Determine the number of levels requiring surgery (typically fusion) in patients with multilevel disease.
Source: Guyer and Ohnmeiss DD Anderson MW. Lumbar discography: an update. Sem Roentgen 2004;39:52–67.

Two components of preprocedure evaluation are essential to be performed prior to discography: clinical history and radiological imaging. Obtaining a short clinical history prior to performing discography is important for several reasons (Table 2). First, documentation of the distribution of the patient's pain can lead the operator to perform the discogram at the correct level. Second, the duration of the patient's pain can suggest whether or not the disc is likely to produce a positive result at low or high pressures (chemically or mechanically sensitized). Third, surgical history may dictate whether or not a lateral or transdural approach (discussed later) is most practical. Significant information can be obtained in a few minutes with well-directed questions. Reviewing imaging studies prior to discography can also provide important information, such as levels of degenerative disc disease, unsuspected disc herniations, postoperative changes that may preclude discography at certain levels, or potential other causes of the patient's symptoms.

Once the patient is interviewed and the radiographic images reviewed, the procedure is explained to the patient and consents are signed for both the procedure and sedation and analgesia. Whereas some operators prefer to perform the procedure without sedation and analgesia, we prefer to provide light sedation to all of our patients with short-acting intravenous medications (midazolam, with or without fentanyl). A single dose of both medications (50 µg of fentanyl and 1 mg of midazolam) prior to placement of the first needle provides enough sedation and analgesia to make the procedure more bearable and, we feel, does not significantly compromise our diagnostic capability. By the time all of the needles have been placed into the discs, the single dose of sedation and analgesia has largely lost its effect and the patient is fully awake to respond to any provocative measures.

A single dose of intravenous antibiotics is given at least 30 minutes prior to the procedure. The antibiotic chosen must provide excellent gram-positive coverage because the greatest risk of postprocedure discitis comes from skin

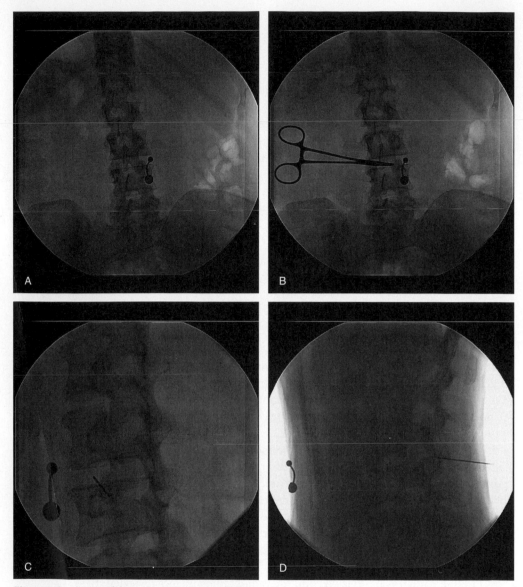

Figure 1. Sequence of discography procedure (disregard overlying jewellry). (A) A preliminary AP image of the lumbar spine is obtained to confirm normal lumbar anatomy. (B) After the overlying skin is prepped and draped, a hemostat is placed over the disc of interest as a marker external to the patient. (C) The C-arm is angled laterally until the familiar Scotty dog appearance of the lumbar vertebra is noted. The superior endplate of the lower vertebral body should be perfectly aligned; the C-arm may have to be angled in a craniocaudal direction to achieve this orientation. The outer (18- to 19-gauge) needle is advanced into the soft tissues parallel to the x-ray beam. (D) The C-arm is moved to the lateral projection to confirm appropriate direction of the needle. (E) Once the outer needle is well seated, the inner 22-gauge needle is advanced into the disc space. This may best be accomplished in the lateral imaging plane. (F) Appropriate placement of the needle should be confirmed in both the lateral and AP planes. The inner needle should be visualized in the inner one-third of the disc space on both projections. (G) In order to gain access to the L5-S1 disc space, the C-arm must be angled in the craniocaudal direction to prevent the needle from hitting the iliac crest. There is typically a small space between the iliac crest and lateral pillar of the spinal column, indicated here by the overlying hemostat. (H) Final image just prior to injection demonstrating all needles in position. Note that the L5-S1 needle is placed more cephalad at the skin site than the L4-L5 needle. This steep angulation is typical in order to gain access into the L5-S1 disc space.

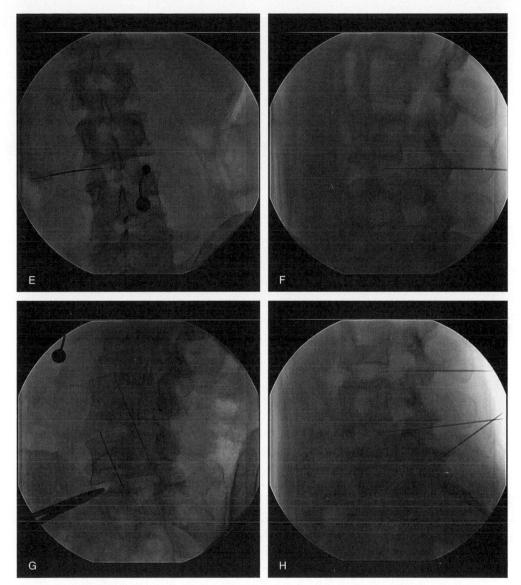

Figure 1. (*continued*)

flora introduced during needle placement. We typically give 1 g of cefazolin; however, in the setting of penicillin or cephalosporin allergy, 1 g of vancomycin can be given instead.

The patient is placed prone on an angiographic table equipped with a rotating C-arm. Rotation of the C-arm is vital to performing the procedure safely and quickly; attempting to perform the discogram on a table with a fixed (nonrotating) tube and image intensifier generally leads to great frustration and a very time-consuming procedure. We do not routinely place bolsters underneath the patient; however, occasionally, small bolsters placed underneath the patients' chest, abdomen, or legs may provide some degree of comfort to patients who otherwise might not be able to undergo the procedure at all.

Table 2. Directed Questions Prior to Performing Discography
For how long have you had back/leg pain?
What is the distribution of your pain?
What is the character of the pain (pins and needles, electrical shock, stabbing, dull, achy, numbness, etc.)?
Is the pain constant or does it come and go? If it comes and goes, is there any activity or position that makes it better or worse?
Do you take medications to relieve the pain? If so, how much and how often?
Have you had any back surgeries?
Do you see a chiropractor or holistic medicine specialist?
Do you have any other medical problems?
Are you on any other medications?
What are your limitations due to your pain?
Do you have any drug or contrast allergies?
Do you have a history of bleeding problems?
When was the last time you took your pain medications?
Have you had any dental work recently, or URI/GI/GU/sinus infection within the past three days?

Although the likelihood of an infectious complication is small (discussed in the following paragraphs), discitis can prove to be a devastating complication in an otherwise relatively healthy patient. For that reason, the procedure is treated as surgical and standard operating procedures for a surgical prep are followed. A wide skin prep is performed twice with betadine scrub and solution, after which an Ioban Antimicrobial Incise Drape (60 × 45 cm) (3M, Minneapolis, MN) is placed across the entire lumbar region. A surgical hand scrub is then performed, and gloves are donned in standard fashion.

A preliminary spot film of the lumbar spine is obtained, and confirmation of normal anatomy (e.g., five lumbar vertebrae) is obtained. Particular attention is paid to osteophytes along the lateral margin of the vertebral bodies, and confirmation of an adequate posterolateral route to the disc space is confirmed. If osteophytes preclude positioning of the needle into the disc space from one side, an approach from the contralateral side may be more advantageous. Rarely, a transdural approach is necessary (discussed later).

Once the appropriate disc levels are determined, the needles can be placed into the disc spaces in anticipation of the provocative testing. Some investigators suggest accessing the disc contralateral to the side of greatest pain; doing so in theory decreases the risk of irritating the affected nerve root during needle placement (4,5). By using a C-arm that can be rotated, appropriate lateral and craniocaudal angulation can be obtained for each disc space. The authors place needles into all the disc spaces prior to performing the first provocative test. In the vast majority of cases, a total of two or three disc spaces (L3L4, L4L5, L5S1) are accessed during the procedure. The reason for using multiple levels is in an attempt to decrease the likelihood of a false-positive examination by evaluating the disc space of interest and one or two control levels (6). In our practice, one of the authors routinely uses one control disc space, whereas the other routinely uses two.

Oblique Extradural Approach

There are several methods by which the disc space can be accessed. The authors use a combination of a rotating C-arm and a "down-the-barrel" technique. The disc space to be accessed is placed in the middle of the visualized field, in order to decrease the amount of parallax. The C-arm is then angled laterally so the "Scotty dog" configuration of the vertebral body below the targeted disc space to be accessed is best visualized, and the superior articular facet is positioned in the middle of the endplate. The C-arm is subsequently rotated in a craniocaudal direction so that the superior endplate of the vertebral body below the disc space is aligned parallel to the x-ray beam. Only after all three of these positions are confirmed is the patient adequately positioned for the procedure.

The two-needle technique is described here, although a single-needle technique can also be performed with a 22- to 25-gauge spinal needle. With the exception of using the outer needle, the single-needle technique is identical. For the two-needle technique, an entry needle (18- to 20-gauge) is placed through the skin and advanced to within a few centimeters of the disc space margin, after which a thinner gauge needle (20- to 22-gauge) is advanced in a coaxial fashion into the disc space itself. The second needle may be curved by the operator prior to advancement into the disc space, which may help to facilitate appropriate positioning of the second needle. The purpose of the two-needle technique is twofold. First, it may decrease the risk of infection, because the same needle that is puncturing the skin site does not enter the disc space directly (7). Other authors dispute this decreased risk of infection (8). Second, because the inner coaxial needle is often curved to circumvent the articular pillar (4,9,10), it is easier to advance the curved needle through the soft tissues of the back if it is passing through an outer introducer needle than it would be without the coaxial system. Although a curve on the needle may be helpful, using the bevel to "steer" the needle is typically enough to guide the thinner needle into the disc space. In the absence of definitive evidence, whether to use a single- or two-needle technique remains largely at the discretion of the operator.

A skin entry site is chosen that lies superimposed to the junction of the superior endplate and superior articulating process ("ear" of the Scotty dog) of the lower vertebral body. Lidocaine is used to anesthetize the skin site, but care is taken to not place the local anesthetic too deep into the anticipated needle path because this could result in inadvertent anesthesia of a potentially affected nerve root. By frequently alternating between lateral and anteroposterior (AP) fluoroscopy while advancing the entry needle, the appropriate angle and needle depth are confirmed. Using intermittent fluoroscopy, the entry needle is slowly advanced to the level of the pedicle on the lateral view; at this point, the needle tip should be equally as far from the disc margin on the lateral view as on the AP view.

A gentle curve (30°–45°) is placed on the inner, thinner gauge needle to facilitate placement into the disc space. If access to the disc space is deemed to be straight forward, simply using the bevel of the inner needle to give direction to the needle tip may be adequate. The authors place the curve so the bevel of the needle is on the inner margin of the curve, allowing both the bevel and the curve to work in concert to direct the needle. When a 22-gauge needle is used, the curve can be made simply by stripping the needle between thumb and forefinger, or by using a hemostat and thumb. Once the curve is made, the inner needle is advanced under fluoroscopic guidance until a popping sensation is felt by the operator, indicating puncture of the annulus. It has been recommended that lateral fluoroscopy be used during advancement of the inner needle to preclude advancement of the needle beyond the ventral margin of the disc space (4); these authors find it most helpful to alternate between AP and lateral fluoroscopy to confirm the appropriate curve on the inner needle. Generally speaking, the distance to the midpoint of the disc should be equal on both the AP and lateral views during needle advancement. If the distance is greater for one projection than the other, recurving the needle may be necessary. The final needle position should be in the middle third of the disc on both projections. Once adequate needle position is confirmed on both the lateral and AP projections, the subsequent disc spaces are accessed in similar fashion.

Special mention must be made of the L5S1 disc space. Rarely is it possible to line up the disc space in the abovementioned fashion because the iliac wing projects into the expected needle path. A much more severe craniocaudal angulation is necessary in order to access this lower disc space; in fact, it is usually the case that the skin entry site for the L5S1 disc space is significantly more cephalad than the skin entry sites for the other disc spaces. In order to adequately position the needle for the approach to the L5S1 disc space, the authors first angle the C-arm laterally to again visualize the Scotty dog appearance. Superimposition of the iliac wing over the transverse process (nose of the Scotty dog) is almost always seen at this point. Using continuous fluoroscopy, the C-arm is subsequently angled in a craniocaudal direction until the iliac wing and transverse process are no longer superimposed. A skin entry site superimposed over the disc space (approximately half way between the inferior endplate of the upper vertebral body and the superior endplate of the lower vertebral body) is then chosen. Using the technique described earlier, the outer needle is advanced just beyond the medial margin of the iliac wing on AP fluoroscopy, after which the inner needle is advanced into the disc space. It is often the case that the inner needle must be manipulated in multiple different projections (including many that seem to make no sense!) before entering the disc space. On occasion, the inner needle simply cannot slide between the vertebral endplates and by the articular pillars; in this case, the contralateral approach should be attempted.

Transdural Approach

On very rare occasions, it may prove impossible to place a needle into the disc space from the oblique extradrual approach described earlier. This is particularly true in patients who have undergone surgical interventions (4). In this instance, a transdural approach may be used. This technique is exactly analogous to performing either a lumbar puncture or an epidural spinal injection, and may be performed with midline or paramedian needle entry sites. The authors prefer to perform transdural punctures from a paramedian approach, again using down-the-barrel imaging guidance. To accomplish this, the C-arm is angled laterally, approximately 10° (in either direction, but typically toward the operator), and craniocaudally until the anticipated thecal sac puncture site and disc space are superimposed. The outer 18- to 20-gauge needle is advanced to the level of the pedicle (on lateral fluoroscopy), and the inner needle is advanced entirely through the thecal sac until the disc space is entered. Confirmation of placement of the needle into the middle third of the disc space is confirmed with both lateral and AP fluoroscopy. Once the needle is adequately placed, the provocative testing is performed identical to the external oblique approach.

Provocative Testing

Once all the needles have been placed in the disc spaces, the diagnostic and provocative tests can be performed. The following describes the authors' preferred method of performing the procedure, although it is recognized that many iterations on the theme exist.

Provocative testing is the mainstay of diagnosis with discography, and care should be taken to perform this portion of the examination fastidiously. The patient should not be given verbal or visual cues as to when the injections are taking place and at which level, but broad and general statements should be given. "Tell me if you feel anything, and what you feel" is a more appropriate statement than "I'm going to inject L4L5 now – tell me if it hurts." It is particularly vital to have the patient describe their pain during the provocative portion. A significant minority of healthy individuals with no back symptomatology will complain of pain on injection of their presumed normal discs, although oftentimes imaging studies confirm an occult abnormality within the disc itself (11–14). Because of this, the response that the operator is most interested in is pain on injection that is concordant with the patient's underlying pain. If the patient complains of pain on injection, it is imperative that the operator asks about the type of pain and whether it simulates the patient's baseline pain. Without this concordance, the false-positive rate will be unacceptably high.

Whether to use a manometer to inject fluid during the provocative test is a question of significant debate (2,8,15–22). The authors use a manometer for all procedures, and use of such a device is recommended by the International Spine Injection Society (ISIS) (6). If a manometer is used, the "opening pressure" of the disc should be measured, and this opening pressure should be subtracted from the manometer reading during injections to determine the true postinjection disc pressure. There are several commercially available devices.

There are three endpoints for discography – pain, pressure, and volume endpoints (2) (Table 3). The first endpoint is a positive pain response. As

---

Table 3. Discography Endpoints

Pain

Any significant pain response, regardless of whether the pain mimics the patient's symptomology.

Pressure (above opening pressure)

Pain response that mimics the patient's symptoms:

<15 psi	chemically sensitive disc
15–50 psi	mechanically sensitive disc
>50 psi	nondiagnostic

Volume

>3.5 cc injected without a pain response: nondiagnostic provocative test, suspect annular tear

---

discussed earlier, a positive pain response is not adequate to consider the discogram positive, but rather the pain must simulate the patient's underlying symptoms. Once pain occurs, the injection should be stopped and the next level assessed – this is true even if the pain response does not mimic the patient's underlying pain. The second endpoint is pressure. Pain can occur at any time during the fluid injection but can generally be separated into an early (low-pressure) and a late (high-pressure) pain response. This distinction of early and late pain response is believed to correlate with chemically or mechanically sensitized discs, respectively. The early pain response typically occurs with very low pressures (<15 psi above the disc opening pressure) and correlates with a chemicially sensitive disc. A pain response that occurs between 15 and 50 psi correlates with a mechanically sensitive disc, whereas pain that occurs after a pressure of greater than 50 psi is considered a nondiagnostic pain response (2). The final endpoint is the total volume injected. The normal disc will accept approximately 1–2 cc of fluid; however, degenerative discs will accept significantly larger volumes (2). In the scenario of a disc that has undergone an annular tear, fluid will leak out of the disc space and the injected volume is nearly limitless. We use 3.5 cc of injected volume as our endpoint; this indicates that the disc is disrupted, and regardless of how much fluid is injected the examination is likely to be negative because intradiscal pressure will never be high enough to elicit a pain response.

Once the needles are in appropriate position, the provocative test may be performed. A baseline measurement of the patients underlying pain level is obtained prior to placing the needles – a visual analog scale is helpful here, as is using a numerical scale. A second baseline measurement of pain is obtained prior to the provocative test but after placement of the needles into the disc spaces. The two baseline measurements are often different. The authors always start the provocative test at one of the control levels because eliciting a pain response at the first level may compromise the findings at the control levels (Anderson, Kinard). The manometer is filled with nonionic contrast that can be used for intrathecal injection. The authors use full-strength Omnipaque-240, which is dense enough to visualize well under fluoroscopy but not so dense that the computed tomography (CT) images obtained after the procedures are nondiagnostic. After the stylet is removed from the inner needle, the manometer is connected. Depending on the device used, a short connecting tube may be beneficial. A small amount of contrast is used to fill the needle hub, and the connection between the inner needle and the manometer is made. A very small turn (a few degrees) on the manometer handle is performed until contrast is first visualized, which gives a pressure measurement on the manometer gauge – this initial reading represents the opening pressure, and the value should be subtracted from all pressure measurements postinjection to obtain a true value for the pressure during injection. The handle of the manometer is turned, constantly watching the pressure, until one of the three endpoints discussed above (pain, pressure, and volume) is achieved. The same procedure is duplicated at the other two levels.

If a pain response is elicited, some investigators have advocated injecting a local anesthetic at that level prior to proceeding to the next level in order to decrease the likelihood of a false-positive response at the following levels (5). We do not do this routinely.

Although neither of the authors use the ISIS scoring system for response to disc stimulation, the reader should be aware that such a scoring system exists.

Imaging Findings

Most operators now use the pain response during the provocative testing to definitively call the discogram positive or negative. Some operators routinely perform CT scans following discography (Anderson, Min, McCutcheon, Anderson 2000, Tehranzadeh), whereas others do not do so. Without a doubt, CT scans post discography identify significantly more morphologic abnormalities than fluoroscopic images alone (e.g., spondylolysis, hpoplastic pars, lateral discs, foraminal stenosis, etc.). The question is raised, however, with what to do with morphologically abnormal discs in the absence of an invoked pain response. The debate rages not only in the literature but during preparation of this chapter as well (one author routinely performs postdiscography CT scanning, whereas the other does not).

In an attempt to standardize discography interpretation and reporting, the Dallas Discogram Scale was invented (23). This scoring system has undergone many modifications and describes both pain responses and findings on CT postdiscography. The scale is useful in an attempt to standardize the nomenclature of CT discograms, and operators are advised to use it when describing postprocedure findings (Table 4).

Fluorsocopically, following contrast injection, normal discs have a collection of contrast within the middle of the disc, with little dispersion of contrast away from the needle tip (Figure 2). The appearance has been termed "cloud-like" or "cotton-ball." If the contrast assumes more of a discoid appearance, it is referred to as "hamburger in a bun." Regardless of the moniker, the important finding is that there is no contrast that extends to the posterior or lateral edge of the disc. When contrast is noted to diffuse posteriorly, one or more annular tears must be present; where contrast diffuses in all directions, severe

Table 4. Dallas Discogram Description	
Type	*Discogram Description*
Type 1	Normal discography, both by no pain response and normal by CT
Type 2	Positive pain response, but normal CT appearance
Type 3	Annular tears leading to a radial fissure
	A Posterior fissure
	B Posterolateral fissure
	C Lateral fissure (lateral to a line from the center of the disk to the lateral boarder of the superior articulating process)
Type 4	Radial fissure extending to the annulus, with bulging of the annulus but NO extrusion of disc material
Type 5	Rupture of the outer annulus with extrusion of disc material that remains in continuity with the underlying disc
Type 6	Disc extrusion that is no longer in continuity with the underlying disc
Type 7	Multiple annular tears; complete disc disruption

Source: Cohen et al. (2); Saal and Saal (16); Sachs et al. (23).

degenerative disc disease is present (Figures 3–5). Contrast extravasation into the epidural space indicates a complete tear of the annulus.

COMPLICATIONS

Complications following discography are extremely rare. Potential complications include bleeding, infection, long-term worsening of pain, and allergic reactions to contrast or local anesthetic. Other complications, such as meningitis, nerve root damage, and arachnoiditis may be seen following the transdural route but are so rare as to warrant reports in the literature.

Discitis is probably the worst potential complication following discography; however, the incidence is very low and is likely in the range of 0.1–0.2% (3). In a review of infectious complications in nearly 5,000 patients, one study demonstrated an incidence of discitis of 0.25% (7). A separate study demonstrated a significant reduction in rates of infection (from 2.7% to 0.7%) by using the two-needle technique. This is likely due to the fact that the needle that enters the disc space never directly traverses the skin surface. The role of prophylactic antibiotics in preventing infection is unclear. Cohen et al. reported no infectious complications in over 2,000 discograms following the use of prophylactic antibiotics (2). Using a different technique, Osti et al. suggest injecting cefazolin directly into the disc space by mixing it with contrast material (24). One of the authors (LJR) adds 0.2 ml of the cefazolin solution to the 20 ml of contrast used during the discogram.

A small percentage of patients will complain of worsening of their pain following discography. This phenomenon is typically self-limited, and within

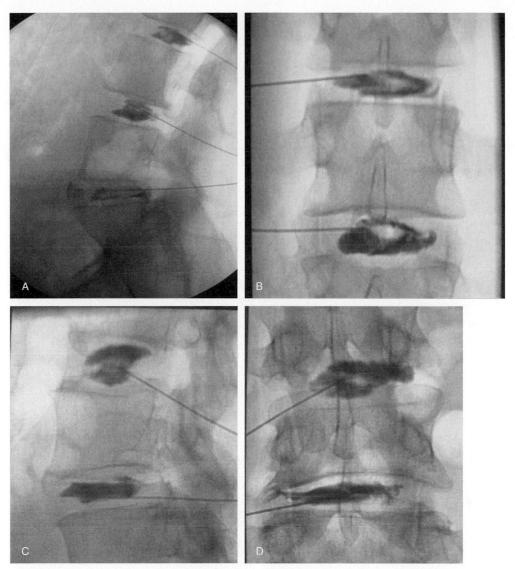

Figure 2. Normal discogram. (A) Lateral view from a discogram at L3-L4, L4-L5, and L5-S1. Notice the normal appearance of the discogram at the upper two levels. The contrast is contained within the nucleus, and there is a cleft in the middle of the contrast giving the classic "hamburger-in-a-bun" appearance of a mature disc. Contrast visualized at L5S1, however, demonstrates contrast diffusion and contrast that is not contained to the nucleus. (B) AP view of the upper two levels from the same patient shown in Figure 2A, redemonstrating contrast containment within the nucleus and the central cleft. (C) Lateral view from a two-level discogram demonstrating two different but normal appearances to the discs. The upper level demonstrates the classic hamburger-in-a-bun appearance, whereas the lower level demonstrates containment of contrast without the central cleft. (D) AP view from the same patient shown in Figure 2C.

hours to days, the patients' symptoms usually return to baseline. A delayed onset of discogenic pain may be due to contrast that slowly infiltrates into the peripheral disc via an annular tear, irritating the pain fibers (4). It has also been postulated that persistent pain following discography may be due to microfractures of the vertebral endplates, particularly if a manometer is used (2).

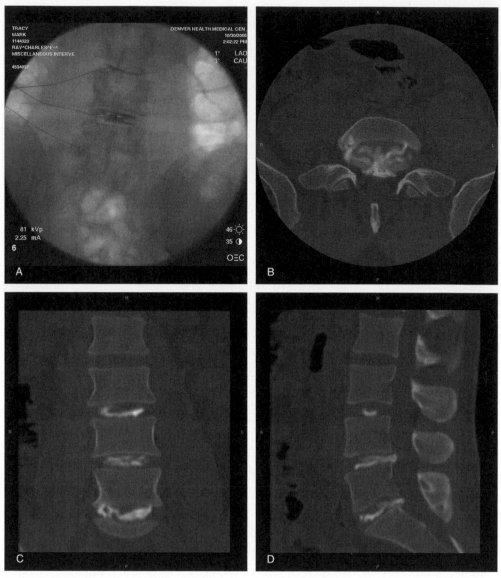

Figure 3. Thirty-four-year-old male with chronic lower back pain for two years. The patient describes polyradiculopathy of the left lower extremity consisting of numbness affecting the entire leg, ankle, and foot. Lumbar epidural steroid injection x2 produced very short-term pain relief. MRI (not shown) demonstrates degenerative disc disease with small protrusions at L4-L5 and L5-S1. During three-level discography, the patient described pain concordant with his underlying pain during the L4-L5 injection, obtained at low pressure (20 psi) and low volume (2.5 cc). (A) AP fluoroscopic image obtained during three-level discography demonstrating degenerative disc disease at the L3-L4 and L4-L5 levels. Similar changes were noted following injection of the L5-S1 space. (B) Axial CT image at the L5-S1 level following discography demonstrating a posterior annular tear with extension of contrast outside the disc space. (C) Coronal reformation of the CT scan in B, demonstrating degenerative disc disease with annular disruption at all three levels. (D) Sagittal reformation of the CT scan in B, demonstrating posterior disc bulges at L4-L5 and L5-S1.

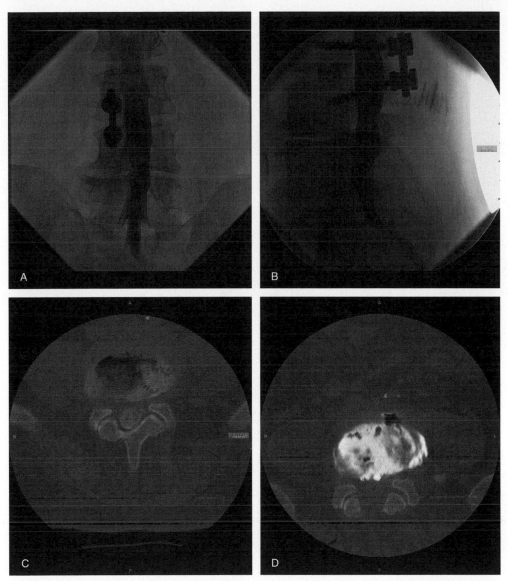

Figure 4. Fifty-year-old male with low-back pain and L4-L5 radiculopathy on the left. The patient has had multiple back surgeries. The patient did not have reproduction of symptoms despite the injection of a large amount (8 cc) of contrast and severe disc disease. This case illustrates the point that reproduction of symptoms can be difficult in patients with severe annular tears because sufficient pressure cannot be generated in the disc space. (A) and (B) AP and lateral images postmyelography (performed due to hardware in the spine following spinal surgery) demonstrate no significant disc bulges or herniations. (C) Axial CT scan postmyelography demonstrates severe degenerative disc disease at L4-L5, but no evidence of significant impingement on the thecal sac. (D) Axial CT scan postdiscography at L4-L5, demonstrating severe degenerative disc disease with multiple annular tears.

Long-term worsening of symptoms is exceedingly rare and is more likely due to progression of disease than caused by the procedure itself (25,26). If the patient describes pain that resolved shortly after the procedure and then progressively worsened, one should be concerned about the possibility of discitis.

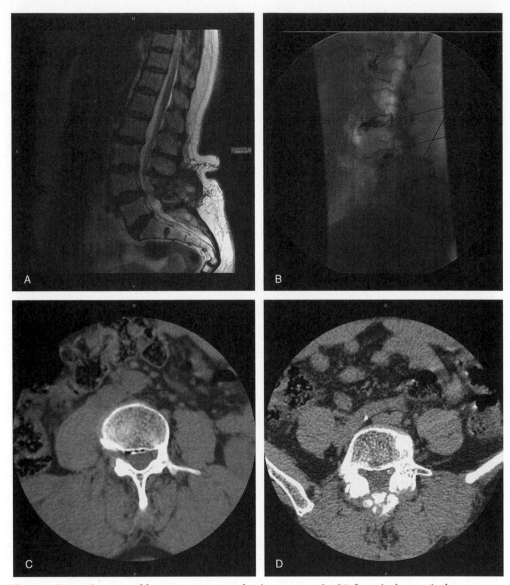

Figure 5. Forty-nine-year-old woman status postlaminectomy at L4-L5 for spinal stenosis due to hypertrophy of the ligamentum flavum, facet arthropathy, and disc bulge. She presented with recurrent symptoms. (A) Sagittal T2-weighted image from an MRI performed postoperatively demonstrates broad-based disc bulges throughout the entire lumbar spine. (B) Lateral image obtained following three-level discography demonstrates annular tears at all three levels. The patient complained of pain during the L3-L4 injection, but the pain was not concordant with her normal pain. Pain was not elicited at the other levels. (C) Axial CT obtained at the L3-L4 level demonstrating contrast extravasation through a full-thickness annular tear into the epidural fat. Gas is also noted, most likely secondary to accidental injection of air during the discogram. (D) Axial CT obtained at the L5 level demonstrating contrast extravasation adjacent to the left L4 nerve root. The contrast extravasation could have occurred from either the L4-L5 or L5-S1 injection.

Bleeding complications are exceedingly uncommon, and the risk of such complications is negligible unless the patient has a bleeding dyscrasia or is on anticoagulation or antiplatelet agents.

CLINICAL RESULTS

Opponents of discography claim, appropriately, that regardless of the attempt at normalizing and quantifying the study results, the end result of the procedure always depends on a subjective response by the patient. This is indeed the case, as it almost always is with both diagnostic and therapeutic procedures dealing with pain. There is likely no way around this obstacle, and understanding this limitation is important for any operator who is interested in performing the procedure. In addition, there will undoubtedly be a subgroup of patients with somatization disorders, both intentional and involuntary, who will make interpretation of the results even more unclear.

False-positive results have been reported to occur in a significant number of patients undergoing the procedure, although the exact incidence is difficult to determine. Possible etiologies include uncontrolled injections that reach too high of a pressure, accidental injection in the annulus, mechanical forces applied to the adjacent endplate, or chemical irritation by the contrast agent itself (2,27,28). In one study, Carragee et al. performed discography in normal volunteers, patients without low-back pain but with a history of cervical spine procedures, and patients with a diagnosis of somatization disorder. Positive results were common in all the groups, including 10% of the volunteers, 40% of the cervical patients, and 75% of the patients with somatization disorders (10). In a separate study, the same investigator performed discography in eight patients without low-back pain but who had undergone iliac bone grafting for nonlumbar spinal procedures (12). Half of the patients experienced severe back pain during discography, which was determined to be concordant with their postoperative pain.

Postoperative patients are often the most challenging patients in whom discography is performed. One reason for this is that spinal hardware and bone grafts may present a physicial obstacle to performing discography. As mentioned earlier, a transthecal approach may prove to be most viable in these patients. A second reason is that, as some authors have suggested, false-positive discograms may occur with more frequency in postoperative patients (2,11). The etiology of false-positive discograms in the postoperative patient is poorly understood; however, the specificity of the examination may improve if both control levels are negative.

Although false-positive examinations are difficult to assess, it should be noted that in the studies described earlier, nearly all of the exams considered as false positive did indeed show some morphological abnormality of the disc itself, whether diagnosed by CT or fluoroscopy. Therefore, although the examination may be considered falsely positive, there exists some abnormality within the disc space that may at least in part account for the findings on the provocative study.

Data concerning discography and success with postdiscography surgical interventions are wide ranging. In one relatively large study, 137 patients demonstrated a positive discogram prior to undergoing surgery (29). In this study, nearly 90% of patients with a positive provocative discogram demonstrated significant relief of symptoms after undergoing their spinal operation. There was a far less impressive response (52%) in patients with no pain response but with abnormal discograms radiologically. In a separate study, Kostuik et al. demonstrated an improvement in surgical success rates when preoperative discography was used (65% vs. 85%) (30). Derby et al. demonstrated an 89% success rates in patients with chemically sensitive discs who underwent surgical procedures (19), while Gill et al. reported a 75% success rates in patients with both a positive discogram and a positive MRI (31).

Other authors have demonstrated far less favorable results regarding the predictive value of successful operations based on discography results. In one study of 35 patients who underwent spinal fixation or fusion, there was essentially no difference in the surgical success rates in patients with positive preoperative discograms when compared to those with negative discograms (32). Other authors have demonstrated similar results (33,34).

A positive discogram should not necessarily indicate that the patient needs surgery. In one study, nearly 70% of patients with a positive discogram demonstrated significant clinical improvement with conservative therapy alone (35).

CONCLUSIONS

Discography remains a hotly debated topic, with spine surgeons and radiologists alike aligned on both sides of the debate. No clear consensus can be made from the available data, and it is highly unlikely that a well-controlled clinical trial will ever be performed to definitively answer the question of the utility of discography. Fastidious attention to detail and standardization of results will likely increase the accuracy and predictive value of the examination, and if the procedure is to be performed at all care must be taken to perform the procedure and interpret the results correctly.

REFERENCES

1. Lindblom K. Diagnostic puncture of intervertebral disks in sciatica. Acta Ortho Scand 1948;17:213–39.
2. Cohen SP, Larkin TM, Barna SA, Palmer WE, Hecht AC, Stojanovic MP. Lumbar discography: a comprehensive review of outcome studies, diagnostic accuracy, and principles. Reg Anesth Pain Med 2005;30:163–83.
3. Guyer RD, Ohnmeiss DD. Contemporary concepts in spine care lumbar discography: position statement from the North American Spine Society Diagnostic and Therapeutic Committee. Spine 1995;20:2048–59.
4. Anderson MW. Lumbar discography: an update. Sem Roentgen 2004;39:52–67.
5. Schellhas KP. Diskography. Neuroimaging Clin N Am 2000;10:579–96.
6. Endres S, Bogduk N. Practice guidelines and protocols: lumbar disc stimulation. Presented at the International Spinal Injection Society 9th Annual Scientific Meeting (2001), Boston, MA, pp. 56–75.

7. Willems PC, Jacobs W, Duinderke ES, De Kleuver M. Lumbar discography: should we use prophylactic antibiotics? A study of 435 consecutive discograms and a systematic review of the literature. J Spinal Disord Tech 2004;17:243–7.

8. Fenton DS, Czervionke LF. Image-guided spine intervention. Philadelphia: Saunders; 2003:227–56.

9. Lander PH. Lumbar discography: current concepts and controversies. Sem Ultrasound CT MR 2005;26:81–8.

10. Kumar N, Agorastides ID. The curved needle technique for accessing the L5/S1 disc space. Br J Radiol 2000;73:655–7.

11. Carragee EJ, Tanner CM, Khurana S, et al. The rates of false-positive lumbar discography in select patients without low back symptoms. Spine 2000;25:1373–80.

12. Carragee EJ, Chen Y, Tanner CM, Truong T, Lau E, Brito JL. Provocative discography in patients after limited lumbar discectomy. Spine 2000;25:3065–71.

13. Carragee EJ, Tanner CM, Yang B, Brito JL, Truong T. False-positive findings on lumbar discography. Reliability of subjective concordance assessment during provocative disc injection. Spine 1999;24:2542–7.

14. Holt EP Jr. The question of lumbar discography. J Bone Joint Surg 1968;50A:720–6.

15. Guyer RE, Ohnmeiss DD. NASS: lumbar discography. Spine J 2003;3(3 Suppl): 11S–27S.

16. Saal JA, Saal JS. Intradiscal electrothermal treatment (IDET) for chronic discogenic low back pain: a prospective outcome study with minimum 2-year follow-up. Spine 2002;27:966–73.

17. Anderson SR, Flanagan B. Discography. Curr Rev Pain 2000;4:345–52.

18. Southern EP, Fye MA, Panjabi MM, et al. Disc degeneration: a human cadaveric study correlating magnetic resonance imaging and quantitative discomanometry. Spine 2000;25:2171–5.

19. Derby R, Howard MW, Grant JM, et al. The ability of pressure-controlled discography to predict surgical and non-surgical outcomes. Spine 1999;24:364–72.

20. Min K, Leu HJ, Perrenoud A. Discography with manometry and discographic CT: their value in patient selection for percutaneous lumbar nucleotomy. Bull Hosp Jt Dis 1996;54:153–7.

21. Bernard TN Jr. Lumbar discography followed by computed tomography. Refining the diagnosis of low back pain. Spine 1990;15:690–707.

22. Perey O. Contrast medium examination of the intervertebral disc of the lower lumbar spine. Acta Orthop Scan 1951;20:237–334.

23. Sachs BL, Vanharanta H, Spivey MA, et al. Dall discogram description: a new classification of CT/discography in low-back disorders. Spine 1987;12:287–94.

24. Osti OL, Fraser RD, Vernon-Roberts B. Discitis after discography. The role of prophylactic antibiotics. J Bone Joint Surg 1990;72B:271–4.

25. Johnson RG. Does discography injure normal discs? An analysis of repeat discograms. Spine 1989;14:424–6.

26. Flanagan MN, Chung BU. Roentgenographic changes in 188 patients 10–20 years after discography and chemonucleolysis. Spine 1986;11:444–8.

27. Almen T. Experimental investigations with iohexol and their clinical relevance. Act Radiol 1983;366S:9–19.

28. Collis JS, Gardner WJ. Lumbar discography. An analysis of one thousand cases. J Neurosurg 1962;19:452–61.

29. Colhoun E, McCall IW, Williams L, Cassar Pullicino VN. Provocation discography as a guide to planning operations on the spine. J Bone Joint Surg (Br) 1988;70: 267–71.

30. Kostuik JP. Decision making in adult scoliosis. Spine 1979;4:521–5.

31. Gill K, Blumenthal SL. Functional results after anterior lumbar fusion at L5-S1 in patients with normal and abnormal MRI scans. Spine 1992;17:940–2.

32. Esses SI, Botsford DJ, Kostuik JP. The role of external spinal skeletal fixation in the assessment of low-back disorders. Spine 1989;14:594–600.

33. Madan S, Gundanna M, Harley JM, Boeree NR, Sampson M. Does provocative discography screening of discogenic back pain improve surgical outcomes? J Spinal Disord Tech 2002;15:245–51.
34. Knox BD, Chapman TM. Anterior lumbar interbody fusion for discogram concordant pain. J Spinal Disord 1993;6:242–4.
35. Rhyne AL III, Smith SE, Wood KE, et al. Outcome of unoperated discogram-positive low back pain. Spine 1995;20:1997–2001.

Facet (Zygapophyseal) Joint Injections

Nick Stence

INTRODUCTION

Back pain due to the many causes is a significant health issue in this country. The annual incidence of lower back pain is at least 5% (1). It affects men and women equally, most often between 30 and 50 years of age. About 85% of patients with isolated back pain cannot be given a diagnosis (2). Finding an association between imaging findings and symptoms is usually difficult or, at times, impossible (1,3).

Given the prevalence of back pain, therapies and interventions treating such processes represent a growing segment of health care spending. For example, spinal injection procedures have expanded significantly since the mid- to late 1990s. The volume of facet joint injections has almost tripled and reimbursements have followed the same trend. The provider profile has changed as well, with anesthesiologists performing the majority of procedures and radiologists share of procedures declining from 1993 to 1999 (4).

Chronic low-back pain is defined as pain persisting longer than three months. Most monotherapies (e.g., analgesics, nonsteroidal anti-inflammatory drugs, muscle relaxants, antidepressants) do not work or have limited efficacy for chronic low-back pain (2). Facet joint pain is thought to be a significant cause of otherwise unexplained chronic low-back pain. In the group of chronic low-back pain patients for whom conventional investigations do not identify a cause of pain, facet joint pain can be diagnosed by facet injections with local anesthetic in 15–40% of patients (5).

Therapy for facet joint pain remains somewhat controversial. Early papers described good short- and long-term outcomes following facet joint steroid injection (6,7). However, the only randomized controlled trials of facet joint steroid injections did not prove they were of value in long-term therapy (4,8). Some of these negative results may be influenced by patient selection; defining true facet joint pain can be difficult, and the percentage of patients with true facet joint pain in these studies is difficult to ascertain (1,3,9).

In this chapter, the normal and pathological anatomy of the facet joints will be discussed. The syndrome of facet joint pain and its diagnosis will be outlined. Various techniques for facet joint injection under fluoroscopy and computed tomography (CT) will be described.

NORMAL ANATOMY

The zygapophyseal, or facet, joint is one of two articulations in the lumbar spine; the intervertebral disc articulation is the second. These joints maintain proper spinal alignment in response to various forces, including axial, flexion/extension, and rotational forces (10). The disc segment is preferentially load-bearing while in forward flexion, and the facet joints are loaded while in hyper-extension and lumbar rotation (11).

The two components of the facet joint are the anterosuperior articular facet from the vertebral body below, and the posteroinferior articular facet from the vertebral body above (Figure 1). The facet joints are true synovial joints. They have hyaline cartilage surfaces, a synovial membrane, and a fibrous capsule. The facet joint in the lumbar spine is oriented vertically in a plane between the sagittal and coronal. This orientation is thought to protect the intervertebral disc from axial rotation and loading (12). The joint space itself is curved from front to back; the inferior facet is convex, whereas the superior facet is concave (13). There are two main articular recesses about the facet joint. The superior recess is located anteriorly and is close to the lumbar canal and neural elements, whereas the inferior recess is posterior and has no contact with neural elements (13).

The innervation of the facet joints is somewhat complex. Medial branches of the dorsal ramus exit the intervertebral foramen, cross the superior border of the transverse process, and then course along the junction of the transverse process and superior articular process prior to turning medially around the zygoapophyseal joint base and under the mamilloaccessory ligament (14). Each zygaphophyseal joint is innervated by the medial branch of the dorsal ramus one level above it and at the same level. For example, the L4-L5 zygaphophyseal joint is innervated by the medial branches of L3 and L4 (15) (Figure 2). At L5-S1, the facet joint is innervated by the dorsal ramus of L5 itself, and not a medial branch (although for practical purposes when performing medial branch blocks, this is often generically referred to as the medial branch) (16). This innervation is different from other components of the lumbar spine. The posterior interverte-bral disc, posterior longitudinal ligament, and the dura are innervated by the sinuvertebral nerve, which arises from the ventral primary ramus (11). This pattern of sensory innervation explains why facet joint pain is an entity distinct from other causes of low-back pain. This also accounts for why facet pain in certain patients may not be specific for a particular spinal level (13).

BACK PAIN RELATED TO FACET JOINTS
Etiology

Low-back pain is a common and often frustrating problem to diagnose and manage. The specific cause of low-back pain remains undetermined in the

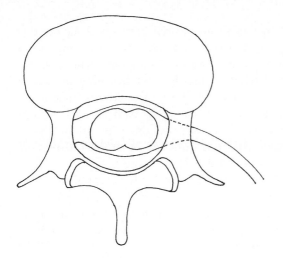

Figure 1. Axial demonstration of the facet joints, and their relationship to the neural foramen, exiting nerve root, and epidural space. [Adapted from Silbergleit et al. (3).]

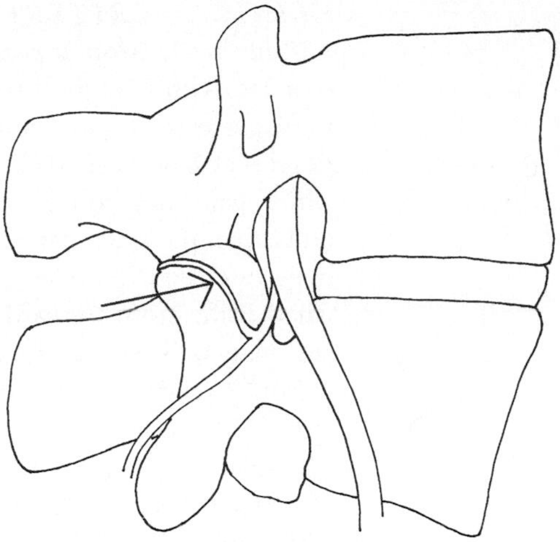

Figure 2. Innervation of the facet joint. The facet joint is innvervated by the medial branch of the dorsal ramus (arrow). [Adapted from Silbergleit et al. (3).]

majority of cases. Low-back pain is a common complaint whose causes are diverse and unrelated, including spinal segment biomechanics, anatomic pathology, neuropathic etiology, and psychological factors (11). Acute back pain resolves in over 70% of patients with less than 25% recurrence (2). As mentioned earlier, facet joint pain is thought to be a significant cause of otherwise unexplained chronic low-back pain. In the group of chronic low-back pain patients for whom conventional investigations do not identify a cause of pain, facet joint pain (as diagnosed by facet injections with local anesthetic) is seen in up to 40% (5,17).

The current understanding of facet joint pain is that it is a referred pain from the nociceptive fibers that innervate the facet joint itself (11), and the pain is most likely secondary to joint degeneration. As discussed earlier, the facet joint has a unique innervation, which allows this syndrome to be selectively diagnosed via anesthetic block of the joint or the nerve fiber innervating the joint (16).

Diagnosis

Making the clinical diagnosis of facet joint pain is difficult for a number of reasons. Back pain can stem from a number of sources, such as discs, ligaments, muscles, sacroiliac joints, as well as the lumbar facet itself. Maneuvers designed to elicit a specific diagnosis are complicated by the fact that they often stress several structures simultaneously, especially the disc, facet joints, and muscles (18). Studies have found no correlation between imaging findings and facet joint pain (19). The only reliable method for diagnosis of facet joint pain as the cause of low-back pain is facet joint block, either by intraarticular injection of anesthetics or by anaesthetizing the medial branches of the dorsal rami (15,20).

CLINICAL CRITERIA

A study by Jackson suggested that there are no reliable clinical factors that correlate with facet joint pain (21). However, routinely using facet joint blocks to diagnose facet joint pain in every patient with low-back pain is not realistic. Revel et al. have devised clinical criteria that can help select that subset of patients whose pain may be relieved by facet joint block (9). The criteria include age older than 65 years, pain not exacerbated by coughing, pain not worsened by hyperextension, pain not worsened by forward flexion, pain not worsened when rising from forward flexion, pain not worsened by extension-rotation, and pain well relieved by recumbency (Table 1). In those patients who have pain well relieved by recumbency, as well as fulfilling at least five of the above criteria, the sensitivity was 92% and the specificity was 80% for facet joint pain (9). Again, use of these clinical criteria should not be used to make the diagnosis of facet joint pain, but they are helpful in selecting patients who should undergo facet joint arthography or diagnostic block.

FACET JOINT BLOCK

Pain that is relieved by facet joint block can be assumed to stem from the facet joint, given its unique innervation (15). However, single, uncontrolled facet joint blocks are complicated by false-positive results of up to 38% of patients (17). For this reason, controlled blocks are recommended to minimize false-positive results. The method for this usually involves initial anesthetic block of the suspected joint. If pain is relieved by this block, two more blocks are performed, one placebo block with saline and one true anesthetic block. If the patient's symptoms are consistent with the injection solution, then the facet joint can be assumed to be the cause of the patient's pain with a low incidence of false-positive results. If only a high degree of sensitivity is desired without concern for false-positive results, pain relief following facet joint block on two separate occasions can be used as the diagnostic criterion (15).

FACET JOINT PROCEDURES

Facet Joint Arthrography

INDICATIONS

Some debate exists regarding the appropriate indications (diagnosis vs. therapy) for facet joint arthrography. As described previously, early studies by Carrerra and Destouet described short- and long-term pain relief following intraarticular injection of local anesthetic and steroids (6,7). Subsequent randomized trials by Lilius and Carette did not find any significant difference in pain relief between patients injected with steroids versus placebo (4,8). Issues regarding technique (whether injections truly were intraarticular) and patient selection (whether patients truly had facet joint pain) may call these results into question (1,3,9). The recommendations of Committee on Nonoperative Care of the North American Spine Society are that the primary role of facet joint injections is to diagnose facet joint pain and that the therapeutic value of intraarticular or periarticular steroid injections is controversial (20). Evidence-based practice guidelines published by Boswell found strong evidence of the usefulness of diagnostic facet joint blocks (22). The same guidelines

Table 1. Clinical Criteria Noted in Patients Who Respond Favorably to a Facet Joint Block

Clinical Characteristic	Percentage Who Respond with Characteristic
Pain well relieved by recumbant position	92
Absence of pain exacerbation	
By coughing	100
By forward flexion	100
When rising from flexion	100
By hyperextension	92
By extension-rotation	77
Presence of at least five of the above characteristics	100

Source: Adapted from Revel et al. (9).

found moderate evidence for short-term pain relief following local anesthetic and steroid injection but only limited evidence for long-term pain relief. Nonetheless, steroid injections are still used in various settings for treatment of facet joint pain, and several recent papers have described techniques involving steroid injections (3,13,23).

TECHNIQUE
General

Absolute contraindications to this intervention include systemic or localized infection, pregnancy or possible pregnancy, and coagulopathy. Relative contraindications include contrast media allergy (for which patient can be premedicated), and use of aspirin.

A relatively dense, nonneurotoxic contrast agent should be used given the small amount of contrast used for joint arthrograms and proximity to neural structures (e.g., Omnipaque 240 or 320; Amersham Health, Inc., Princeton, NJ). Only 0.1–0.3 ml of contrast is required for adequate joint visualization.

Conventional local anesthetic can be used for diagnostic blocks, such as lidocaine 2% or bupivacaine 0.5%; higher anesthetic concentrations are preferred given the small amount of volume injected. For intraarticular injections, no more than 1.5 ml of local anesthetic should be injected to avoid rupture of the synovial lining.

Long-acting steroids can be injected with bupivacaine for therapeutic injections. Compounds used by various authors include triamcinolone acetonide (Kenalog 10 or 40; Apothecon, Princeton, NJ) (3), cortivazol (Altin; Diamant, Paris, France) (24), or 2.5% prednisolone acetate (Hydrocortancyl; Diamant) (13). Injections of up to 1.5 ml of steroid into the joint, after the injection of 0.1 ml of contrast material, is seemingly adequate, although it is felt that total injected volumes of greater than 1.5 ml run the risk of rupturing the joint capsule. Rupture of the joint capsule is probably more of an issue for diagnostic blocks (where the results could be confounded by spread of anesthetic agents) and then for blocks performed for pain management that use steroids. Any injected steroid preparation should be perservative free.

A 25-gauge needle results in less patient discomfort than larger needles. Muscle spasm from procedural pain can sometimes limit the ability to direct the needle. A 22-gauge needle may be used if the 25-gauge needle is difficult to direct.

As with all procedures, informed consent is required. The usual complications of any interventional procedure should be explained, including nominal risks of infection, bleeding, and allergic reaction. Other complications are rare but have been reported in the literature, including spinal anesthesia and chemical meningism (25–27). If the procedure will be used solely for diagnosis of facet joint pain, the patient should be advised about it.

Fluoroscopic guidance is mandatory for these procedures. CT guidance is an alternative but is not commonly employed in general practice due to its relative unvailability (3,28).

The skin should be sterilized, prepped, and draped in the usual fashion, leaving the skin of the lower back and upper buttocks exposed.

Oblique Approach (15)

An oblique view of the lumbar spine may be obtained either by positioning the patient obliquely and supporting them with a cushion, or by rotation of the C-arm while the patient lies prone. Lower lumbar joints are oriented at 45° from the sagittal plane, whereas upper joints are closer to sagittal in orientation, mirroring the thoracic spine. The C-arm is rotated until the joint cavity of the target facet is clearly visualized. The target for injection is the midpoint of the joint cavity. If the joint cavity cannot be clearly visualized fluoroscopically, the alternative techniques such as the posterior approach or a medial branch block should be pursued.

The skin over the target site is infiltrated with local anesthestic in the usual fashion. The skin puncture site will be directly over the target. The needle shaft is positioned at this site along the axis of the x-ray beam (down the barrel). The needle is then directed slowly toward the target along the x-ray beam axis, passing through subcutaneous fat, fascia, and musculature.

The needle tip should be directed initially toward either articular process immediately adjacent to the target; this ensures that the needle is at the appropriate depth (Figure 3). If the needle is instead directed immediately toward the joint cavity, the needle tip may pass through the joint entirely and into the epidural space. Once contact with the bone is made, the needle is redirected toward the joint cavity. Penetration of the joint capsule can usually be perceived by the operator as a subtle loss of resistance as the synovial membrane is penetrated, or by a sensation of the needle being gripped by the articular processes.

Needle placement is confirmed by injection of 0.1–0.3 ml of contrast medium. Contrast within the joint space will initially appear as a small longitudinal line and then expand into a dumbbell shape as contrast fills the superior

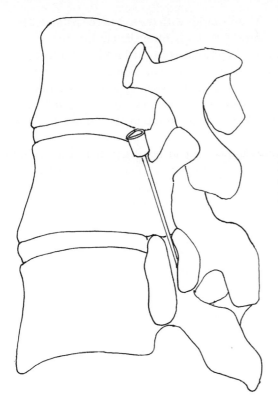

Figure 3. Demonstration of the appropriate needle direction to access the facet joint for injection procedures. [Adapted from Silbergleit et al. (3).]

and inferior articular recesses. If this conformation of contrast is not obtained, the needle is not within the joint space. Contrast will commonly assume a radiate appearance if injected into the tissues outside of the joint space.

Spot images of the joint arthrogram should be obtained to document adequate needle placement. Local anesthetic and/or steroid solution can then be injected. As discussed earlier, injection volumes should be limited to less than 1.5 ml to avoid the possibility of rupturing the joint capsule.

Posterior Approach (13)

The posterior approach to lumbar facet joint arthrography was described in detail in a paper by Sarazin et al. (13). The goal of this technique is to pass the needle into the inferior articular recess of the facet joint, rather than into the obliquely oriented space between the articular facets (Figure 4). Advantages of this technique include ease of reaching the joint space even in the presence of facet joint osteophytosis, and no need to reposition the patient when injecting bilateral joints. Sarazin et al. report success rates of greater than 90% at his institution with the posterior approach, limited in 6% of cases by leakage of contrast from the joint capsule and in 4% of cases by inability to reach the inferior articular recess (13).

For the posterior approach, the patient is placed prone with cushions placed under the abdomen to reverse the lumbar lordosis. This maneuver enlarges the inferior articular recess and decreases the tissue thickness in the area of interest, resulting in better image quality and less tissue to traverse to reach the joint. The skin is prepped and draped as described previously.

The x-ray beam is oriented anteroposterior with respect to the patient. The target site for needle placement for L1 to L5 is immediately inferior to the inferior articular process of the facet joint of interest. At L5-S1, the target site is just below the superior aspect of the sacrum. The skin above this site is anesthetized, then the needle shaft is oriented parallel to the x-ray beam axis. The needle is passed directly downward along the x-ray beam axis until the joint capsule is reached. Again, needle passage through the joint capsule is frequently perceived by the operator.

Following contrast injection, contrast should be observed to flow freely into the superior recess of the joint. A radiate pattern of contrast spread at the needle tip indicates that the joint was not penetrated. Images should be obtained to document correct needle placement. Sarazin et al. recommend injection of 2 ml of contrast into the joint, but as described earlier, a smaller amount (0.1–0.3 ml) may be preferred and can be adequate depending on the indication for arthrography.

FINDINGS
Normal

The normal contrast-filled lumbar facet joint appears as a ring on PA images and has an S-shaped appearance on lateral images. Its margins should be smooth and regular. The superior and inferior recesses should be well demonstrated and communicate freely with one another. Normal total joint volume is between 1 and 3 ml (13).

Pathological

DEGENERATIVE JOINT DISEASE

As mentioned previously, no correlation can be made between degenerative changes at the facet joint and facet joint pain (19). However, degenerative

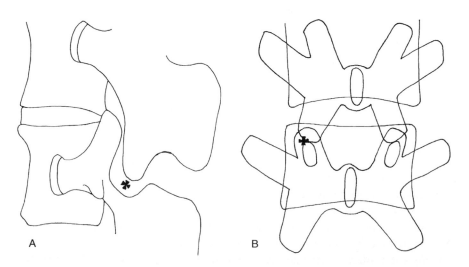

Figure 4. Target location for posterior approach. The location of the inferior recess of the facet joint is demonstrated (asterisks).

changes are frequently seen at arthrography. A dengerated facet joint will have irregular margins and heterogeneous filling of the joint capsule.

SYNOVIAL CYSTS

Synovial cysts are a recognized cause of femoral and sciatic nerve root pain in the elderly (23). They are usually well characterized by CT and magnetic resonance imaging. They can occasionally be seen as protrusions in the spinal canal. Contrast may occasionally leak from these cysts during facet joint injection.

ABNORMAL COMMUNICATIONS

Flow of contrast into an upper or lower ipsilateral facet joint may occur during facet joint arthrography. This is common in patients with spondylosis, as the pars interarticularis is the boundary between adjacent facet joints. Communication between contralateral facet joints is more rare and may occur as a result of spondylosis or advanced facet osteoarthritis with large synovial cysts.

Interpretation of Pain Relief (15)

When arthrography is used to diagnose facet joint pain, evaluation and interpretation of pain relief is essential for accurate diagnosis. The patient should be interviewed within 24 hours of the procedure. The amount of pain relief should be ascertained, as well as the distribution and duration of pain relief.

A positive response to block is defined as greater than 90% relief of pain in the region of the block for a duration expected from the anesthetic used. A patient may still have pain from additional facet joints that were not blocked, so the evaluator will need to ascertain if the pain relief reported is commensurate with the facet joints blocked. If multiple joints are suspected to be involved, these will have to be blocked independently to establish contributions from each level. Once the extent of joint involvement is ascertained, all involved joints should be blocked in an attempt to obtain complete pain relief. If the patient has pain stemming from a structure other than a facet joint, results may be confounded by only partial relief of pain. However, some data indicate that it is uncommon for patients to have pain stemming from multiple sources (15).

Once the patient obtains complete relief after the initial block, controlled blocks should be performed as described previously to eliminate false-positive responses.

Facet Joint Medial Branch Block

INDICATIONS

Whereas facet joint injections are performed alternately for either diagnosis or therapy of facet joint pain, selective block of the medial branch of the dorsal ramus is primarily used for diagnosis of facet joint pain (15). Medial branch blocks have been shown to be a fairly reproducible and reliable means of accurately diagnosing facet joint pain (14,16). Medial branch blocks may be easier to perform than joint injections and are the preferred technique for diagnosis prior to medial branch neurotomy (15); there is, however, no evidence that they actually are superior to joint injection for diagnosing zygapophyseal joint pain (29).

Studies have demonstrated false-negative rates of medial branch blocks of 8–11%. This is attributed to a number of factors, including venous uptake of anesthetic, inadequate concentration of anesthetic about the nerve, and possibly variant innervation of the zygapophyseal joint. A significant false-negative rate of 50% has been associated with injections that demonstrated venous uptake during test contrast administration (16). Because of this, test contrast injections are recommended in all cases, with needle repositioning if venous uptake is observed.

TECHNIQUE
General

General considerations with regard to informed consent, contraindications, anesthetic and contrast composition, and procedure site preparation are similar to facet joint injections. Steroids are not used for medial branch blocks, given the typical indication of diagnosis of facet joint pain.

As discussed in the anatomy section, a given zygaphophyseal joint is innervated by medial branches above and at the target level. Therefore, these two levels must be anesthetized for every joint of interest.

Approach (14,15)

The patient is positioned prone on the fluoroscopy table. Target points vary depending on the level of interest. For L1-L4, the target point is the junction of the superior articular facet and the transverse process that the target nerve crosses. This has also been described as midway between the superior border of the transverse process and the mammiloaccessory ligament. For L5-S1, because the target nerve is the L5 dorsal ramus itself, the target point is the junction of the sacral ala with the superior articular process of the sacrum.

For L1-L4, the skin puncture site is selected superior and lateral to the target point; this is usually just above the tip of the transverse process. The needle should be directed caudad and medial toward the target point. This orientation helps to avoid introduction of the needle into the intervertebral foramen and the epidural space. For L5-S1, the skin puncture site is just lateral to the target point, and the needle should be directed medially toward the target. For this level, care must be taken to keep the needle tip below the superior margin of the sacrum.

Intermittent fluoroscopy should be used to guide the needle as close to the target point as possible. Once the needle contacts bone, it should be readjusted to be as close to the target point as possible; ideally, the needle tip should be slightly medial to the lateral margin of the silhouette of the superior articular process.

Once the needle is in correct position, 0.1–0.3 ml of contrast medium is injected to confirm position at the nerve root and assess for venous uptake. If venous uptake occurs, the needle should be repositioned by 1–2 mm and contrast reinjected. Once no venous uptake is observed, 0.5 ml of anesthetic agent is injected onto the nerve.

Radiofrequency Neurotomy

GENERAL

In patients diagnosed with zygapophyseal low-back pain, an ideal therapy may be a method for permanently disrupting the nociceptive pathways responsible for pain. Radiofrequency neurotomy is a technique that involves raising the temperature of tissues around an electrode tip in order to disrupt nociceptive pathways. When applied to tissue, low-energy, high-frequency alternating current produces heat. Depending on the duration and amount of current applied, as well as electrode size, a thermal lesion can be produced that can denature nerves and thus interrupt pain fibers. A more complete description of the equipment and pathophysiology can be found elsewhere (29).

Shealey first described using this technique to treat facet joint pain in 1973 (30). Others followed suit and began uncontrolled audits using various techniques for diagnosing pain and for performing the neurotomy. The percentage of subjects that experienced a substantial decrease in pain varied from 17 to 82%, although follow-up was rarely more than a year (31).

Three subsequent controlled, double-blinded trials have been performed. Two found moderate evidence that radiofrequency neurotomy is more effective than placebo (32,33), while one found no effect (34). A recent review of these trials, however, demonstrated substantial limitations in these studies' diagnostic criteria (all used only single, uncontrolled diagnostic blocks) and RF technique (35). An open prospective study that did use controlled diagnostic medial branch blocks and preferred RF technique found that substantial pain relief could be achieved in patients appropriately selected for the procedure (36). Nonetheless, a randomized, controlled trial utilizing controlled diagnostic blocks and accepted RF technique has yet to be published.

TECHNIQUE (36)

The technique described and validated by Dreyfuss is felt to most accurately treat the medial branch nerve according to its anatomy (36,37). Patients selected for neurotomy should undergo controlled diagnostic blocks on two separate visits to confirm facet joint pain and decrease the likelihood of false-positive results.

The patient is placed in the prone position on the fluoroscopy table. For each target nerve, a 22- or 25-gauge, 90-mm spinal needle is used as a guide for radiofrequency electrode placement. This needle is introduced in a similar fashion as for medial branch blocks described earlier; however, the target point for neurotomy is more proximal along the course of the nerve. This translates radiographically to the superior edge of the transverse process at the junction of the transverse process and superior articular process.

Once the guide needle is placed, the C-arm is rotated laterally 15° and caudad 20° to allow visualization of the target region from below. This view allows visualization of the guide needle tip as it rests on the bone in the groove of the transverse process and superior articular process.

A skin puncture point is selected over the target point and anesthetized with lidocaine. A 16-gauge electrode with a 5-mm exposed active tip is introduced through the puncture point toward the target point. The electrode should lie along the superior and dorsal margin of the transverse process, and its tip should abut the root of the superior articular process. Confirmatory lateral and oblique views should be obtained to ensure that the needle lies parallel to the course of the nerve and does not enter the intervertebral foramen.

Once needle position is confirmed radiographically, 0.75 ml of lidocaine is injected through the guide needle to anesthetize the tissues to be ablated. After this, the guide needle should be withdrawn to avoid it acting as a conductor for the RF electrode. An ablation is performed by raising the electrode tip temperature to 85° for 90 seconds. The electrode is withdrawn along the nerve course approximately 4–5 mm, and a second burn is performed.

This procedure should be repeated for both levels of innervation of the facet joint in question. After the procedure, pain medication should be provided for postprocedural pain from the thermal lesion and electrode insertion.

REFERENCES

1. El-Khoury GY, Renfew DLl. Percutaneous procedures for the diagnosis and treatment of lower back pain: discography, facet-joint injection, and epidural injection. *AJR Am J Roentgenol* 1991; 157:685–91.
2. Bogduk N. Management of chronic low back pain. *MJA* 2004; 180: 79–83.
3. Silbergleit R, Mehta BA, Sanders WP, Talati SJ. Imaging-guided injection techniques with fluoroscopy and CT for spinal pain management. *Radiographics* 2001; 21: 927–42.
4. Lilius G, Laasonen EM, Myllynen P, Harilainen A, Gronlund G. Lumbar facet joint syndrome: a randomized clinical trial. *J Bone Joint Surg* 1989; 71-b:681–4.
5. Schwarzer AC, Aprill CN, Derby R, Fortin J, Kine G, Bogduk N. Clinical features of patient with pain stemming from the lumbar zygapophyseal joints. Is the lumbar facet syndrome a clinical entity? *Spine* 1994; 19:1132–7.
6. Destouet JM, Gilula LA, Murphy WA, Monsees B. Lumbar facet injection: indication, technique, clinical correlation and preliminary results. *Radiology* 1982; 145:321–5.
7. Carrerra GF. Lumbar facet injection in low back pain and sciatica: preliminary results. *Radiology* 1980; 137:65–6.
8. Carette S, Marcoux S, Truchon R, et al. A controlled trial of corticosteroid injections into the facet joints for chronic low back pain. *NEJM* 1991; 325:1002–7.
9. Revel ME, Listrat VM, Chevalier XJ, et al. Capacity of the clinical picture to characterize low back pain relieved by facet joint anesthesia: proposed criteria to identify patients with painful facet joints. *Spine* 1998; 23(18):1972–6.
10. Anderson GBJ. Intradiskal pressure, intra-abdominal pressure and myoelectric back muscle activity related to posture and loading. *Clin Orthop* 1977; 129:156–64.
11. Bervan S. The lumbar zygapophyseal (facet) joints: a role in the pathogenesis of spinal pain syndromes and degenerative spondylolisthesis. *Semin Neurol* 2002; 22:187–95.
12. Adams MA. The mechanical function of the lumbar apophyseal joints. *Spine* 1983; 8:327–30.
13. Sarazin L, Chevrot A, Pesis E, et al. Lumbar facet joint arthrography with the posterior approach. *Radiographics* 1999; 19:93–104.
14. Dreyfuss PH. Specificity of lumbar medial branch and L5 dorsal ramus blocks: a computed tomography study. *Spine* 1997; 22(8):895–902.
15. Bogduk N. International spinal injection society guildelines for the performance of spinal injection procedures: Part 1: Zygapophyseal joint blocks. *Clin J Pain* 1997; 13(4):285–6.
16. Kaplan M, Dreyfuss P, Halbrook B, Bogduk N. The ability of lumbar medial branch blocks to anesthetize the zygapophyseal joint: a physiologic challenge. *Spine* 1998; 23(17):1847–52.

17. Schwarzer AC, Aprill CN, Derby R, Fortin J, Kine G, Bogduk N. The false-positive rate of uncontrolled diagnostic blocks of the lumbar zygapophyseal joints. *Pain* 1994; 58:195–200.

18. Revel ME, Listrat VM, Chevalier XJ, et al. Facet joint block for low back pain: identifying predictors of a good response. *Arch Phys Med Rehabil* 1992; 73:824–8.

19. Schwarzer AC, Wang SC, O'Driscoll D, Harrington T, Bogduk N, Laurent R. The ability of computed tomography to identify a painful zygapophyseal joint in patients with chronic low back pain. *Spine* 1995; 20:907–12.

20. Dreyfuss PH. Lumbar zygapophyseal (facet) joint injections. Contemporary Concepts in Spine Care. Rosemont, IL: North American Spine Society; 1994.

21. Jackson RP. The facet syndrome: myth or reality? *Clin Orthop* 1992; 279:110–21.

22. Boswell MV. Interventional techniques in the management of chronic spinal pain: evidence-based practice guildlines. *Pain Phys* 2005;8(1)1–47.

23. Parlier-Cuau C, Wybier M, Nizard R, Champsaur P, Le Hir P, Laredo JD. Symptomatic lumbar facet joint synovial cysts: clinical assessment of facet joint steroid injection after 1 and 6 months and long-term follow-up in 30 patients. *Radiology* 1999; 210:509–13.

24. Gangi A, Dietemann JL, Mortazaui R, Pfleger D, Kauff C, Roy C. CT-guided interventional procedures for pain management in the lumbosacral spine. *Radiographics* 1998; 18:621–33.

25. Goldstone JC, Pennant JH. Spinal anaesthesia following facet joint injection. *Anaesthesia* 1987; 42:754–6.

26. Marks R. Spinal anaesthesia after facet joint injection. *Anaesthesia* 1988; 43:65–6.

27. Thomson SJ, Lomax DM, Collett BJ. Chemical meningism after lumbar facet joint block with local anaesthetic and steroids. *Anaesthesia* 1991; 46:563–4.

28. Aguirre DA, Bermudez S, Diaz OM. Spinal CT-guided interventional procedures for management of chronic back pain. *J Vasc Interv Radiol* 2005; 16:689–97.

29. Lord SM, Bogduk N. Radiofrequency procedures in chronic pain. *Best Pract Res Clin Anaesthesiol* 2002; 16(4):597–617.

30. Shealy CN. Percutaneous radiofrequency denervation of spinal facets: treatment for chronic back pain and sciatica. *J Neurosurg* 1975; 43:448–51.

31. North RB, Han M, Zahurak M, Kidd DH. Radiofrequency lumbar denervation: analysis of prognostic factors. *Pain* 1994; 57:77–83.

32. Gallagher J. Radiofrequency facet joint denervation in the treatment of low back pain: a prospective controlled double-blind study to assess its efficacy. *Pain Clinic* 1994; 7:193–8.

33. Van Kleef A, Barendse GA, Kessels A, Veets HM, Weber WC, De Lange S. Randomized trial of radiofrequency lumbar facet denervation for chronic low back pain. *Spine* 1999; 24(18):1937–42.

34. Leclaire R, Fortin L, Lambert R, Bergeron YM, Rossignot M. Radiofrequency facet joint denervation in the treatment of low back pain. *Spine* 2001; 26(13):1411–7.

35. Hooten WM, Martin DP, Huntoon MA. Radiofrequency neurotomy for low back pain: evidence based procedural guidelines. *Pain Medicine* 2005; 6(2):129–38.

36. Dreyfuss PH. Efficacy and validity of radiofrequency neurotomy for chronic lumbar zygapophyseal joint pain. *Spine* 2000; 25(10):1270–7.

37. Bogduk N, Macintosh J, Marsland A. Technical limitations to the efficacy of radiofrequency neurotomy for spinal pain. *Neurosurgery* 1987; 20:529–35.

Articular Interventions in Pain Management: A General Approach

Blaze Cook

INTRODUCTION

In the early 16th century, Paracelsus described the joint as a fluid-filled space. However, it was not until the early 20th century that aspiration and injection of the joint for the treatment of maladies was attempted. Today, articular injections are a common outpatient procedure (1). However, in contrast to the common and well-accepted articular interventions performed, the data supporting such interventions are sparse. In general, most intraarticular interventional research is performed on the knee and then extrapolated to other joints. Additionally, most research is focused on the treatment of osteoarthritis pain and then extrapolated to other disease processes, such as rheumatoid arthritis, crystal deposition disease, athletic injuries, and other arthropathies. A further confounding factor in interpretation of the literature on articular interventions is that there is a profound placebo effect (2), a complicating factor that accompanies interpretation of procedure outcomes.

Inherent in any study involving pain is the general difficulty in quantifying what is generally a very subjective outcome. Many different markers have been used in an attempt to quantify outcomes such as pain scales, range of motion, and time performing a given exercise. All are imperfect and add an additional level of complexity. Finally, and perhaps most importantly from an interventional radiology standpoint, few studies verify needle or agent location. This creates considerable confusion when interpreting the literature and exploring patient outcomes involving articular/periarticular interventions. In some cases, a significant percentage of interventions are performed and evaluated in a nontarget or inconsistent location.

There are many advantages to compartment-directed therapy, and there is a large range of disease severity in which intraarticular interventions may be of benefit. Perhaps the most commonly cited with intraarticular therapy is to circumvent the reliance on excessive nonsteroidal anti-inflammatory drugs, which are associated with considerable adverse effects (3). Disadvantages include the relatively invasive nature of articular injection, and the cost and time associated with such injections.

This chapter will review some of the currently accepted intraarticular interventions and describe general approaches for image-directed joint access.

JOINT PAIN

Although a detailed description of pain pathways is beyond the scope of this chapter, a rudimentary understanding of pain sensation and transmission is helpful before exploring ways to decrease the subjective sensation of pain. The description of joint pain may be arbitrarily divided into two separate sensations, which may coexist in the same patient. *Spontaneous pain* is pain at rest with no inciting factor (4). Spontaneous pain may, for example, be an aching sensation when the patient is lying down or a sharp pain when the patient is sitting. The second type of abnormal pain sensation is *hyperalgesia*, or a painful response that is out of proportion to the stimulus. This stimulus may be normal stresses on the joint or relatively mild stimuli that would go unnoticed in a normal joint (4). This stimulus causes an increased perception of pain, for example, joint pain when walking or climbing stairs.

Joint inflammation causes an increase in both peripheral and central nocioception. Peripherally, there is an increase in nocioceptive transmissions from small myelinated and unmyelinated neurons. These small (Aδ and C) fibers normally have a high threshold before firing; however, with inflammation, the threshold lowers and the firing activity increases with joint motion. Additionally, larger type A fibers, which are normally involved with proprioception, begin to show increased activity with pressure and movement of the joint. A last set of nocioceptive fibers, fibers that normally do not activate, also begin to fire as inflammation continues. There is evidence that inflammation-induced nocioceptive responses in one joint may hypersensitize other joints to pain. In rats, upregulation of pain reception in one joint also causes an upregulation in the contralateral joint (4). The mechanisms of this effect in humans are not well studied and may have an additive or synergistic effect.

Centrally, the receptive nocioceptive fibers become hyperexcitable (4). Initially, this response resembles the hyperexcitibility of the peripheral nerves described earlier. However, expansion of excitability to sites adjacent to the affected joint may ensue, expanding the receptive field of the affected neuron. The various mechanisms of upregulating and maintaining the hyperexcitibility occur within the spinal cord.

A GENERAL APPROACH TO JOINT INJECTIONS

At the most general level, intraarticular interventions are conceptually straightforward. The affected joint space (or periarticular space) is accessed using an instrument such as a needle and an intervention performed, which may include withdrawal of fluid or instillation of a therapeutic agent. However, the technical aspects of joint intervention are complicated. Details such as actual location of the needle tip are often overlooked in blind injections, postintervention maneuvers such as joint cooling and immobilization are inadequately studied and inconsistently used, and yet injections remain a very common procedure. It should be noted that intentional injections into the periarticular space, without intraarticular communication, have been shown by some authors to provide benefit (5,6), which implies that supporting structures of the joint may contribute to pain in patients with osteoarthritis (2) and perhaps other causes of a painful joint.

The availability of imaging guidance during procedures has the potential to change the way intraarticular interventions are studied and performed. It is now possible to definitively state where the intervention is being performed, removing a significant confounding variable in both investigation and treatment. With imaging guidance, not only are intraarticular interventions more accurate, but there is also a documented better response (7).

As a general guide to technique, the risks and benefits of the proposed intervention should be described to the patient in detail. The patient should then be positioned in a comfortable position that they can maintain for the entire procedure. Adequate supportive padding to allow the joint or limb to be completely passive in a comfortable position may be beneficial. This may include positioning that is specific to the imaging modality being utilized.

Depending on the demands of the modality, sterile draping and technique may not be necessary. Chlorhexidine is not required because a simple swab with alcohol has been shown to be equally effective (8). Sterile technique including drapes, gloves, and instruments may be required depending on the imaging modality and anatomic location of the proposed intervention. If a blind approach is used, an alcohol swab after noting the landmarks and a sterile needle may be all the preparation needed.

Large joints are generally accessed with a 20 to 22-gauge needle. At our institution, we use 3-inch, 22-gauge spinal needles for accessing the shoulder and hips. Smaller needles may be appropriate for smaller joints; however, a larger gauge needle may be required to drain debris or thick synovial fluid. As will be discussed later, aspiration is recommended before injection. At the conclusion of the procedure, a sterile dressing is applied.

Many postinjection management strategies have been described, again most without rigorous investigation. Perhaps the most intensive rest regimen report included three days of bed rest followed by a period of limited weight bearing using crutches, which nearly doubled the benefit-response period of the intervention in the knee to 9.5 weeks (from 5.5 weeks) for patients with rheumatoid arthritis (9). Another investigation demonstrated a significant difference with 24 hours of bed rest following intraarticular steroid injection for knee synovitis (10). Studies utilizing yttrium in radiosynovectomy (discussed later) also show an advantage to postprocedure rest. In a seemingly opposite approach, gently flexing and extending the joint to mix the agent in the joint space has also been reported to be beneficial (9). Resting the joint for 24–48 hours by prescribing complete rest or decreased activity has been suggested, although the success of this strategy is debated (10,12). Avoidance of strenuous activities that may place excessive stress on the injected joint, such as running, has been suggested for prolonged intervals. There have, however, been no studies examining rest after corticosteroid joint injection for osteoarthritis (2), and another randomized trial demonstrated no benefit to resting. Cooling the joint with ice has been suggested to decrease diffusion of and prolong exposure to the injected agent. Icing the joint also has been thought to decrease the incidence of postinjection corticosteroid flares. In summary, after injection, it is probably beneficial to ice the joint and counsel the patient to ambulate as little as possible for 24–48 hours and to avoid strenuous exercise for at least 72 hours, with the understanding that there are no concrete data to validate this specific regimen.

A NOTE ABOUT IMAGE GUIDANCE

There is little emphasis about the role of image guidance in intraarticular therapy in the available literature. Although a large portion of the published research was performed before the widespread availability of ultrasound, fluoroscopic and radiographic verification was available. In studies that directly compare blind versus image-guided procedures, a clear benefit to image guidance is demonstrated. Up to one half of "intraarticular" knee injections are, in fact, extraarticular or in an uncertain location (12). As another example, only 27% of anterior approach glenohumeral injections were intraarticular in an investigation using MRI to evaluate actual agent localization (13).

Some authors have found the presence of a knee effusion to be predictive of a superior outcome. There have been many proposed theories as to why (and if) this predicts a favorable outcome including active synovitis or a short-term "inflammatory burst" of osteoarthritis (2). Another potential benefit is that the effusion expands the joint space, making the targeted synovial compartment larger and, perhaps, precise intraarticular delivery of the agent easier.

Few authors address the technical success of precise compartment localization of the studied agent, and yet, it is seemingly so important. The exact location of the agent should be considered critical in evaluating the efficacy, outcome, and complication of any joint procedure. It follows that determining the outcome in any individual patient may also depend heavily on concrete knowledge of the precise location of the intervention to determine expected outcome or to anticipate complications. At the very least, imaging guidance should be considered in patients who do not respond to blindly injected therapy (7).

JOINT ASPIRATION AND LAVAGE

Joint aspiration before injection is recommended by the American College of Rheumatology (14). The benefits of this strategy are to relieve articular hypertension, reduce the concentration of inflammatory mediators, and decrease the crystalline concentration in the synovial fluid (15). Aspiration before injection of corticosteroids has proven to be more effective than injection alone in both rheumatoid arthritis and osteoarthritis (16). Aspiration may also be the only intervention required for relief of pain from a traumatic effusion or hemarthrosis when the source of bleeding has resolved (16). In osteoarthritis, aspiration alone may provide some benefit (17). Aspiration also has the additional effect of decreasing the effective dilution volume of the agents, thereby increasing the final concentration of corticosteroid in the synovial fluid as well as creating room for the volume of agent required. However, decreasing the joint volume will also make loss of access more likely and reaccessing the joint space more difficult.

Although no specific technique for aspiration has been studied or compared to another, the general technique of aspiration is probably universally applied. The syringe (with or without extension tubing) is connected to the needle before the needle is advanced into the skin. If a syringe using an anesthetic solution, such as lidocaine, is attached for needle advancement, the syringe should be removed without displacing the needle tip from the articular space. This can be facilitated by attaching the syringe to the needle with as little torque as necessary to provide a good seal. Many clinicians tighten the needle on a Luer lock syringe with excessive torque, making detachment difficult and needle tip displacement more likely. An empty syringe is attached, and using mild negative pressure, the fluid from the joint space is slowly aspirated. A gentle tapering of flow should be observed and the fluid visually inspected (Table 1). Smooth, consistent, easy flow of synovial fluid implies correct needle placement. If the flow of synovial fluid stops or slows abruptly prior to the expected withdrawal volume, obstruction of the needle by debris, synovial fronds, loculations, septations, or displacement of the needle should be suspected (18). Repositioning the needle or injecting sterile saline may resume flow through the needle. If the needle position continues to be in doubt, reimaging and/or injecting contrast may verify location. In most cases, as much synovial fluid as possible should be removed (18). Routine culture of the joint fluid is not necessary if there is no clinical suspicion of infection. If on inspection the synovial fluid appears atypical, the fluid should be sent for laboratory analysis, which includes a white blood cell count with a differential of polymorphonuclear neutrophilic leukocytes, crystal analysis, Gram staining, and culture (19) (Table 1). After complete aspiration of the joint, injection of material may be performed with or without appropriate contrast material for the imaging modality to verify intraarticular location. It should be noted that if there is clinical suspicion of debris or infection in a joint before accessing it, it is prudent to use a larger diameter needle (lesser gauge) to facilitate the removal of debris without clogging.

Table 1. Synovial Fluid Inspection

	Normal	*Noninflammatory*[a]	*Inflammatory*[b]	*Septic*
Color	Clear	Straw yellow	Yellow	Variable
Clarity	Transparent	Transparent	Hazy opaque	Opaque
Viscosity	High	High	Low	Variable
WBCs/mm^3	<200	200–2k	2k–75k	>50k

[a] Osteoarthritis, trauma, avascular necrosis, Charcot's arthopathy, hemochromatosis, pigmented villonodular synovitis.
[b] Septic arthritis, crystal-induced arthritis, rheumatoid arthritis, spondyloarthropathy, systemic lupus erythematosus.

Source: Chokkalingam et al. (19).

The theoretical benefit from joint aspiration is carried further with joint lavage. Complete removal of infectious agents, crystalline substances, and inflammatory mediators are thought to be the primary source of pain relief. There are two distinct techniques of joint lavage: the tidal (single-needle) and continuous (double-needle) lavage. There have been no rigorous studies evaluating the volume needed for adequate lavage or the size of needle sufficient to remove sometimes thick debris, although there is a general consensus that volumes must be sufficient to expand the joint space. As a benchmark, volumes for knee joint lavage should be greater than 1 l (16). Selection of an appropriate-sized needle is also important. Larger needles may be required to drain thick debris or purulent material; for this purpose, needles at least 14 gauge in diameter are recommended.

With the single-needle technique, the joint is accessed and an alternating pattern of fluid aspiration and fluid injection is made. The lavage agent is generally normal saline. The continuous lavage technique is similar to the tidal technique except two access points are utilized to continuously flush the joint using one needle for influx and one needle for efflux. The advantages of the continuous technique are that it is less time consuming and a greater volume can be used (typically 2–10 l).

The effectiveness of joint lavage is debated. A blinded, randomized, controlled trial failed to find any significant difference in outcomes between tidal joint lavage and a sham procedure (20). However, other less rigorous studies describe variable benefits with lavage (21–23). Joint lavage combined with intraarticular corticosteroid therapy has shown effectiveness, although it is unclear if there is additional benefit to lavage with corticosteroid injection as compared with simple aspiration and subsequent injection.

INJECTION AGENTS

The options for intraarticular medical interventions fall into one of four categories: corticosteroids, hyaluronic acid, osmic acid, and yttrium. All agents seek to decrease inflammation and decrease pain by a variety of pharmacological methods. The two primary agents that have demonstrated efficacy in the treatment of articular and bursal pain are corticosteroids and hyaluronic acid, although osmic acid shows promise.

Corticosteroids

Corticosteroids are the workhorses of intraarticular interventions. These agents have been used widely since the 1950s (24). During the 1960s, intraarticular corticosteroids began use in professional athletes in the treatment of sports-related injures, and in the 1970s fell into disfavor due to attributed tendon injury. Today, corticosteroids continue to be used extensively for multiple indications and are described by the American College of Rheumatology as "... safe and effective when administered by an experienced physician (25)." Ninety percent of orthopedists and 95% of rheumatologists use corticosteroid injections as a component of their therapeutic strategy (24). The typical dosing regimen is an interval schedule, generally with three months between treatments, although there are little data supporting this interval.

The end goal of corticosteroid injection is to decrease inflammation, effusion, and pain, which they perform with variable success. For the majority of patients, the duration of relief is brief, so a reasonable goal for intervention should be in treating short-term flares of disease such as exacerbation of pain, nocturnal pain, painful effusions, and bridging to other therapies (such as antirheumatic drugs) (26,27). A single injection is almost never sufficient to provide relief from pain for a duration longer than approximately 1–2 months in the majority of patients.

DOSAGE/SPECIFIC AGENTS

The prototype drug, cortisone, has been modified to reduce solubility by esterification, theoretically reducing the systemic absorption and increasing therapeutic time in the joint. The cortisone derivatives that have been studied in humans include hydrocortisone, prednisolone, triamcinolone hexacetonide, methylprednisolone, and cortivazol. These drugs have not been directly compared in a controlled trial (27). Many dosing recommendations have been made with few direct comparisons. The most commonly used agent is methylpredinisolone acetate. In general, for an equivalent dose, decreasing solubility will increase effect. Actual dosage recommendations have not been thoroughly studied, and rigorous dosage comparisons are not available. All corticosteroids should be compared using an equivalency number, with most operators using hydrocortisone to compare potency (Table 2). A general guideline for dosages and injection volumes is presented in Table 3.

Some physicians find it useful to mix a local anesthetic with the corticosteroid prior to injection. This is for both patient comfort and diagnostic purposes. If the patient reports immediate relief of pain (due to the local anesthetic), the needle is likely localized in the correct anatomic compartment for the corticosteriod to be effective. When mixing agents in the same syringe, it is always prudent to check for drug compatibility to ensure that there is no

---

Table 2. Corticosteroid Preparations

Generic Name	Trade Names	Potency (hydrocortisone equivalents/mg)	Concentration (mg/ml)	Anticipated Duration (days)
Betamethasone	Soluspan, Celestone	25	6	9
Dexamethasone	Decadron	25	4–8[a]	6–8[a]
Triamcinolone	Aristospan, Aristocort, Kenalog	5	10–40[a]	7–21[a]
Methylprednisolone	Solu-medrol	5	20–80	8
Prednisolone	Hydeltra-TBA, Predalone TBA, Prednisol TBA	4	20	10–14[a]
Hydrocortisone	Hydrocortisone	1	25	8

[a] Varies by formulation.

Source: Genovese (26).

Table 3. Suggested Dosages and Volumes

Target	Dose (mg × hydrocortisone equivalents)	Volume (ml)
Knee	200–450	1–4
Shoulder	150–300	1–4
Elbow	100–150	1–4
Ankle	100–150	0.5–1
Wrist	100	0.5–1
Interphalageal	25–50	0.025–0.5
Metacarpophalangeal	25–50	0.025–0.5
Metatarsophalangeal	25–50	0.025–0.5

Source: Genovese (26).

precipitation reaction. Additionally, patients should be warned that the analgesic effect eventually declines and that a subjective recurrence in pain is expected when this occurs.

ACTIONS

Corticosteroids are all lipid soluble and cross the cell membrane and react with cytoplasmic receptors before moving to the nucleus to affect change in cell physiology and modify two responses. The anti-inflammatory response results in decrease of macrophage activation, leukocyte adherence to capillary walls, and diapedisis. Additionally, the capillary leak effect seen with inflammation is modulated by corticosteroids through poorly understood mechanisms (28). The second major effect of corticosteroids is an immunomodulatory effect; corticosteroids decrease the response of cell-mediated immunity as well as reducing the concentration of T-lymphocytes, monocytes, and eosinophils (28).

INDICATIONS

Intraarticular corticosteroids have been described as treatment in a wide variety of disorders. Essentially, if inflammation is considered to play a role in the pathophysiology, steroids have been found to be useful. The inflammatory-suppressive effect is useful in a wide range of pathologies, from inflammatory arthritis to athletic injuries. Osteoarthritis continues to be the most common indication, and the best studied, although both acute and chronic inflammatory conditions are treatable with intraarticular corticosteroids. The injections modulate inflammation that may improve the underlying pathophysiology of the disease process, or they may simply decrease the inflammation of the joint tissues and decrease pain while improving range of motion. There is no regeneration or reversal of the underlying disease process when corticosteroids are used.

CONTRAINDICATIONS

There are few absolute contraindications to corticosteroid injection. Prior hypersensitivity reaction to the proposed agents, severe coagulopathy, and active infection (including cellulitis or infection of the proposed injection tract) should preclude injection. However, in the event of an accidental injection of a joint that is infected, there is evidence that corticosteroids may be protective if proper antibiotic therapy is initiated rapidly (16). If there is any concern that the target joint is infected, it is prudent to send an aspirate of the joint for analysis and reschedule the procedure for a later date.

Relative contraindications include the possibility of avascular necrosis of the adjacent bone. Rarely seen relative contraindications that have been described to include ocular herpes, active tuberculosis, and acute psychosis, all of which are theoretically complicated by systemic steroids.

Systemic absorption of the injectate does occur and is proportional to the potency, dose, and total synovial surface area of the joints injected. The maximum systemic blood pool corticosteroid concentration is inversely proportional to solubility, although agent time in the blood pool is prolonged when compared to more soluble agents. Plasma cortisol levels may be affected for four or more weeks following injection (29) (including transient suppression of endogenous cortisol). There is no net effect on bone resorption (30), and there is no significant effect on blood glucose control in patients with diabetes mellitus (16). Interestingly, there may be a benefit to other noninjected joints, due to systemic absorption (31) or from placebo effect.

EXPECTED COURSE

After the injection of corticosteroids, pain relief from the injection has been reported to range in duration from immediate to years. More commonly, onset of relief can be expected in the range of 24 hours, with duration of approximately one month. Reported clinical experience has identified patients who report relief for a substantially longer period (32); however, there are no predictive factors to identify these responders before intervention. A review by Courtney and Doherty states, "... none of the following correlated with the efficacy of intraarticular corticosteroids – disease duration, radiological scores, inflammatory markers, and signs of inflammation (18)."

Attempts to predict patients who will demonstrate a better response to corticosteroid articular injection have largely been unsuccessful (33,34). This is confounded by the multiple interventions that are simultaneously performed at the time of intervention, such as joint aspiration, rest, ice, and the injection of other agents. The presence of a joint effusion has been described as a possible predictor of a good outcome (11). Again, this may be due to easier access to the joint space with fewer complications and a better delivery of the agent. Variables that have been found not to be predictive of outcome are radiographic severity, duration of disease, presence of crystals, and raised synovial cell count.

COMPLICATIONS/ADVERSE REACTIONS

Although not a complication, patients should be counseled that the duration of benefit is finite and that it is an expected outcome for the symptoms to return and another injection be performed. Known complications of intraarticular corticosteroids are surprisingly rare and often overstated, and again it is important to note that complications from corticosteroid injections may be from injection into surrounding or supporting structures. Use of strict image-guided techniques will decrease nontarget injections and presumably decrease the complication rate. Additionally, some complications have been reported using a specific corticosteroid agent, and generalization may not be applicable to all agents. Table 4 provides an overview of the most common and/or serious potential complications of intraarticular corticosteroid injections.

The most common local postinjection complication is a painful local reaction in the joint. This has been described as a "postinjection flare," which commonly begins 6–12 hours after injection and resolves after one to three days (2). Approximately 2–10% of patients will complain of this complication, which may be due to a reactive or chemical synovitis in response to the agent itself or preservatives within the injectate (24,35). However, postinjection flares have also been reported after the injection of normal saline (36). Whatever the underlying cause, future injections should avoid the offending agents. The patient should be counseled that this is a self-limited reaction and that analgesics such as acetaminophen are helpful, along with cold or warm compresses. The primary consideration before dismissing a postinjection flare is missing the much more rare septic joint. Any joint pain that persists beyond the three-day expected course should be investigated further.

Skin depigmentation or atrophy of the subcutaneous tissues may occur and is reported to be a complication that occurs approximately 1% of the time (37,38). These periarticular or nontarget complications occur more frequently with the longest acting corticosteroids, such as triamcinolone hexacetonide (2).

The most common systemic reaction to intraarticular corticosteroids is facial flushing. Although disconcerting for the patient and the physician, facial flushing is reported to occur with up to 40% of injections, with severe flushing in 12% (39). This flushing reaction should not be confused with an anaphylactic reaction, which is rare (40). Although commonly perceived (and reported) to increase glucose levels in diabetics, at least one study has demonstrated no significant effect on serum glucose in this population (41). Furthermore, there is no net change on bone density to suggest acceleration of osteoporosis (42).

Table 4. Reported Complications of Corticosteroid Injections

Facial flushing (40%) (24,39)

Post injection flare/pain (2–10%) (24,35)

Skin depigmentation (1%) (37)

Septic arthritis (rare) (24)

Nerve/blood vessel damage (rare) (24)

Tendon weakening/rupture (rare) (24)

Anaphylaxis (very rare) (24)

Steroid arthropathy (debated) (24)

Hyperglycemia (debated) (24)

Joint sepsis (<<1%) (2)

Steroid arthropathy/charcot degeneration (debated) (32)

The most detrimental complication is introducing an organism into the joint space, creating a septic joint. However, the frankly septic joint after injection is exceedingly rare and is reported to be on the order of 1 in 25,000 injections (38,43,44). Even with this very low rate, it is still prudent to counsel the patient to be observant of joint pain that persists past 72 hours or increases over a week.

In a review by Nichols, complications related to corticosteroid injections in athletes were reported at a rate of 15% (35). Of these, postinjection pain accounted for nearly two-thirds of the reported side effects and complications. Therefore, if postinjection pain is removed from consideration, the complication rate drops to 1 in 20. Of the remaining adverse reactions, the most common were skin atrophy, skin depigmentation, localized erythema, and facial flushing. Interestingly, the same review was unable to find published studies that "... provide unequivocal scientific evidence that corticosteroid injections do or do not cause damage to human musculoskeletal structures."

Long-term joint or supporting tissue damage has been a long debated issue with corticosteroid use, and prospective studies in humans have demonstrated no detrimental effect (45,46). Studies in rabbits suggest that corticosteroids may decrease cartilage strength and increase the number of cartilage fissures (47). However, studies in guinea pigs, dogs, and primates have failed to reproduce these results and may instead show a protective effect (48–50). There have been case reports of tendon rupture following corticosteroid injection; however, documented location of the injected agent was not described and may have been intratendonous or extraarticular. Steroid arthropathy or charcot-like joint destruction may be a result of underlying pathology and not a direct result of corticosteroid injection (32). Osteonecrosis, a devastating complication, has not been reported with injection of joints for common athletic conditions (51); a causal relationship of corticosteroids inducing osteonecrosis in any population remains open for debate (37).

Hyaluronic Acid

Hyaluronic acid is a polysaccharide chain composed of repeating disaccharide units of *N*-acetylglucosamine and glucuronic acid (51). It is a naturally occurring molecule found in human synovial fluid, produced by type B syonviocytes that secrete hyaluronic acid directly into the joint space where it is thought to augment viscous and elastic properties of the fluid (51). One theory holds that the longer chains and higher molecular weight molecules may enhance the viscous properties, perhaps making synovial fluid more effective. At high shear forces, the elasticity of hyaluronic acid is increased and the viscosity reduced, acting as a "shock absorber" during fast movements. At low shear forces, hyaluronic acid has increased viscosity and decreased elasticity, thereby acting as a lubricant during slow movements.

Injection of hyaluronic acid is termed viscosupplementation, implying that the injection is augmenting the viscous properties of the synovial fluid, which should enhance the lubrication and protection of the articular cartilage as well as the joint space (11,12). Viscosupplementation for human clinical use began in Japan and Italy in 1987, and was used in Canada and Europe before approval in the United States in 1997 (56). It was used in race horses for some time prior to its use in humans (13). Currently, hyaluronic acid is only FDA-approved for use in osteoarthritis; however, benefit has been shown in rheumatoid arthritis (14). As with corticosteroids, most of the literature is focused on osteoarthritis, and osteoarthritis of the knee is the most studied joint. These data are then extrapolated to other joints and disease processes. As a benchmark, the human knee contains a concentration of 5–8 mg of hyaluronic acid dissolved in approximately 2 ml of synovial fluid (51).

In osteoarthritis, hyaluronic acid is reduced in concentration and molecular interactions are decreased, in some cases by up to one-half of the normal concentration (15). The reasons that this induces joint pain are at least twofold. First, there is a decrease in cushioning of the joint by synovial fluid and increasing stress forces on the adjacent tissues. Second, lower viscosity decreases the filtering function of the synovial fluid that normally bathes the articular cartilage, thereby reducing the nutrient availability (51).

DOSAGE/SPECIFIC AGENTS

The FDA classifies hyaluronic acid as a medical device; therefore, the rigorous requirements of FDA drug testing are not applicable (51). Two classes of hyaluronic acid derivatives are available for use in the United States. The first, hyaluronan (Hyalgan, Supartz in USA; Orthovisc, Neovisc in Canada) is naturally occurring and purified from rooster comb derivatives, with the exception of Neovisc, which is produced by bacterial culture (61). The second, G-F 20 (Synvisc, Genzyme Corp., Cambridge, MA), is the only synthetic hyaluronic acid that is available in the United States (51). G-F 20 is a cross-linked hyaluronic acid, increasing the molecular weight and viscoelastic properties of the molecule. There is evidence of increased effectiveness of this agent over non-cross-linked hyaluronic acid, although the data are conflicting (52).

Hyaluronic acid is administered in a weekly sequence of three to five injections. Hyglan is supplied in 2-ml vials or 2-ml prefilled syringes. The contents of the injectant include inert substances and are detailed in the package insert. Synvisc is also supplied in 2-ml prefilled syringes, again with inert substances, given once a week in a three-week regimen. Supartz, also mixed with inert ingredients in 2.5-ml prefilled syringes, is administered weekly for three to five weeks. All agents are formulated for use in osteoarthritis of the knee.

ACTIONS

Originally it was thought that the beneficial effects of viscosupplementation were solely due to the synovial fluid augmentation effects of increased viscosity. However, the actual indwelling time of injected hyaluronic acid is on the order of days, but the beneficial effects are highly variable and last from months (53) to years (54). Theorized explanations for this discordance are possible anti-inflammatory effects of the molecule (not well elucidated), antinociceptive properties of the molecule, or stimulation of endogenous hyaluronic acid production (54). Hyaluronic acid has been described to have several direct anti-inflammatory effects by inhibiting phagocytosis, adherence of leukocytes, and reducing inflammatory mediators (51). An analgesic effect has been demonstrated in mice, producing a similar effect as indomethacin in reducing pain (55). A large placebo effect, as found in all joint injections, almost certainly plays a significant role.

There have been no human trials that demonstrate a chondroprotective effect of hyaluronic acid (51). Studies in animals are mixed. Investigations in sheep (62) and Pond-Nuki dogs (63) have demonstrated a chondroprotective effect. However, other studies in dogs have also shown no significant effect on the progression of osteophyte formation and cartilage degeneration (51).

INDICATIONS

The most studied indication for hylauronic injection is osteoarthritis of the knee, which is the only FDA-approved indication. Benefits include general reduction of pain for all affected populations as well as delay of surgery for middle-aged persons (64). Benefit in rheumatoid arthritis of the knee has been demonstrated, and evidence of improvement in other joints for other indications is likely forthcoming.

CONTRAINDICATIONS

Contraindications to hyaluronic acid injection are similar to corticosteroid injection. Prior hypersensitivity reaction to a previous injection and injection through or into an infected space are absolute contraindications. Coagulopathy is a relative contraindication.

EXPECTED COURSE

There have been many studies assessing the effectiveness of hyaluronic acid for pain relief, usually in comparison to corticosteroids or placebo. The results are mixed, and the majority of studies are single-blind or single-arm trials. A meta-analysis of the available data did show a small but significant benefit (65). An additional meta-analysis that examined only double-blind trials of patients with knee osteoarthritis demonstrated a moderate improvement in pain relief at 5–7 and 8–10 weeks, with benefit ending by 15–22 weeks (53). In counseling patients, it is safe to say that benefit onset is slow, likely beginning after 24 hours. Patients who have had previous corticosteroid injections may note that the onset of pain relief is delayed, perhaps up to five days postinjection (2). The duration of benefit will likely last approximately three months, and perhaps longer. At the time the relief wears off, another series of injections may be considered.

COMPLICATIONS/ADVERSE REACTIONS

Table 5 summarizes the potential complications following hyaluronic acid injection. The only significant adverse reaction to intraarticular hyaluronic acid

---

Table 5. Reported Complications from Hyaluronic Acid Injections

Local painful reaction (3%)

Pseudoseptic joint (rare)

Granulomatous inflammation (rare)

Septic joint (rare)

Anaphalaxis (rare)

injection is local joint pain. In a large series of 1,537 patients, postinjection pain occurred in 2.7% of injections (in 8.3% of patients); of these, all but one-fifth resolved without long-term sequelae (66).

Pseudoseptic reactions have been reported following injections (67). Clinically, these resemble a septic joint and should be distinguished from a true septic joint, a rare but significant differential consideration. A pseudoseptic joint presents as a painful joint, with an effusion, generally 1–3 days after the injection of hyaluronate. The primary differential considerations are septic joint and granulomatous inflammation (which may be a variation of the same entity). Fluid analysis will demonstrate a cellular infiltrate, predominantly monocytic, without organisms or crystals (68). Should organisms or other markers of a septic joint be discovered (see Table 1), appropriate treatment should begin immediately.

A granulomatous inflammatory reaction may be due to an inability of the synovium to absorb or degrade the injected molecule. The underlying pathophysiology of a granulomatous inflammatory reaction is macrophage consumption of the molecule that releases inflammatory mediators in a foreign-body type reaction, with formation of multinucleated giant cells around undegradable material with resultant granuloma formation (61). Currently, the largest published case series occurred in six patients injected with cross-linked hyaluronic acid (61). It should be noted that granulomatous inflammatory reactions have been reported with many other common intraarticular interventions, such as metal prosthetics, polyethylene prosthetics, and cement debris (61). Clinically, this presents with development of swelling and warmth of the joint within 48 hours after viscosupplementation. The symptoms peak at day 5, and gradually resolve over the course of one to two weeks (61). After the acute phase, one-third of patients report no difference in their pain, and two-thirds reported their pain to be worse than before injection. NSAIDS have little effect on the symptoms. In the previously noted series (69), none of the patients had an elevated sedimentation rate, elevated C-reactive protein level, fever, or joint erythema that may distinguish a granulomatous inflammatory reaction from a septic joint. Of course, if there is clinical suspicion that a joint may be infected, or an atypical presentation, joint aspiration and analysis should be performed. Four aspirates from the series of the six cases noted earlier demonstrated a white blood cell (WBC) count of less than 10,000/mm (3) and no organisms (61).

There has been at least one case report of a septic joint after hyaluronic acid injection (69), and this is almost certainly attributable to the injection itself. In the previously discussed large series, not a single case of sepsis due to product contamination was reported.

Osmic Acid and ⁹⁰Yttrium

Volkman introduced the concept of surgical synovectomy in 1877 (70), and the methods of reducing synovium by other means seek to duplicate the response of this commonly practiced method. Synovectomy is a broad term that implies removal of the synovium, by surgery (surgical synovectomy), chemical (chemosynovectomy), or radiopharmaceutical (radiosynovectomy) means. Many agents have been described for chemical/radiosynovectomy. Chemotherapeutic agents, aspirin, antibiotics, and alternative radiopharmaceuticals have been used (27). All of these agents work with the same underlying principle.

Treatment of the joint with osmic acid and [90]yttrium affect the joint by direct modification of the synovium, either by chemical or radioactive means. These modifications are termed synovectomy and synoviorthesis interchangeably in the literature. Chemical or medical synovectomy, now most commonly performed with osmic acid, was first used in 1951 for the treatment of a knee effusion (71). Radiosynovectomy was also first described in the 1950s. The term medical synovectomy is imprecise and may refer to either chemosynovectomy or radiosynovectomy. The term synoviorthesis was coined in the late 1960s with the literal meaning of restoring the synovium (*ortheis*, to restore) (70). For the remainder of the chapter, the term chemosynovectomy will be understood to refer to osmic acid synovectomy/synoviorthesis and the term radiosynovectomy will refer to [90]yttrium synovectomy/synoviorthesis.

The data supporting radiosynovectomy are sparse, and serious thought should be given before performing radiosynovectomy. It is discussed here for completeness. Histological examination of tissue after radiosynovectomy have shown a reduction in the size and number of synovial villi with decreased hyperemia acutely, eventually progressing to fibrosis (70). A review of the literature published in 2000 found only two well-designed studies comparing radiosynovectomy with placebo, and the results were conflicting (70). A follow-up, randomized placebo-controlled trial in 2005 failed to find a significant difference between radiosynovectomy with intraarticular corticosteroids versus intraarticular corticosteroids alone (72). Chemosynovectomy, in contrast, has shown promise in clinical use but data are insufficient to recommend widespread use. Osmic acid is a strong oxidizing agent that has a direct caustic effect on the synovium. It is theorized that the necrotic synovium will be replaced by production of synovial tissue by underlying tissues, as has been shown in mice (73). A 2003 retrospective analysis of 105 consecutive osmic acid injections for chronic knee synovitis (due to varying causes) demonstrated complete freedom from pain postinjection for a period lasting from months to years (71). Reported complications included postinjection pain (12%) and skin burns (2%). No rigorous double-blind trials have been performed using osmic acid.

In both chemosynovectomy and radiosynovectomy, agents are injected in combination with a local anesthetic and a corticosteroid. The local anesthetic is necessary to blunt the pain response from the direct destruction of synovial tissue. The corticosteroid is used to modulate the inflammatory response that normally ensues. The corticosteroid injection also has an effect on the underlying inflammatory process, a fact that also complicated interpretation of response to these agents. What portion of benefit to the underlying articular inflammatory process is directly attributable to corticosteroids, and if the effect is additive or synergistic, is poorly understood.

OVERVIEW OF IMAGE-GUIDED TECHNIQUES

The majority of articular interventions are performed without imaging guidance. However, there are advantages to image-guided intraarticular interventions for managing pain. First, there is verification and documentation that the injected agent is within the appropriate space. For example, there are reports of an accuracy of less than 30% for a blind anterior approach shoulder injection (74). This complicates shoulder intervention by both invalidating intraarticular intervention research performed using this approach and confusing the interpretation of patient response. Both of these issues are laid to rest with imaging verification of intracompartmental injection. Direct imaging guidance is also very useful in rapidly accessing the joint space in patients with distorted landmarks, such as the severely obese or postoperative patients.

Any radiographic modality may be used for articular interventions, the most common being ultrasound and fluoroscopy. However, cross-sectional techniques such as computed tomography (CT) and possibly, in the future, magnetic resonance may be the optimum imaging guidance in certain cases. With each modality, there are advantages and limitations, and each method should be considered with the individual patient and involved area in mind. Many specific techniques, approaches, and methods have been described and are in current practice. The ideal procedure would be accurate in localization, quick in access, painless, and minimize the radiation dose to the patient and the operators.

A central tenet in any image-guided procedure is that the patient should be carefully positioned. This is important to make certain that the patient does not move and inadvertently change the location of the procedure. To this end, the patient should be positioned comfortably with the joint positioned so that they can maintain the position passively for a prolonged period of time. A comfortable patient will allow the physician to take appropriate steps to successfully complete the procedure without rushing.

As a general guide to anatomic location, it may be helpful to refer to cross-sectional imaging of the appropriate joint from the patient that may be on record, to review the location of the synovial capsule and the location of vital structures.

General Ultrasound Technique

The ultrasound-guided technique confers many advantages. It is relatively low in cost, less cumbersome, and faster than fluoroscopy or CT. There is also greater anatomic detail, and the window or viewing angle can be changed at will. The entire procedure may be performed by a single physician, and contrast material is not necessary for location verification as agitated injection agent often has enough tiny air bubbles to create an effective contrast agent. Finally, there is no exposure to ionizing radiation to either the patient or the physician.

The use of local anesthetic is optional because ultrasound guidance allows a swift definitive needle advancement. If, however, there is concern that the procedure may be difficult or prolonged, a local anesthetic is advised. As a general rule, ultrasound-guided articular access mirrors the access routes recommended for blind access, and many potential routes can be quickly evaluated before the procedure to determine which route is best in any individual patient. The real-time ease of selecting pathways to the joints adds significant flexibility to ultrasound guidance, and the physician should not necessarily feel limited to described access routes as long as anatomic precautions are strictly followed. Before beginning the procedure, it is prudent to interrogate the proposed area using both grayscale and Doppler imaging.

Vessels should be noted and avoided. A general site of approach is then approximated using bony landmarks or the skin may be marked.

Needle and syringe selection is joint specific and the agent should be prepared prior to injection. A larger gauge needle should be selected if aspiration of debris is anticipated. A syringe suitable to contain the volume of the agents should be used. The patient should be placed in a comfortable position so that movement is minimized. The target joint should be well supported, providing ample back cushioning to accommodate significant pressure from the ultrasound probe while allowing the patient to keep the joint completely passive.

The skin is prepped and draped in the usual sterile fashion. If real-time guidance is used, a sterile ultrasound probe cover is used; however, some physicians prefer to directly sterilize the head of the transducer. Once the precise site is selected, the ultrasound probe should be positioned with the long axis of the beam in line with the needle entry site. The beam should be directed obliquely at the needle and advancement directly visualized. A special ultrasound visible needle may be used to improve visualization, although scoring the shaft of the distal needle with a scalpel has a similar effect. If no large debris is anticipated, the joint may be aspirated and injected using the same needle that is used to infiltrate the anesthetic. Care should be taken not to attach the needle too tightly to the syringe, as disconnecting the needle may dislodge the tip from the joint space. If a second (larger gauge) needle is required, it is advanced using the same method.

Once the needle is in the joint space, the procedure may continue as with any other technique. Generally, if the synovial space is well visualized, the agent can be seen flowing into the space as echogenic material flowing from the needle tip. If desired, the solution may be agitated to encourage the formation of small air bubbles to accentuate this effect. Some physicians advocate vigorous massage of the needle tract to break down a possible communication in the soft tissue planes. After the procedure, a sterile dressing should be placed over the access site and postinjection maneuvers and instructions (such as ice, immobilization, activity restriction, etc.) given to the patient.

General Fluoroscopic Technique

Fluoroscopy has been used for large joint interventions for some time, particularly the hip and shoulder. Specific procedures may be tailored to the imaging equipment available. For example, an adjustable-angle image intensifier will make patient positioning less of an obstacle, whereas a fixed-angle image intensifier will require a great deal of care in patient positioning to assure that the needle is viewed end-on and can be advanced perpendicular to the table.

Once the patient is positioned, the area is marked with a radiopaque object (Figure 3A–D). Intermittent fluoroscopy can be used to appropriately place the marker. Once the marker is in satisfactory position, a mark is made on the skin, and the area is cleansed and draped. The selected area should be anesthetized with a 1% solution of lidocaine buffered with bicarbonate in a roughly 10:1 concentration. The anesthetic agent should be deeply infiltrated, near the joint space itself. If unsure, intermittent fluoroscopy can be used to inspect the trajectory of the anesthetic needle. If the joint is entered and the needle is in the appropriate size, the needle may be left in place.

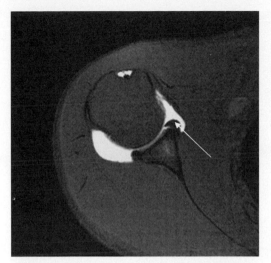 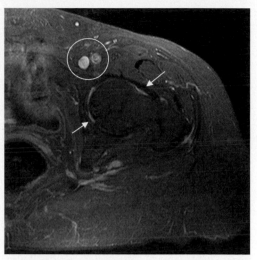

Figure 1. Axial magnetic resonance arthrogram image of the right shoulder demonstrating a distended joint capsule and associated anatomy. The fibrocartilaginous portion of the glenoid is demonstrated (arrow).

Figure 2. Axial magnetic resonance of the left hip demonstrating location of vessels (circle) and location of synovial space (arrows).

Using a connecting tube between the syringe and needle confers two major advantages. First, it allows freedom to remove the operator's hand from the direct x-ray beams of the fluoroscope while watching the injection real time. Second, it allows minor movements of the hand holding the syringe without greatly affecting the needle position. If desired, a small amount (2 cc) of water-soluble contrast agent may be used to fill the tubing and the air bled, so that there is undiluted contrast in the needle to verify the needle tip location (75).

Consideration should be made before beginning the procedure as to how the fluoroscopic unit will be operated. If an assistant is available for nonsterile tower operation, or if a sterile control panel is a possibility, the intermittent fluoroscopic technique may be considered. Using either technique, the needle should always be viewed end-on, ensuring accurate localization in two planes. If there is doubt to the needle location in the third plane, the image intensifier may be moved 90° or a cross-table image should be obtained.

Once the basic setup is complete, using sterile technique the needle is advanced over the marked area. Once there is enough purchase in the superficial tissues to support the needle, the position should be verified using fluoroscopy. If the needle trajectory is satisfactory, further advancement may be made using intermittent fluoroscopy as needed. Minor adjustments to the needle trajectory may also be made using this approach; however, the needle should be viewed as closely to end-on as possible.

The direct fluoroscopic advancement technique is similar to the intermittent technique. However, instead of intermittent verification of the needle path, direct observation is used. Using a pair of long-handled hemostats or needle drivers, the needle is advanced to the joint space under direct fluoroscopic observation while taking care to keep the physician's hands out of the direct fluoroscopic beam.

Once the target joint space is accessed, verification of location may be made by direct aspiration of synovial fluid or injection of contrast if prepared as in

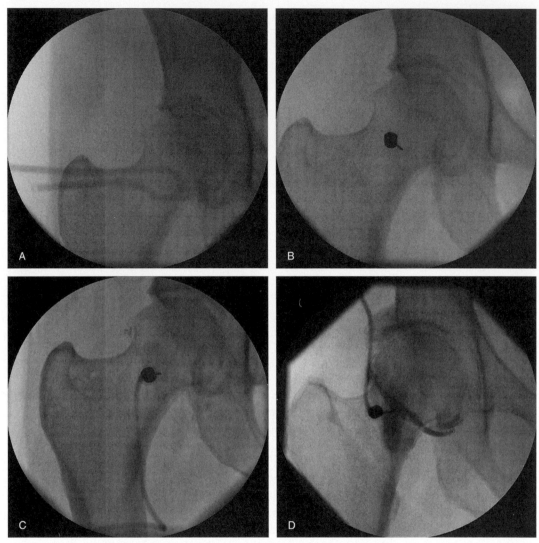

Figure 3. (A) Localization. A radiopaque object is placed over the skin to determine an appropriate access point. (B) The needle selected for intervention is advanced to the joint margin using intermittent fluoroscopy to verify location. The needle is centered in the image, to reduce parallax, and the needle is viewed closely to end-on. (C) The extension tubing is attached, and the physician's hands are outside of the field. (D) Contrast is used to verify location. Note that the position of the operator has changed by 180° (as evidenced by the injection tubing), without significant movement of the needle.

the earlier paragraph. It is possible that the joint is successfully accessed without significant return of synovial fluid. If this situation is suspected, injection of contrast will help determine the intraarticular location of the needle. The agent is then injected and the needle removed. A dressing is applied and postinjection instructions are given to the patient.

General Computed Tomography Technique

CT also offers unique advantages. First and foremost is the excellent spatial resolution, which comes at a cost of temporal resolution. In an obese patient, or a patient with significant osseous degenerative disease, CT may be the only modality that practically may be considered. However, CT guidance for articular access takes considerably longer than other modalities, is more expensive, and is limited to medium to large joints. CT also uses ionizing radiation. Local anesthetic is generally used because needle advancement is almost always a multistep process in part because it is generally difficult anatomy that selects patients for CT guidance.

Needle and syringe selection is joint specific and the agent should be prepared prior to injection. The patient should be placed comfortably and essentially immobilized using tape to ensure that after the scout scan the patient does not move. If CT fluoroscopy is to be used, less immobilization may be required. The patient should be made as comfortable as possible because these procedures tend to be longer than those using ultrasound or fluoroscopy.

The patient is placed in the gantry and a scout projection obtained. The localizing laser is then activated for skin marking. Using the slice position data from the bed registration system, a row of metallic markers or grids are placed as close to centrally over the target as possible to mark the entry position in the axial plane. The patient is placed back in the gantry and an additional image obtained, with the grid in position for localization. These data are used to select a final entry site. Some physicians prefer a direct vertical approach for needle advancement, which may necessitate moving or rotating the patient to create a window avoiding vital structures. Another technique is to visually estimate the angle required to access the joint, which requires no patient repositioning but may require more frequent scanning. Whatever the preferred method, a site is marked between metal markers (note that one cannot exactly mark beneath a metal marker), again using the slice position selected during the final scout scan. The patient is removed from the gantry. The area is prepped and draped with great care to avoid moving or repositioning the patient.

A small-gauge needle, loosely attached to a syringe of local anesthetic, is used to raise a skin wheal at the proposed entry site and advanced while infiltrating local anesthetic into the superficial tissues. If desired, an additional scan may be performed after disconnecting the syringe and using the infiltrating needle to verify the angle and plan repositioning for the final access needle. If multiple corrections to the needle course are made, it can prolong the procedure considerably. If the anatomy is difficult or the approach near vital structures, multiple repositionings of the needle course may be necessary. This increase in procedure length is a necessary trade-off for accurate anatomic localization. If CT fluoroscopy is used, needle location verification may be done intermittently throughout the procedure, or the needle may be advanced under direct observation using hemostats (to avoid exposure of the hands) in the same manner as the direct fluoroscopic technique described earlier.

After sufficient anesthetic infiltration, the joint specific needle is advanced in a similar manner as using fluoroscopy, with CT localization when required. It is advisable to obtain at least one image when the needle has enough purchase to be self-supporting to verify the approach. Once the joint spaced is accessed, the interventions may proceed.

CONCLUSIONS

Intraarticular interventions to manage pain are common, safe, simple procedures. The data currently support the use of corticosteroids and hyaluronic acid, although chemosynovectomy shows promise. There are no data to suggest a specific corticosteroid dose or dosing regimen; however, traditional standard of practice suggests an interval of three months. Hyaluronic acid is administered in a weekly sequence. After the injection, there are multiple maneuvers that may be tried to maximize the effect of the agent. Duration of either agent may last from weeks to years, with a common duration of corticosteroids benefit lasting a few weeks and hyaluronic acid benefit lasting a few months.

Imaging guidance allows knowledge of the precise anatomic location of the agent, an important factor in both investigation and interpreting patient response. Ultrasound guidance is flexible and inexpensive, and should be the preferred method for intervention. Fluoroscopic and CT guidance are additional options, and referring to previous cross-sectional imaging may be helpful in planning an approach to the articular space.

REFERENCES

1. Wise C. Arthrocentesis and injection of joints and soft tissues. In: Ruddy S, Harris EDJ, Sledge CB, Kelley WN eds. Kelly's Textbook of Rheumatology, 7th ed. St. Louis: W.B. Saunders; 2005.
2. Aryal X. Injections in the treatment of osteoarthritis. Best Prac Res Clin Rheumatol 2001:15(4):609–26.
3. Smalley WE, Griffin MR, Fought RL, Ray WA. Excess costs from gastrointestinal disease associated with nonsteroidal anti-inflammatory drugs. J Gen Intern Med 1996;11:461–9.
4. Schiable HG, Ebersberger A, Segond Von Banchet G. Mechanisms of pain in arthritis. Ann NY Acad Sci 2002:966:343–54.
5. Lequesne M, Bensasson M, Kemmer C, Amouroux J. Painful juxtamensical areas in certain arthropathies of the knee and their treatment by juxtameniscal cortisone infiltration. Ann Rheum Dis 1970;29:689.
6. Sambrook PN, Champion GD, Browne CD, et al. Corticosteroid injection for osteoarthritis of the knee; peripatellar compared to intraarticular route. Clin Experimental Rheumatol 1989;7:609–13.
7. Naredo E, Cabero F, Beneyto P, et al. A randomized comparative study of short term response to blind injection versus sonographic-guided injection of local corticosteroids in patients with painful shoulder. J Rheumatol 2004;31:308–14.
8. Cawley PJ, Morris IMA. Study to compare the efficacy of two methods of skin preparation prior to joint injection. Br J Rheumatol 1992;31:847–8.
9. Neustadt DH. Intra-articular therapy for rheumatoid synovitis of the knee: effects of the post-injection rest regimen. Clin Rheumatol Prac 1985;3:65–8.
10. Chakravarty K, Pharoah PDP, Scott DGI. A randomized controlled study of post-injection rest following intra-articular steroid therapy for knee synovitis. Br J Rheumatol 1994;33:464–8.
11. Chatham W, Williams G, Moreland L, et al. Intraarticular corticosteroid injections: should we rest the joints? Arthritis Care Res 1989;2:70–4.
12. Jones A, Regan M, Ledingham J, et al. Importance of placement of intra-articular steroid injections. BMJ 1993;307:1329–30.
13. Sethi PM, Kinstone S, Elattrache N. Accuracy of anterior intra-articular injection of the glenohumeral joint. Arthroscopy 2005;21(1):77–80.

14. American College of Rheumatology Subcommittee on Osteoarthritis Guidelines. Recommendations for the medical management of osteoarthritis of the hip and knee: rheumatologists in the United States. Arthritis Rheum 2000;43:1905–15.

15. Owen DS Jr. Aspiration and injection of joints and soft tissues. In: Ruddy S, Harris EDJ, Sledge CB eds. Kelley's Textbook of Rheumatology. Philadelphia: W.B. Saunders; 2001:583–603.

16. Schumacher HR. Aspiration and injection therapies for joints. Arthritis Rheum 2003;49:413–20.

17. Dawes PT, Kirlew C, Haslock I. Saline washout for knee osteoarthritis: results of a controlled study. Clin Rheumatol 1987;6:61–3.

18. Courtney P, Doherty M. Join aspiration and injection. Best Prac Res Clin Rheumatol 2005;19:345–69.

19. Chokkalingam S, Velazquez C, Mody A, Brasington R. Diagnosing acute monoarthritis in adults: a practical approach for the family physician. Am Fam Physician 2003;68(1):83–90.

20. Moseley JB, O'Malley K, Peterson NJ, et al. A controlled trial of arthroscopic surgery for osteoarthritis of the knee. New Engl J Med 2002;347(2):81–8.

21. Ike RW, Arnold WJ, Rothschild E, Shaw HI. The Tidal Irrigation Cooperating Group. Tidal irrigation versus conservative medical management in patients with osteoarthritis of the knee: a prospective randomized study. J Rheumatol 1992;19:772–9.

22. Chang RW, Falconer J, Stulberg SD, Arnold WJ, Manheim LM, Dyer AR. A randomized, controlled trial of arthroscopic surgery versus closed-needle joint lavage for patients with osteoarthritis of the knee. Arthritis Rheum 1993;36:289–96.

23. Ayral X, Dougados M. Joint lavage. Rev Rheum 1995;62:281–7.

24. Schumacher HR, Chen LX. Injectable corticosteroids in treatment of arthritis of the knee. Am J Med 2005;118:1208–14.

25. American College of Rheumatology Subcommittee on Rheumatoid Arthritis Guidelines. Guidelines for the management of rheumatoid arthritis: 2002 update. Arthritis Rheum 2002;46:328–46.

26. Genovese MC. Joint and soft-tissue injection. Postgrad Med 1998;103(2):1–11.

27. Gossec L, Dougados M. Intra-articular treatments in osteoarthritis: from the symptomatic to the structure modifying. Ann Rheum Dis 2004;63:478–82.

28. Drug information for the health care professional. Copyright 2006, Thompson Micromexed (ISBN 1-56363-539-9).

29. Laaksonen AL, Sunnell JE, Westeren H, Mulder J. Adrenocorticoal function in children with juvenile rheumatoid arthritis and other connective tissue disorders. Scand J Rheumatol 1974;3:137–44.

30. Emkey RD, Lindsay R, Lyssy J, et al. The systemic effect of intra-articular administration of corticosteroid on markers of bone formation and bone resorption in patients with rheumatoid arthritis. Arthritis Rheum 1996;39:277–82.

31. McDonald AG, Land DV, Sturrock RD. Microwave thermography as a non invasive assessment of disease activity in inflammatory arthritis. Clin Rheumatol 1994;13:589–92.

32. Creamer P. Intra-articular corticosteroid treatment in osteoarthritis. Curr Opin Rheumatol 1999;11:417–21.

33. Jones A, Doherty M. Intra-articular corticosteroids are effective in osteoarthritis but there are no clinical predictors of response. Ann Rheum Dis 1995;54:379–81.

34. Friedman DM, Moore ME. The efficacy of intraarticular steroids in osteoarthritis: a double blind study. J Rheumatol 1980;7:850–6.

35. Nichols AW. Complications associated with the use of cortosteroids in the treatment of athletic injuries. Clin J Sport Med 2005;15:E370.

36. Gaffney K, Ledingham J, Perry JD. Intra-articular triamcinolone hexacetonide in knee osteoarthritis: factors influencing the clinical response. Ann Rheum Dis 1995;54:379–81.

37. Caldwell JR. Intra-articular corticosteroids. Guide to selection and indications for use. Drugs 1996;52:507–14.

38. Seror P, Pluvinage P, d'Andre FL, et al. Frequency of sepsis after local corticosteroid injection (an inquiry of 1 160 000 injections in rheumatological private practice in France). Rheumatology 1999;38:1272–4.

39. Pattrick M, Doherty M. Facial flushing after intra-articular injection of bupivicaine and methylprednisolone. BMJ 1987;295:1380.

40. Jones A, Doherty M. Intra-articular therapies in osteoarthritis. In: Brandt KD, Doherty M, Lohmander LS eds. Osteoarthritis. Oxford: Oxford University Press; 1998:299–306.

41. Slotkoff A, Clauw D, Nashel D. Effect of soft tissue corticosteroid injection on glucose control in diabetics [abstract]. Arthitis Rheum 1994;37(Suppl 9):S347.

42. Emkey RD, Lindsay R, Lyssy J, et al. The systemic effect of intraarticular adminis-tration of corticosteroid on markers of bone formation and bone resorption in patients with rheumatoid arthritis. Arthritis Rheum 1996;39:277–82.

43. Gray RG, Gottlieb NL. Intra-articular corticosteroids: an updated assessment. Clin Ortho Relat Res 1983;177:235–63.

44. Hollander JL. Intrasynovial corticosteroid therapy in arthiris. Maryland Med J 1970;19:62–6.

45. Roberts WN, Babcock EA, Breitbach SA, et al. Corticosteroid injection in rheumatoid arthritis does not increase rate of total joint arthoplasty. J Rheumatol 1996;23:1001–4.

46. Raynault JP, Buckland-Wright C, Tremblay JL, et al. Clinical trials: impact of IA steroid injections on the progression of knee osteoarthritis. Osteoarthritis Cartilage 2000; 8(Suppl A):S16.

47. Verify Behrens F. Alterations of rabbit articular cartilage by intra articular injections of gulcocorticoids. J Bone Joint Surg (Am) 1975;57(1):70–6.

48. Williams JM, Brandt KD. Triamcinolone hexacetonide protects against fibrillation and osteophyte formation following chemically induced articular cartilage damage. Arthritis Rheum 1985;28(11):1267–74.

49. Pelletier JP, Martel-Pelletier J. Protective effects of corticosteroids on cartilage lesions and osteophyte formation in the Pond-Nuke dog model of osteoarthiris. Arthitis Rheum 1989;32(2):181–93.

50. Gibson T, Burry HC, Poswillo D, et al. Effect of intra-articular corticosteroid injec-tions on primate cartilage. Ann Rheum Dis 1977;36(1):74–9.

51. Snibbe JC, Gambardella RA. Use of injections for osteoarthritis in joints and sports activity. Clin Sports Med 2005;24:83–91.

52. Karlsson J, Sjogren LS, Lohmander LS. Comparison of two hyaluronan drugs and placebo in patients with knee osteoarthritis. A controlled, randomized, double-blind, parallel-design multicentre study. Rheumatology 2002;41:1240–8.

53. Modawal A, Ferrer M, Choi HK, Castle JA. Hyaluronic acid injections relieve knee pain. J Fam Pract 2005;54(9)758–67.

54. Cohen MD. Hyaluronic acid treatment (viscosupplementation) for OA of the knee. Bull Rheum Dis 1998;47:4–7.

55. Balazs EA, Denlinger JL. Viscosupplementation: a new concept in the treatement of osteoarthritis. J Rheumatol 1993;20(Suppl 39):3–9.

56. Marshall KW. Viscosupplementation for osteoarthritis: current status, unresolved issues and future directions. J Rheumatol 1998;25:2056–8.

57. George E. Intra-articular hyaluronon treatment for osteoarthritis. Ann Rheum Dis 1998;57:637–40.

58. Watterson JR, Esdaile JM. Viscosupplementation: therapeutic mechanisms and clinical potential in osteoarthritis of the knee. J Am Acad Orthop Surg 2000;8(5):277–84.

59. Goto M, Hanyu T, Yoshio T, et al. Intra-articular injection of hyaluronate (SI-6601D) improves joint pain and synovial fluid prostaglandin E2 eels in rheumatoid arthritis: a multicenter trial. Clin Exp Rheumatol 2001;19:377–83.

60. Watterson JR, Esdaile JM. Viscosupplementation: therapeutic mechanisms and clinical potential in osteoarthritis of the knee. J Am Acad Orthop Surg 200;8:277–84.

61. Pathogenesis and Clincal Management of Osteoarthritis. Presentation from sanofi aventis. http://www.hyalgan.com/download/professional/pdf/pathogenesis.pdf (accessed June 2006).

62. Ghosh P. The role of hyaluronic acid (hyaluronan) in health and disease: interactions with cells, cartilage, and components of synovial fluid. Clin Exp Rheumatol 1994; 12:75–82.

63. Armstrong S, Read R, Ghosh P. The effects of intraarticular hyaluronan on cartilage and subchondral bone changes in an ovine model of early osteoarthritis. J Rheumatol 1994;21:680–8.

64. Schiavinato A, Lini E, Guidolin D, et al. Intraarticular sodium hyaluronate injections in the Pond-Nuki experimental model of osteoarthritis in dongs. II. Morphological findings. Clin Orthop 1989;241:286–99.

65. Cefalu CA, Waddell DS. Viscosupplementation: treatment alternative for osteoarthritis of the knee. Geriatrics 1999;54:51–7.

66. Lo GH, LaValley M, McAlindon T, Felson DT. Intra-articular hyaluronic acid in treatment of knee osteoarthritis. JAMA 2003;290:3115–21.

67. Lussier A, Cividino AA, McFarlane CA, et al. Viscosupplementation with hylan for the treatment of osteoarthritis: findings from clinical practice in Canada. J Rheumatol 1996;23:1579–85.

68. Goldberg VM, Coutts A. Pseudoseptic reactions to hylan viscosupplementation: diagnosis and treatment. Clin Orthop Relat Res 2004;419:130–7.

69. Chen AL, Desai P, Alder EM, DiCesare PE. Granulomatous inflammation after hylan G-F 20 viscosupplementation of the knee: a report of six cases. J Bone Joint Surg 2002;84-A(7):1142–7.

70. Bessant R, Steuer A, Rigby S, Gumpol M. Osmic acid revisited: factors that predict a favourable response. Rheumatology 2003;42:1036–43.

71. Morshed S, Huffman GR, Ries MD. Septic arthritis of the hip and intrapelvic abscess following intra-articular injection of hylan G-F 20. A case report. J Bone Joint Surg Am 2004;86(4):823–6.

72. Heuft-Dorenbosch LLJ, de Vet HC, van der Linden S. Yttrium radiosynoviorthesis in the treatment of knee arthritis in rheumatoid arthritis: a systematic review. Ann Rheum Dis 2000;59:583–6.

73. Jahangier Z, Jacobs JW, Lafeber FP, et al. Is radiation synovectomy for arthritis of the knee more effective than intraarticular treatment with glucocorticoids?: results of an eighteen-month, randomized, double-blind, placebo-controlled, crossover trial. Arthritis Rheum 2005;52(11):3391–402.

74. Okada Y, Nakanishi I, Kajikawa K. Repair of the mouse synovial membrane after chemical synovectomy with osmium tetroxide. Acta Pathol Jpn 1984; 34(4):705–14.

75. Sethi PM, Attrache N. Accuracy of anterior intra-articular injection of the glenohumeral joint: a cadaveric study. Arthroscopy 2005; 21:77–80.

Percutaneous Management of Visceral Pain

Frank Morello

INTRODUCTION

Pain from the abdominal and pelvic viscera is difficult to manage because it is often secondary to a malignancy or a chronic inflammatory process. A patient with such chronic pain usually needs narcotics to reduce the severity. When tolerance to the medication develops, increasing doses of narcotics are necessary for further pain relief. In addition to the physiological impairment this causes, increasing doses of narcotics can lead to mental and emotional impairment, all of which can significantly reduce a person's quality of life (1). Any therapy that can reduce such dependence while lessening the severity of the underlying pain will be favorable to the overall well-being of the patient.

First described by Kappis in 1919 (2), various methods of percutaneous visceral pain control have been employed since Moore (3) popularized the classic posterolateral approach to the celiac plexus using fluoroscopic guidance. The success of either temporary or permanent pain relief from these methods, along with the relatively low complication rates, justify their mention as viable pain control options for patients with severe or poorly controlled symptoms. Interventional radiologists who understand the anatomy and physiology of visceral pain can use their percutaneous skills to offer an effective and minimally invasive therapy for a disease process that otherwise has a less-than-optimistic course.

VISCERAL PAIN PATHWAYS

Visceral pain can be caused by any process that causes visceral nerve fiber irritation. The classic example is midabdominal pain caused by either pancreatitis or a pancreatic neoplasm (4). Abdominal or pelvic pain of visceral origin is usually described as vague, poorly localized, dull, crampy, pulling, squeezing, or colicky. If the offending process can be relieved, the pain usually resolves as well.

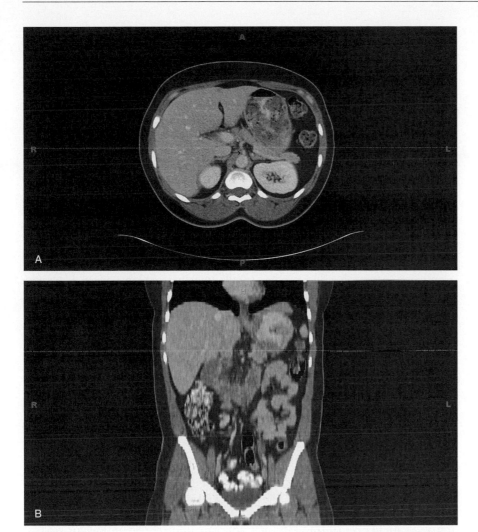

Figure 1. (A) Axial CT at the level of the celiac ganglion. Axial contrast-enhanced CT demonstrates the level of the celiac ganglion in a normal patient. The ganglion lies just beneath and lateral to the celiac artery origin (arrow). (B) Coronal reconstruction of CT image from figure A. The level of the celiac ganglion is indicated by the line traversing the image.

Unfortunately, such pain is seldom relieved, even with narcotics, for a variety of reasons. The underlying disease often cannot be controlled, the irritating process is diffuse and involves more than one nerve distribution, and there is frequently associated somatic and neuropathic pain as well. Fortunately, most of the visceral pain pathways travel through a few key anatomic "nerve centers," which makes it easier to plan an approach for percutaneous therapy. Understanding the anatomic distribution and location of these pain pathways will help predict the necessary area to target in a percutaneous procedure.

The main innervation pathways for the abdominal viscera travel through the celiac plexus, which lies in the retroperitoneum just anterior to the crura of the diaphragm between the T12 and L1 levels (Figure 1A, B). This plexus surrounds the celiac and superior mesenteric arteries and is composed of a network of sympathetic and parasympathetic nerve fibers from which several secondary abdominal plexuses arise. The two large ganglia of the celiac plexus receive parasympathetic fibers from the vagus nerve and sympathetic fibers from the three splanchnic nerves (greater, lesser, and least). The greater splanchnic nerve arises from the T5-T9 paravertebral ganglia and passes through the crura of the diaphragm to end in the celiac ganglion of the celiac plexus. Fibers from the celiac plexus also join the lesser splanchnic nerve (arising from the T10 and T11 ganglia) to form the aorticorenal ganglion and plexus. The least splanchnic nerve arises from the T12 ganglion and enters the abdomen with the sympathetic trunk to end in the renal plexus.

The secondary plexuses that arise from the celiac plexus travel along the course of the aorta and its branching arteries. Of note are the superior and inferior mesenteric plexuses that provide fibers for the majority of the intestines. Whether through secondary plexuses or directly to the end organs, the celiac plexus is responsible for postganglionic fibers that innervate the distal esophagus, stomach, duodenum, small intestine, colon, adrenal glands, kidneys, proximal ureters, pancreas, spleen, liver, biliary system, and major blood vessels (5). This network of postganglionic sympathetic organ innervation is also thought to carry pain sensation from the same locations.

In similar fashion, a rich network of plexuses also provides innervation to the pelvic viscera (Figure 2). The majority of these are connected to the superior hypogastric plexus. This plexus is situated anterior to the last lumbar vertebra and the promontory of the sacrum, between the two common iliac arteries. The superior hypogastric plexus is composed of the lumbar sympathetic chains, branches of the aortic plexus, and parasympathetic fibers of the S2-S4 roots. It is the major pathway for innervation of the distal ureters, gonads, sigmoid colon, vagina, rectum, bladder, perineum, vulva, prostate, uterus, and the major pelvic blood vessels (5).

At the termination of the paired paravertebral sympathetic chains, just anterior to the sacrococcygeal junction, lies the ganglion of Walther (ganglion impar). Pain fibers that travel through this ganglion are responsible for visceral

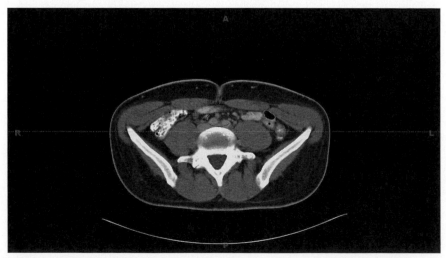

Figure 2. Axial CT at the level of the superior hypogastric plexus. Axial contrast CT demonstrates the level of the superior hypogastric plexus in a normal patient (circle).

perineal pain of sympathetic origin. This tends to be a vague, poorly localized pain with sensations of burning or urgency.

METHODS OF VISCERAL PAIN CONTROL
Patient Selection

Visceral nerve blockade has been a long-practiced method to achieve pain relief from visceral origin (6). When considering a percutaneous approach, one must first determine the location and etiology of the pain. Timing of an intervention is also important. If the source of the pain can be treated either medically or surgically, an attempt to do so may lessen, or even relieve, the symptoms making a percutaneous blockade unnecessary. Conversely, if the disease has reached an advanced stage, the effects of a neurolytic blockade may not be satisfactory (7). Finally, a differentiation must be made between somatic pain and visceral pain because somatic pain is not controlled by percutaneous visceral nerve blockade. A temporary blockade can often help differentiate somatic from visceral pain before a more permanent neurolytic blockade is attempted, and it may also predict the success of a permanent neurolysis (6).

Imaging Guidance

The traditional choice of imaging guidance has been fluoroscopy (3). As with many classic percutaneous therapies, the advent of computed tomography (CT) has allowed a cross-sectional and perhaps more accurate means of needle placement that has replaced fluoroscopy as the imaging guidance of choice for many procedures. CT imaging during visceral nerve blockade has been emphasized not only for the accuracy of needle placement but also for an estimation of the procedure's efficacy by the cross-sectional analysis of pretreatment contrast diffusion (8). This has also led to the introduction of nonstandard approaches to the celiac plexus, such as a posterior transaortic approach (9) and an anterior approach (10). As with most procedures, the use of CT as an imaging guidance tool allows one the license to choose the most direct pathway to the target with the least amount of danger to surrounding structures. A percutaneous approach to visceral nerve blockade involves placing a needle under radiological guidance into one of the common "nerve centers" previously discussed. Confirmation can be made by image-guided visualization of needle placement and further confirmed through the distribution of injected contrast.

Medications

If temporary pain relief is desired, such as for a self-resolving inflammatory process, the medication choice is an anesthetic and steroid mixture. The most commonly used local anesthetic for temporary blockade is 5–10 ml of 0.25% bupivicaine, which has the longest effect of the local anesthetics currently available. The use of a local anesthetic in a temporary block serves two purposes. First, it lessens the pain caused by the procedure itself. Second, it provides temporary visceral pain relief until the steroid can reach full effect. There is no consensus on which steroid is optimal for visceral nerve blockade. Commonly used steroids are similar to that used for joint injections – triamcinolone, methylprednisolone, and betamethasone. As such, no consensus exists on the usual dosages, and these are also derived from their use in other musculoskeletal applications: 40–80 mg each of triamcinolone and methylprednisolone and 6–12 mg of betamethasone.

Permanent blockade is usually reserved for palliation of the severe pain of malignancy. This is achieved by the injection of a substance that causes local neurolysis. The two commonly applied medications include 10% phenol and 50–100% absolute alcohol. The mechanism of action for phenol is to denature the proteins in the neural tissue. It is painless on injection, so a concomitant local anesthetic is usually not necessary. Absolute alcohol works by extracting phospholipids, cholesterol, and cerebroside from neural tissues and precipitating mucoprotein and lipoprotein (11). Because alcohol is a caustic substance that causes pain on injection, it is commonly diluted by 50% with 0.25% bupivacaine.

Results

The success of percutaneous visceral nerve blockade depends on a variety of factors. The most important is the complete medication diffusion and coverage of the target area. For example, it has been shown that if the celiac ganglion is divided into four quadrants around the celiac axis, adequate pain relief was not achieved unless there was contrast diffusion and subsequent medication coverage of at least three of the four quadrants (12). Obviously, ideal results would be achieved if all four quadrants were covered. Usually, a total volume of 20–40 ml of medication mixture is required to achieve full coverage.

The severity of the offending process certainly affects the success of a procedure. If concurrent therapy is to primarily treat the underlying disease process, a percutaneous blockade may be more effective.

The appropriate choice of medication is dictated by the extent of pain relief desired. A short- to long-term anesthetic and steroid combination is used if temporary pain relief is desired; alcohol or phenol must be used if permanent neurolysis is the objective. In large part, this also depends on the realistic expectations for pain relief agreed on by the operator, patient, and consulting physicians. If more pain relief was expected than was realistically possible, even a small degree of pain relief may not matter to the patient if the expectation was not fulfilled.

The success of percutaneous visceral nerve blockade is directly measured by the reduction of perceived pain and indirectly by the reduction of narcotics necessary for pain relief. Because of the multifactorial nature of the pain, the goals of performing a neurolytic blockade of the sympathetic axis are to maximize the analgesic effects of opioid or nonopioid analgesics and to reduce the dosage of these agents in order to alleviate side effects (13). Using these criteria, a range of success between 50% and 74% has been reported (14,15). As previously discussed, meticulous needle placement and adequate medication diffusion over the target area are the main indicators of success. Poor success rates have been mainly attributed to the advanced nature of the underlying disease once a decision has been made to attempt percutaneous therapy (15). Despite the relatively good success rates in some investigators, experience, visceral nerve blockade has not been found to significantly increase quality of life or life expectancy (16).

Complications

Fortunately, major complications of percutaneous visceral nerve blockade are extremely rare. Major complications of needle placement include retroperitoneal hemorrhage, aortic dissection, pneumothorax, and major infection. Major complications of the actual sympathetic nerve blockade include paraplegia that is thought to occur from spasm of the lumbar segmental arteries that perfuse the spinal cord. Over a five-year time period, Davies (17) found that the incidence of major complication from a celiac plexus block was 1 in 683 procedures (0.15%). Other complications are diarrhea and loss of autonomic organ function. For the most part, these latter complications can be controlled with anticholinergics and supportive medication such as antidiarrheals.

Common side effects from visceral nerve blockade are usually controlled with supportive measures. These are direct results of needle placement and/or irritation from the medication used. Back pain is self-resolving but can be relieved with anti-inflammatory medication. Diaphragmatic irritation can cause pain, hiccups, or pleuritic pain and can also be relieved with supportive measures until resolution. Orthostatic hypotension may occur up to five days after the block in 1–3% of patients. Treatment includes fluid replacement and bed rest while avoiding sudden changes in position. Thigh-high lower extremity compression stockings can also provide support to vascular structures until compensatory vascular reflexes are fully activated and this side effect disappears.

VISCERAL NERVE BLOCKADE PROCEDURES
Celiac Plexus Block

It is the traditional method of choice for controlling the pain from pancreatitis or a terminal pancreatic cancer. Any irritative process that offends the upper abdominal viscera likely has pain fibers that travel through the celiac plexus. Often, a temporary blockade can be utilized to test the potential success of a permanent neurolysis. Before the advent of CT as an image guidance tool, the needle placement for a celiac plexus block was always performed under fluoroscopic guidance using bony landmarks. As stated earlier, this traditional technique utilizes the posterolateral approach (3). With the patient in prone position, bilateral (usually 22 g) needles are placed into the back 7–8 cm lateral to the T12 vertebral body (18). A 45° medial angle directs the needles toward the T12-L1 area. Once the needle tips are about 1.5 cm anterior to the vertebral body, a careful inspection is made to eliminate the possibility of intravascular needle placement. The injection of 20–25 ml solution through each needle completes the procedure. Care must be taken to ensure that the pleural space is not traversed (Figure 3).

An anterior fluoroscopic approach has also been described (10), particularly to lessen the pain involved with complex percutaneous biliary procedures. For this approach, a 20-g needle is inserted through the abdomen directly on to the right side of the L1 vertebral body half-way between its superior and inferior endplates. The needle is retracted 1–3 cm, and, after aspiration, a few milliliters of contrast is injected. As long as there is no free return of blood on aspiration, filling of a blood vessel on contrast injection, or direct resistance to injection, the needle position is considered satisfactory and 40 ml of 0.5% lidocaine is injected for temporary neural blockade. If these maneuvers demonstrate an

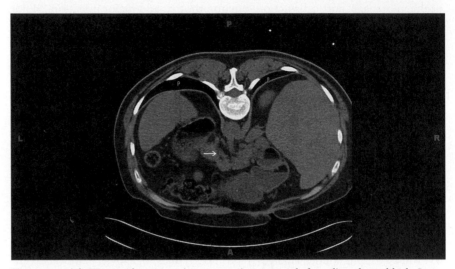

Figure 3. Axial CT scan demonstrating a posterior approach for celiac plexus block. In this patient, the posterior approach for a celiac plexus (arrow) block proved to be contraindicated because of the hyperinflation of the posterior pleural space (P) upon positioning the patient prone. This approach may be particularly difficult in patients with underlying hyperinflation of the lungs, such as patients with chronic obstruction pulmonary disease.

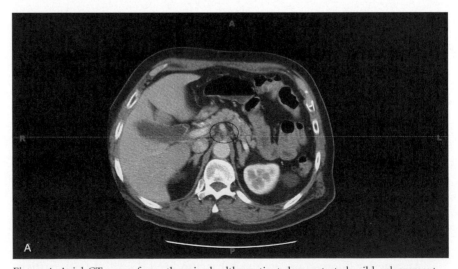

Figure 4. Axial CT scan of an otherwise healthy patient demonstrated mild enlargement of the celiac plexus, particularly on the patient's left side (circle). In most patients, the celiac plexus is not visualized during CT scanning.

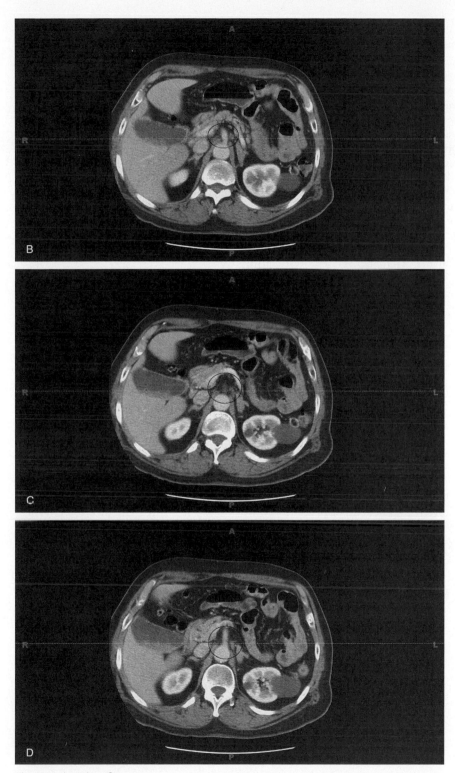

Figure 4. (*continued*)

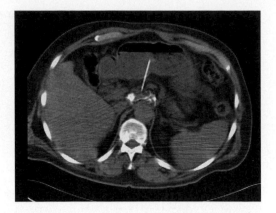

Figure 5. Contrast injection following an anterior approach for celiac plexus ablation. Axial CT scan following placement of a single needle demonstrates contrast outlining the space surrounding the celiac plexus. Note the contrast pooling outside the intravascular space. This contrast configuration confirms appropriate needle placement, and sclerotherapy can then be safely performed.

inadequate needle position, the tip is repositioned for another series of confirmatory maneuvers before final injection.

An anterior approach can also be used with CT guidance. The celiac plexus can often be visualized, particularly in the setting of a chronic visceral process (Figure 4A–D). If the celiac plexus cannot be visualized, the needle is placed paramedian to the origin of the celiac plexus. Traversal of many organs (liver, stomach, duodenum, pancreas) typically causes neither discomfort nor complications.

Complications from a fluoroscopic-guided procedure such as renal trauma, pneumothorax, and inadvertent puncture of the aorta/cava were lessened, or even eliminated, with the use of CT as an imaging modality of choice for this procedure. With CT, whether an anterior or posterior approach is utilized, a more precise needle placement can be made. The objective is the same as when performed with fluoroscopy – to place the needle tips anterior to the crura of the diaphragm on each side of the celiac axis. As previously discussed, CT also gives the advantage of predicting a more complete response to therapy through pretreatment analysis of contrast diffusion as a measure of medication coverage (8) (Figure 5). Finally, ultrasound guidance can be used in an endoscopic approach to the celiac plexus, and this has shown success as an alternative method of performing a celiac plexus block (19). Despite the recent application of this approach, success rates have been similar to percutaneous approaches.

Superior Hypogastric Plexus Block

This has recently become popular for treatment of chronic pelvic pain. To perform this visceral block, CT or fluoroscopic guidance is used to place a needle anterior to the L5-S1 junction. Unlike celiac plexus blockade, there is no evidence to support diffusion of a pretreatment contrast injection as a measure of success. A test injection with local anesthetic, however, can predict the success or failure of a more permanent neurolysis.

Ganglion Impar Block

It can be performed to treat pain from a rectal or perineal location. The ganglion is located just anterior to the sacrococcygeal junction (Figure 6A, B).

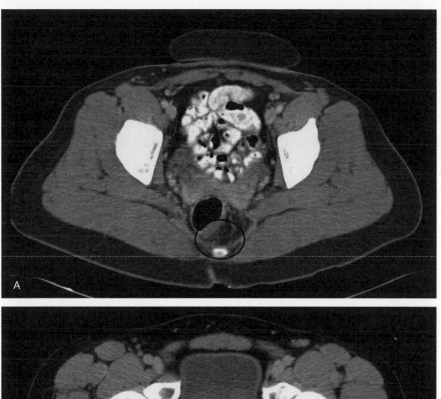

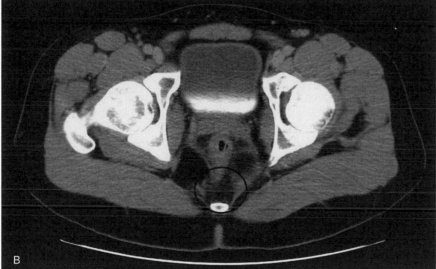

Figure 6. (A and B) Axial CT scans at the level of the ganglion impar (circle), which lies just anterior to the sacrococcygeal junction. Notice that the level varies from patient to patient, as evidenced by the difference in the femoral head-acetabulum appearance between the two patients.

As with the other blockades, CT offers the most precise method of imaging guidance. Given the difficult location of this ganglion, CT is recommended as the imaging tool of choice, not only to maximize procedure efficacy but also to minimize potential complications.

REFERENCES

1. Levy MJ, Wiersema MJ. EUS-guided celiac plexus neurolysis and celiac plexus block. Gastrointest Endosc 2003; 57:923–9.

2. Kappis M. Sensibilitat und lokale Anasthesie im chirurgischen Gebiet der Bauchhohle mit besonderer Berucksichtigung der splanchnicus-Aasthesie. Beitrage zur klinischen Chirurgie 1919; 115:161–75.

3. Moore DC. Celiac (splanchnic) plexus block with alcohol for cancer pain of the upper abdominal viscera. In: Bonica JJ, Ventafridda V, eds. Advances in pain research and therapy, Vol. 2. New York: Raven, 1979; 357–71.

4. Wong GY, Schroeder DR, Carns PE, et al. Effect of neurolytic celiac plexus block on pain relief, quality of life, and survival in patients with unresectable pancreatic cancer: a randomized controlled trial. JAMA 2004; 291:1092–9.

5. Ross E, Hynes WL, Janfaza DR, et al. Sympathetic blocks. Harvard Medical School, Brigham and Women's Hospital Pain Management Center. Available at http://ether-web.bwh.harvard.edu/pmc/padmin/sympathetic.html. Accessed May 15, 2006.

6. Yuen TS, Ng KF, Tsui SL. Neurolytic celiac plexus block for visceral abdominal malignancy: is prior diagnostic block warranted? Anaesth Intensive Care 2002; 30:442–8.

7. Rykowski JJ, Hilgier M. Efficacy of neurolytic celiac plexus block in varying locations of pancreatic cancer: influence on pain relief. Anesthesiology 2000; 92:347–54.

8. Iki K, Fujita Y, Inada H, Satoh M, Tsunoda T. Celiac plexus block: evaluation of injectate spread by three-dimensional computed tomography. Abdom Imaging 2003; 28:571–3.

9. Lieberman RP, Waldman SD. Celiac plexus neurolysis with the modified transaortic approach. Radiology 1990; 175:274–6.

10. Leiberman RP, Nance PN, Cuka DJ. Anterior approach to celiac plexus block during interventional biliary procedures. Radiology 1998; 167:562–4.

11. Noble M, Gress FG. Techniques and results of neurolysis for chronic pancreatitis and pancreatic cancer pain. Curr Gastroenterol Rep 2006; 8:99–103.

12. De Cicco M, Matovic M, Bortolussi R, et al. Celiac plexus block: injectate spread and pain relief in patients with regional anatomic distortions. Anesthesiology 2001; 94:561–5.

13. de Leon-Casasola O. Critical evaluation of chemical neurolysis of the sympathetic axis for cancer pain. Cancer Control 2000; 7:142–8.

14. Gress F, Schmitt C, Sherman S, Ikenberry S, Lehman G. A prospective randomized comparison of endoscopic ultrasound- and computed tomography-guided celiac plexus block for managing chronic pancreatitis pain. Am J Gastroenterol 1999; 94:900–5.

15. Rykowski JJ, Hilgier M. Efficacy of neurolytic celiac plexus block in varying locations of pancreatic cancer: influence on pain relief. Anesthesiology 2000; 92:347–54.

16. Wong GY, Schroeder DR, Carns PE, et al. Effect of neurolytic celiac plexus block on pain relief, quality of life, and survival in patients with unresectable pancreatic cancer: a randomized controlled trial. JAMA 2004; 291:1092–9.

17. Davies DD. Incidence of major complications of neurolytic coeliac plexus block. J R Soc Med. 1993; 86:264–6.

18. Ischia S, Ischia A, Polati E, Finco G. Three posterior percutaneous celiac plexus block techniques – a prospective, randomized study in 61 patients with pancreatic cancer pain. Anesthesiology 1992; 76:534–40.

19. Arcidiacono PG, Rossi M. Celiac plexus neurolysis. J Pancreas (Online) 2004; 5:315–21.

Embolization of Painful Neoplasms

Jennifer R. Huddleston and Stephen P. Johnson

One of the most devastating aspects of advanced cancer is the development of metastatic lesions to the bone. Approximately one-third of all adenocarcinomas will result in osseous metastases and an overwhelming 70% of patients who die of cancer show osseous metastases at autopsy (1). In particular, adequate pain management continues to be an unresolved issue in a majority of these patients. Fortunately, new endovascular techniques are currently being developed in an attempt to alleviate pain associated with metastatic disease. In this chapter, we will review some of the fundamental aspects of osseous metastases and the sources of cancer pain. We will then describe the various endovascular treatments that have been used to date including the most common therapeutic agents and their applications, benefits, and side effects.

PATHOLOGY OF OSSEOUS METASTASES

With over 300,000 cases each year, secondary metastases to bone are 15 times more prevalent than primary bone tumors (1). The most common carcinomas to metastasize to bone are prostate, breast, kidney, thyroid, and lung. Some studies report that up to 90% of these cancers result in bony lesions at autopsy (1). Less common sources also include skin, cervix, and various organs of the gastrointestinal tract (see Table 1).

Metastases to bone most often occur due to hematogenous spread in what has been described as a "seed-and-soil" mechanism (1,2). It is postulated that a single cell enters the vasculature via enzymes and proteases of tumor origin. From there, the cell circulates throughout the body and is preferentially deposited at remote sites. The location of these deposits is due to the attraction of local tissue factors such as integrins for the metastatic cell. Secondary lesions to bone, particularly the axial skeleton, are thought to occur due to the presence of such factors in the red marrow. Once deposited, the metastatic cell produces angiogenesis factors and promotes neovascularization and further growth of the cancerous focus. Ironically enough, despite the large number of cases of

Table 1. Types of Metastatic Bone Lesions

	Osteoblastic	*Osteolytic*
Associated cancer types	Prostate	Renal cell
	Carcinoid	Melanoma
	Gastrinoma	Non-small-cell lung cancer
	Small-cell lung cancer	Thyroid
	Breast[a]	Breast[a]
	Other GI[a]	Other GI[a]
Cellular process	Activated osteoblasts	Activated osteoclasts
	Bone formation	Bone resorption
Painful	Less often	Most often
Pathological fractures	Lower frequency	High frequency

GI – gastrointestinal.
[a] Propensity for lesions with mixed type of cellular processes.

metastatic disease, some estimate that only 1 in 10,000 neoplastic cells ultimately present in the circulation are capable of this process (1).

Of the two types of bony lesions, osteolytic and osteoblastic, most metastatic lesions tend to be osteoblastic in nature (2). Blastic lesions are associated with new bone formation, whereas lytic lesions are associated with bone breakdown and resorption. Tumors resulting in mostly blastic metastases include prostate, carcinoid, gastrinoma, and small-cell lung cancer (see Table 1). Research with prostate tumor cells suggests this process is likely due to excess activation of osteoblasts by the growth factor endothelin from bone stroma. When the endothelin signaling pathway is pharmacologically blocked, bone formation and the progression of bone metastases in prostate cancer patients is inhibited (3,4). These lesions are mostly associated with bone formation; thus, bone integrity is maintained, and they are less frequently associated with severe pain. Similarly, they are also less frequently associated with pathological fractures.

In contrast, renal cell cancer, melanoma, non-small-cell lung cancer, and thyroid cancer tend to be osteolytic in nature (see Table 1). Stimulating factors such as macrophage colony-stimulating factor, parathyroid hormone-related protein, and interleukins are thought to activate osteoclasts and cause an increased rate of bone resorption, turnover, and destruction (3). This breakdown of bone in turn leads to a higher incidence of pathological fracture and are frequently a source of bone pain. In addition, osteolytic metastases have a higher association with neovascularity and hemorrhagic response (1). Postoperative bleeding can be significantly reduced by prophylactically embolizing the area of the tumor prior to surgery (1).

Meanwhile, the possible spectrum of disease and progression between osteoblastic and osteolytic metastases remains unclear. Although the primary cancers listed earlier show a predominant pattern of bone response, some variants also exist. Not all prostate metastases are blastic in nature, and some types of cancer can even display both types of lesions simultaneously. Breast and gastrointestinal cancer tend to display a mixed array of osteoblastic and osteolytic lesions (2).

Whether osteoblastic, osteolytic, or both, the majority of metastatic cases in bone involve more than one lesion. Only 10% of cases are restricted to a solitary lesion. The most common site is the spine and affects up to 70% of all cancer patients (5,6). Other common sites in order of descending frequency include the pelvis, femur, ribs, proximal humerus, and skull (1). The local factors in red bone marrow attract circulating metastatic cells; hence, the predilection for skeletal metastases for bones with more red marrow. In addition, the location of skeletal metastases is also associated with the location of the primary tumor. Whereas breast, lung, prostate, lymphoma, multiple myeloma, and renal cancers are often associated with spinal metastases (6), metastases of the more distal appendicular skeleton are most often associated with lung cancers (1).

PATHOLOGY OF PAIN ASSOCIATED WITH MALIGNANCY

Over two-thirds of all patients with metastatic cancer have associated pain syndromes (7). This number rises to over 80% in the terminal stages of metastatic disease (8). Of the many factors affecting cancer related pain including type of cancer, stage of disease, and presence of metastases, the last one is one of the most determinant factors of pain severity. In particular, those with metastatic involvement of bone have shown significantly higher severity of pain. Over 85% of patients with bony metastatic lesions require analgesic medication such as opioids while only 5% of patients without bony metastases require such treatments (9).

The source of pain in these patients can originate from a variety of different pathways. These include direct effects from the tumor itself invading bone or compressing nerves as well as complications of previous radiation, chemotherapy, or surgical treatment. By far, the most common source of bone pain is direct tumor involvement (10). In absence of any pathological fracture or nerve disruption, this pain is purely somatic in nature and most likely sensed from cellular activity of osteoblasts and osteoclasts in the periosteum and synovium (11). This somatic pain is oftentimes described as focal and constant although it can also ache, throb, and/or be referred to another site. Most often bone pain secondary to malignancy worsens gradually over days to weeks, as opposed to an acute increase in pain more indicative of fracture or nerve damage.

The process by which metastatic tumors produce pain has yet to be completely elucidated. One source suggests that the tumors themselves may activate nociceptors, or pain receptors, by pressure, ischemia, or secretion of pain-causing substances such as prostaglandin E2 and osteoclast-activating factor (12). Others propose that these tumor secretions may sensitize the pain-sensing nociceptors and make them more susceptible to activation by previously non-activating stimuli (11). Regardless of the source of stimulus, once the nociceptors are activated, the neural signal of pain is conducted through the local A and C pain fibers to the dorsal horn of the spinal cord and up the spinothalamic and spinoreticular tracts to the thalamus and reticular formation.

Other types of pain found in cancer patients, although less likely to be directly associated with metastatic lesions of bone, include visceral and neuropathic pain. Visceral pain is dull in nature and vaguely localized and inconsistent compared to somatic pain. It is usually due to direct noxious stimuli such as ischemia, inflammation, or compression of internal organs. Most often it is associated with pancreatic cancer and other abdominal cancers with mass effect. Although it is not entirely impossible, extensive reviews of previous literature do not reveal any cases of visceral pain associated with osseous metastases.

In contrast, although small in number, there have also been reported cases of neuropathic pain associated with osseous metastases. Neuropathic pain is described as being more prolonged and burning in nature and associated with focal neurological deficits and referred pain to the skin. There are several hypotheses that attempt to describe the origin of neuropathic pain including previous sensitization and overactivation of cutaneous nerve fibers (13), peripheral nerve destruction with disorganized repair and resultant independent depolarization (14), and demyelinated axons with resultant ectopic activity (15). Neuropathic pain is not uncommon in cancer patients and, like somatic bone pain, most often arises from direct infiltration of neurons by tumor, radiation fibrosis, or injury during surgery. With similar sources, similar natures, and the potential for referral, it is possible that neuropathic pain is misinterpreted as or coincides simultaneously with somatic bone pain.

Regardless of whether it is somatic, neuropathic, or both, the predilection for metastatic lesions to the vertebrae also results in most common site of bone pain (Figure 1). Up to 98% of known cancer patients presenting with back pain have underlying metastases (14). Although cancerous lesions are the overwhelming majority of sources of back pain in previously diagnosed patients, it is important to note that less than 1% of back pain in the general population is due to cancer (16). Other sites of pain include the pelvis, femur, rib, proximal humerus, and skull, depending on the distribution of metastatic lesions and previous treatment exposures. In addition to destruction of bone by direct tumor processes, there are also several iatrogenic sources that contribute to pain symptoms in cancer patients. Avascular necrosis of the femoral and humeral heads can occur secondary to steroid treatment. Pseudorheumatism can occur with the rapid withdrawal of corticosteroids. Radiation treatment can result in osteoradionecrosis of any exposed bone, particularly the mandible, after radiation treatment for head and neck cancers (9).

As can be seen here, pain syndromes related to metastatic disease in bone affect a significantly large number of cancer patients. Unfortunately for some of these patients, the extent of this pain far exceeds the standard treatments of chemotherapy, radiation, and analgesics. As conventional treatments fail, researchers and physicians are looking to a new realm of direct application of treatment through interventional and intravascular techniques. Next, we will discuss the role of embolization in cancer pain management. We will look at the various agents and techniques currently being used, their indications, contraindications, benefits, and risks, as well as discuss some of those currently under development.

EMBOLIZATION AGENTS (17,18)

Some of the earliest embolization techniques can be dated back to France in the early 1970s when neurosurgeons injected materials to occlude vessels prior to

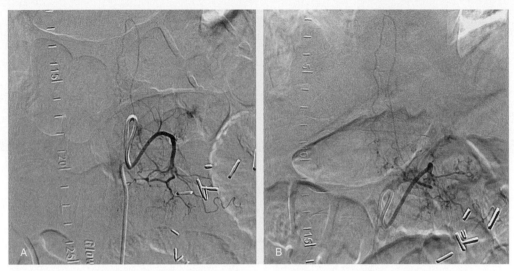

Figure 1. AP (left) and lateral (right) view displaying the classic "hairpin turn" of the artery of Adamkiewicz.

removing spinal hemangiomas (19). Since then, the process has gained in popularity and been adapted and applied to numerous clinical treatments. With such great advancements, and widespread application of embolotherapy, has also come the development of several different agents to suite each specific treatment's needs and requirements. The most common agents used today in the treatment of tumors are steel or platinum coils, gelfoam pledgets or powder, polyvinyl alcohol and acrylic particles, and ethanol. Other agents such as cyanoacrylate adhesive glue, other sclerosants, and detachable balloons are also available but not currently being used widely in cancer therapies.

Coils of stainless steel or platinum are the largest of the agents (Figure 2). They are available in a wide variety of lengths from 1 to 150 mm as well as diameters 2 to 40 mm and require delivery catheters with 0.010- to 0.050-inch inner diameters. They provide permanent occlusion of medium- to large-sized vessels and are thus effective at occluding more proximal vessels. Coils are also available with attached polyester fibers for promoting platelet activation and thrombosis. Their delivery is fast and relatively easy to facilitate. Due to the possibility for collateral vessels distal to the occlusion, coils have a somewhat limited use in tumors. They are more often used to occlude the larger vessels in trauma and adjunctly utilized following particulate embolization therapy.

Another agent used for occlusion of larger vessels is gelfoam or gelatin sponge. This versatile material is supplied as a dry sheet or fine 50-μm grain powder. Sheets are cut into smaller pieces or pledgets depending on the size needed to occlude the vessel and the catheter through which they must fit. Either the pieces or powder is then injected into the vessel via the transcatheter system where they expand to a larger size. Dilute contrast can be added prior to injection in order to better visualize the distribution of the material under fluoroscopy. Coils, thrombin, or other sclerosing agents can also be added to aid in a more complete occlusion.

One needs to be cautious, particularly with gelfoam powder, small particulate agents, and sclerosants, to prevent any reflux of the agent into undesired

203

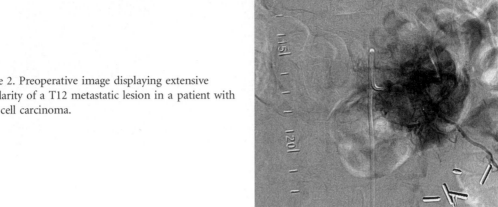

Figure 2. Preoperative image displaying extensive vascularity of a T12 metastatic lesion in a patient with renal cell carcinoma.

vessels. Due to the small size of the particles, gelfoam powder will cause distal ischemia and necrosis of downstream tissues. Inadvertent embolization of normal tissue can be devastating and result in skin ulceration, soft tissue necrosis, and nerve damage. Unlike metal coils, though, gelfoam is a temporary means of occlusion. The material is absorbed and degraded and recanalization of the vessel occurs within 2–6 weeks. For this reason, gelfoam can be used to protectively embolize adjacent vessels during selective tumor embolization with particulates or sclerosants. Similarly, it is generally a poor choice for strict tumor embolization when complete and permanent tumor necrosis is desired.

For occlusion of more distal small arteries and arterioles, the predominant agent is polyvinyl alcohol (PVA) (Figures 3–6). PVA particles are spherically shaped with diameters ranging 50–1200 µm, with the majority between 150 and 200 µm. In addition to occluding the vessel, PVA also produces an inflammatory reaction within the vessel walls that causes sclerosis and further occlusion. Dry particles of PVA are suspended and expand in dilute contrast to enable visualization under fluoroscopy. Albumin can also be added to prevent particle clumping. The suspension is delivered through the catheter system by slowly injecting 0.5-ml pulses under fluoroscopic guidance. The endpoint of embolization occurs when vessel flow slows and delivery of the agent becomes difficult. Care must be taken to prevent injecting beyond the endpoint, which leads to reflux of embolization materials out of the target vessel. Unlike gelfoam, PVA particles are considered a permanent agent. This permanence combined with its ability to occlude small arteries and arterioles, such as those found in collateral vessels, PVA is an ideal agent for restricting the blood supply to tumors. Earlier versions of PVA were prone to clumping with more proximal and less predictable embolization. The recent introduction of spherical PVA has resulted in a more uniform shape and more fluid and predictable delivery of the agent. The authors further stress the need for caution against overinjecting with these newer agents due to their decreased susceptibility for clumping and possible propensity to reflux into nontargeted vessels .

Similar to PVA, acrylic spheres (Trisacryl Embospheres; Biosphere Medical, Rockland, MA) have also been developed for permanent occlusion of small

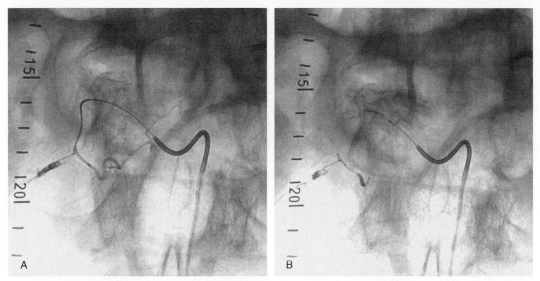

Figure 3. (Left) Example of a 5F guide catheter, microcatheter, and liquid coil in the right intercostal artery prior to embolization. (Right) The microcatheter is then slightly withdrawn and the embolization agent is injected.

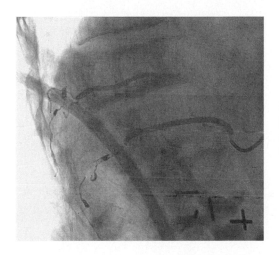

Figure 4. Lateral unsubtracted view status postembolization with coil, particulate, and adhesive glue. The linear opacifications seen are due to the adhesive agent filling the feeding arteries.

arteries and arterioles. They range in size from 40 to 1200 μm in diameter and compress by up to 20%. This unique property allows for more complete occlusion but makes them susceptible to cracking and biodegrading if compressed through a catheter that is too small. Compared to PVA, they are smoother and have fewer tendencies to clump but similarly must be used with contrast in order to visualize their distribution under fluoroscopy.

Absolute (95%) ethanol is a liquid sclerosing agent that causes permanent occlusion at the level of the capillary. This highly toxic substance not only causes death to the previously perfused tissue but also denudes the endothelium of the vessel wall and causes an immediate inflammatory reaction, which results in thrombosis. This property makes ethanol a very effective, although painful, technique for tumor ablation and subsequent pain control. Due to the painfulness of alcohol embolization, the procedure is usually performed under general anesthesia.

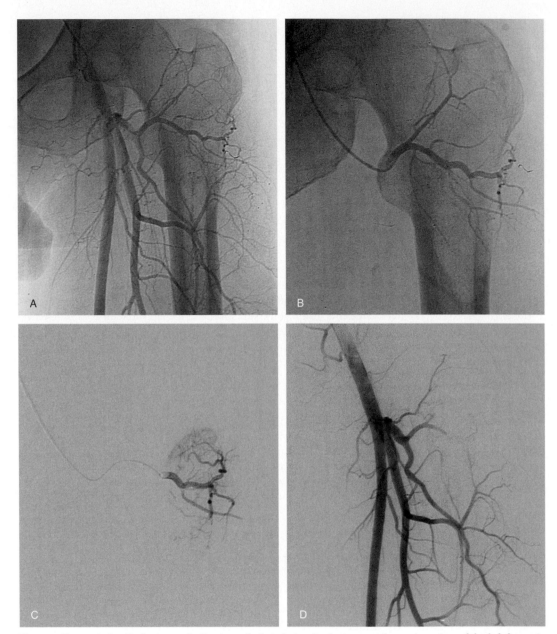

Figure 5. Image series displaying embolization of a lytic lesion in the intertrochanteric region of the left femur in a patient with renal cell carcinoma. The majority of the tumor is being supplied by a branch of the left profunda artery (A). A 5F catheter was used to select the lateral branch of the profunda artery (B). A microcatheter was then used to subselect the primary vessel feeding the tumor (C). The result was near obliteration of the tumor vasculature with preservation of the muscular branches of the artery (D).

Extreme caution must be taken when working with ethanol. Inadvertent embolization can lead to devastating complications. The volume needed to fill the vascular bed should be estimated by first injecting contrast to the desired level of embolization. Small increments of this amount are then slowly delivered through the lumen of an occlusion balloon placed just proximal to the desired delivery site. Not only does the occlusion balloon prevent reflux of

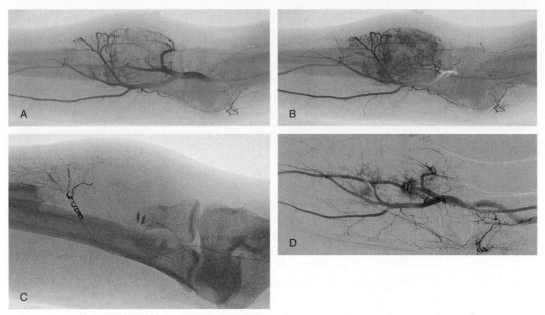

Figure 6. Preoperative embolization of a renal cell metastases to the right radius. The arterial (A) and capillary (B) phases of the arteriogram display an extensive hypervascular mass with severe destruction of the proximal radius. Subselective catheterization of the interosseous artery was performed with subsequent treatment using PVA particles and steel coils (C). Postembolization arteriography displays a successful 90% devascularization of the tumor (D).

the toxic substance into nontargeted vessels but it also diminishes flow into the targeted vessel, thus delaying washout of the agent. In addition to being a powerful tool for cancer treatment, ethanol is also used to treat arteriovenous malformation by essentially eliminating the conduit between the artery and the vein. Other sclerosing agents such as sotradecol are also available but have extremely limited use in tumor embolization according to their frequency in the literature.

Finally, there is the highly viscous ethiodol. This iodinated oil is capable of occluding small vessel but is most often used as a vehicle for chemoembolization of liver tumors. In particular, hepatomas have a specific affinity for ethiodol. The combined agents are injected into the vasculature and drawn to the site of the hepatic tumor. Due to the iodination, this process can easily be monitored and managed under fluoroscopy.

Now that we have had a brief overview of embolization agents, let us now turn to their specific techniques and applications for pain management of skeletal metastases.

APPLICATIONS OF EMBOLIC AGENTS IN PAIN MANAGEMENT

The proposed mechanisms by which embolization therapy provides pain relief in patients with metastatic disease are twofold. Dramatic direct and indirect effects can ultimately result in decreased pain and suffering for these patients.

Directly, by cutting off the feeding blood supply to a metastatic lesion, embolic therapies can lead to a reduction in tumor size, growth, and ultimate mass effect. Indirectly, by restricting blood flow to cancerous tissue preoperatively, researchers have seen a significant reduction in intraoperative blood loss as well as associated postoperative complications. Although most research has been done on patients with metastatic lesions of the spine and pelvis, the concepts and applications of embolic therapy have been applied for osseous lesions throughout the body.

Direct Palliative Therapy

Embolization has become a key component for patients seeking direct palliative therapy for pain relief. As both a primary treatment for symptomatic lesions and a secondary treatment for those who have failed other modalities, embolization is providing treatment to patients previously refractory to surgery, radiation, or chemotherapy as well as those who are poor operative candidates or have recurrent, multiple, or unresectable lesions (20). The exact mechanism by which pain relief occurs in these patients is not completely clear. It is suggested that a reduction in tumor size results in a decrease in the expansion pressure and stretching of the periosteal nerves that cause somatic pain (21). One study showed an 80% reduction in tumor size and an associated complete relief of pain in 100% of patients (22).

Another more recent study reports a mean tumor reduction of only 50%, but this, too, was associated with complete relief of pain in all patients (23). In this same study, of those with unresectable bone metastases strictly treated for pain and not tumor reduction, 64% were completely free of pain following embolization, 27% were significantly free of pain, and 9% had some relief of pain. None of the patients needed further pain management by opiates following embolization.

Throughout these studies, a variety of embolic agents have been used. These include PVA, gelfoam, coils, and sclerosants used either independently or in various combinations. Provided successful embolization, symptomatic relief occurs regardless of agent in the majority of patients. Successful embolization is defined by most studies as hypoattenuation on CT or low-intensity signal on MR resembling necrosis and/or a decrease in tumor perfusion of less than 25% (23). Although there have been successes with individual agents, there have been few studies comparing various agents in patients with metastases to bone. One study did do a comparison of PVA and acrylic microspheres in patients with meningiomas and found no significant difference in the amount of tumor necrosis and size reduction between the two agents (24).

The majority of these studies report immediate pain relief within the first 12 hours to a few days of embolization (17–23). Delay of pain relief is most frequently attributed to postembolic pain syndrome. This collection of symptoms includes nausea, vomiting, fever, ileus, leukocytosis, as well as transient pain and discomfort, but typically resolves within 1–2 weeks. The duration over which patients remain symptom free ranges from 2 to 9 months (17–23). Some researchers relate this temporary relief to the completeness of occlusion and availability of collateral circulation (21). Fortunately for these patients, embolization can be repeated as needed for palliation provided there is no contraindication for intervention (25). However, proximal coil embolization should be utilized judiciously due to the possible need for access to more distal vessels supplying the tumor during later treatments.

In addition to pain relief from the mass effect of tumors within bone, patients who have undergone embolic therapy have also gained relief of pain from neurological compromise (25,26). Similar to the relief of osseous pain, these neurological symptoms may be relieved for several months to years. In addition, embolization may obviate the need for surgical management. There is even a case report of a patient with acute spinal cord compression from metastatic lesion being primarily treated with embolization without previous surgery or radiation (27). The patient not only had decreased pain but also decreased spinal compression on MRI and improved movement, sensation, and neurological function.

The direct delivery of chemotherapy drugs in addition to the embolic agents has also been described. This method of tumor treatment has been used for several years in the treatment of secondary hepatic tumors and has expanded its applications to also include osseous metastases. There are two main purposes of using this combination of therapies (28). Primarily, the embolic agent causes a decrease in arterial flow, thus decreasing washout of the chemotherapy agent applied. In addition, the anoxic environment created by embolization impedes a tumor cell's ability to actively pump the chemotherapeutics out of their intracellular environment. These two mechanisms ultimately result in a higher concentration of the chemotherapy drug acting on the target tumor.

Various combinations of embolic and chemotherapy agents have been used in this technique. The most common embolic agents have included gelfoam, microspheres, ethiodized oil, and PVA particles. Again, there is no literature to suggest any one material is superior to any other. The temporary agents like gelfoam and ethiodized oil have the advantage of allowing for recanalization and thus repeat treatments via the same vessel. When using permanent acrylic microspheres or PVA, repeat treatment is also possible but must be done through collateral vessels downstream of the initial occlusion (Tables 2, 3).

In addition to embolization alone, chemotherapy agents have also been used in conjunction with occlusive agents. The type of chemotherapy used is dependant on type of primary tumor involved as well as any response or lack thereof to previous chemotherapy attempts. A small study out of Japan was performed with mitomycin-C in patients with bone metastases. The endpoints here were tumor response and decrease in pain. Objective tumor response and a complete remission of pain were seen in 75% of the lesions examined. These effects were then maintained for the mean follow-up period of 17 months (29). A similar study in Europe looked at carboplatin and pirarubicin mixed with PVA for palliative therapy in patients with inoperable pelvic and spine metastases. Eighty-three percent of these patients who had previously failed general chemotherapy and radiotherapy had significant pain relief following chemoembolization. These effects then lasted a mean duration of 12 months. Moreover, none of these patients studied encountered postembolization syndrome as has been seen in so many others treated with embolic therapy.

Table 2. Endovascular Embolization Agents

Agent	Sizes	Permanence	Occlusion Site	Other
Coils	Length: 2–30 mm, width: 2–40 mm, diameter 0.010–0.050 inch	Permanent	Medium-large arteries	Available with attached polyester fibers for activating further thrombosis
Gelatin sponge	Dry sheet or fine 50-µm diameter powder	Temporary, recanalize within 2–6 weeks	Medium-Large	Caution with powder due to increased risk of reflux
PVA	50- to 1200-µm diameter particles (most 150–200 µm)	Permanent	Small arteries and arterioles	Most commonly used
Acrylic microspheres	200- to 1200-µm diameter particles	Permanent	Small arteries and arterioles	Compressible, less tendency to clump compared to PVA
Absolute (95%) ethanol	Liquid, limit use to <25 ml	Permanent	Small arteries and arterioles	Highly toxic, painful
Ethiodol	Iodinated oil	Permanent	Small arteries	Most often used with chemoembolization

Table 3. Common Agent Manufacturers

Agent	Manufacturer
Coils	Platinum; Boston Scientific, Fremont, CA
	Gianturco, Tornado, nester stainless steel; Cook, Bloomington, IN
	Hilal microcoils; Cook, Bloomington, IN
Gelatin sponge	Gelfoam; Upjohn, Kalamazoo, MI
PVA	Invalon; Nycomed Medical Systems, Paris, France
	Contour SE; Boston Scientific, Fremont, CA
	Bead Block; Terumo, Sommerset, NJ
Acrylic microspheres	Embospheres; Boston Scientific, Rockland, MA

The method of delivery of the embolic and chemotherapy agents is a multistep process. After the feeding artery is identified by superselective angiography, the chemotherapy agent combined with the embolic agent is delivered via the transcatheter system until blood flow is static. If the embolization agent is ethiodized oil, the artery is often then embolized with an additional particulate such as gelfoam or PVA. In some cases, additional chemotherapy agents are also added after the initial chemoembolization injection in order to provide an additional dose of chemotherapy agent. As with all embolization procedures, special care must be taken to ensure there is no reflux of embolic or chemo agent into nontargeted vessels. With the positive results currently encountered in this area of research, combination therapy with embolization and chemotherapy will undoubtedly lead to further use and application in the future.

Indirect Palliative Therapy

Whereas some patients encounter pain relief by the direct effects described earlier, many also benefit from other indirect means as well. Neovascularity in tumors is quite common (23). In particular, renal cell carcinoma, thyroid cancer, and multiple myeloma are prone to high levels of vascularization and characteristic hemorrhagic response. In those with renal cell and thyroid carcinoma, 30–45% are estimated to have bone metastases and of these lesions, 65–75% are hypervascular (21–23,30). Other tumors with this vascular propensity include angiosarcoma, leiomyosarcoma, hepatocellular carcinoma, and some neuroendocrine tumors (20). For patients with these types of tumors that require surgical resection, technical difficulties involving excessive hemorrhage are of great concern. Fortunately, due to interventional techniques, preoperative embolization of these tumors has lead to a dramatic decrease in intraoperative blood loss as well as a significant decrease in various postoperative complications (21–23,30).

Preoperative embolization is the most frequent indication for transcatheter embolization. Over 70% of these embolic therapy procedures are performed with the purpose of optimizing surgical procedures and results (23). It is suggested that the best candidates for such intervention are those with intermediate-sized metastatic lesions of bone with planned intralesional resection or curettage. There is little to no indication for small lesions when expected intraoperative blood loss is very low. In constrast, for cases of large lesions requiring wide radical resection, embolization is relatively contraindicated due to the extensive hypervascularity it promotes in the tissue surrounding the tumor and risk of high-volume hemorrhage during a large surgical resection.

Similar to the technical success of palliative therapy, preoperative embolization is considered successful when less than one-quarter of the tumor remains perfused following treatment and blood loss during surgery is less than 1,500 ml (23). Early studies report losses as low as 450–750 ml in 75% of patients with technically successful occlusion (30). Other studies report mean losses between 1,000 and 2,000 ml. This is significantly lower than those in control groups without embolization who typically lose between 2,000 and 18,000 ml (20,30–38). Even partially embolized lesions have been shown to have a significantly lower blood loss than nonembolized lesions (36).

In a case performed by the author, a patient with renal cell carcinoma metastatic to the right radius underwent embolization prior to surgical resection (see Figure 6). The estimated blood loss by the orthopaedic team was a mere 150 ml and postoperative pain was reported to be minimal.

This dramatic decrease in operative blood loss has also contributed to greater intraoperative clarity and less complicated surgical course (35). Other benefits of preoperative embolization indirectly contributing to improved patient pain and morbidity are decreased operative time (39), decreased number of transfusions (34,37), as well as some cases of decreased hospital stay (32).

Various agents have been used in cases of preoperative embolization, though some have been shown to have greater efficacy than others. Coils, ethanol, and gelatin are less often used when compared to PVA. Coils alone, which can be equated to proximal surgical ligation, have been found to have no significant effect on intraoperative blood loss in hypervascular spinal metastases (40). Similarly, coils have not shown any additional benefit when combined with other agents such as PVA. One study indicates coils might be more useful preoperatively in the protective embolization of arteries distal to the origin of tumor feeders (37). Such use reduces the need for superselective catheterization of the tumor feeders themselves and eliminates inadvertent embolization of downstream tissues. Due to their increased rates of neurological complications, liquid agents such as ethanol and adhesives are also less often used (41).

Timing of surgery after treatment is of particular of concern when it comes to the efficacy of gelfoam. In one study, patients undergoing surgery three days after embolization suffered substantial blood losses intraoperatively due to the rapid revascularization of the tumor via collateral vessels (32). As an easily degradable and temporary agent, gelfoam use is recommended only for cases where surgery will be performed within 24 hours (32). In addition, other studies also suggest that gelfoam might be less reliable at decreasing intraoperative blood loss when compared to PVA particles (34,42).

Due to these issues and complications with various other agents, a large number of preoperative embolizations are performed using PVA. As mentioned previously, PVA particles are available in a range of sizes from 50 to 1200 μm. Some studies indicate there is no significant difference in intraoperative blood loss when larger (250–500 μm) diameter particles are used when compared to smaller (<250 μm) diameter particles (36). In one report, even cases of incomplete embolization with particles of either size had a significantly lower mean blood loss of 2,000 ml compared to controls with losses of 5,000 ml. This number was further reduced to 1,500 ml in patients with complete occlusion. With the increased risk of occluding end arteries associated with smaller particles, and comparable occlusion rates, many physicians prefer the using larger particles. This is especially true when treating spinal metastases and there is risk of compromising the vascular supply to the spinal cord (36). The authors prefer to use particles smaller than 250 μm if subselecting the vasculature of the tumor only. Smaller particles lead to more tumor cell necrosis. However, if there is any risk of embolizing adjacent tissue, particles larger than 250 μm are indicated to prevent possible necrosis of nontargeted tissue.

TECHNICAL CONSIDERATIONS

In general, subselective embolization of tumors is preferred. This safer delivery of agent to the tumor with minimal embolization of the adjacent tissue may require microcatheter selection of individual feeding branches of tumors. Approximately 75–80% of the authors' embolizations are performed using a combined system of a microcatheter placed through a standard guide catheter. Microcatheters also help limit catheter-induced vasospasm, which can result in inadequate tumor embolization. If microcoils are a part of the procedure, standard microcatheters (RapidTransit, Cordis; Renegade, Boston

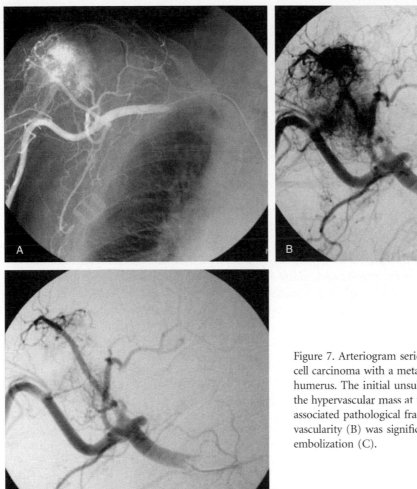

Figure 7. Arteriogram series of patient with renal cell carcinoma with a metastatic lesion in the right humerus. The initial unsubtracted view displays the hypervascular mass at the surgical neck and an associated pathological fracture (A). The extensive vascularity (B) was significantly reduced following embolization (C).

Scientific; Tracker, Boston Scientific) are usually used. If PVA or acrylic microspheres are the primary agents being used, the author typically utilizes high-flow microcatheters (Renegade HI-FLO; Boston Scientific) that have a largen lumen diameter and are less prone to particulate occlusion. However, these microcatheters are not recommended for use with microcoils due to the propensity for the microcoils to become lodged within the lumen of the microcatheter.

It is important to note there is one anatomic area of particular concern and need for increased caution. When treating lesions of the spine, it is important to perform a thorough preprocedure angiogram to identify not only the vessels feeding the tumor but also any contribution of these vessels to the arterial supply of the spinal cord. The radiculomeduallary branch of the anterior spinal artery, also known as the major anterior segmental medullary artery or artery of Adamkiewicz (see Figure 7), has many anatomical variants and can arise as a branch of the aorta, an intercostal, or a lumbar artery. Typically, this occurs on the left side (80%) between T8 and L4. This crucial vessel supplies the lower two-third of the spinal cord. Any unintended embolization would have devastating consequences. The suggested angiographic protocol includes the bilateral examination of the intercostal or lumbar arteries at the affected level of the metastatic lesion as well as the vessels at least two levels superior and inferior to the level of the lesion (20,33). The segmental vessels supplying the spinal cord, particularly the artery of Adamkiewicz that demonstrates a classic "hairpin course" (see Figure 7), should also be specifically identified. If an anterior spinal artery shares the same pedicle of the feeding artery of the tumor, embolization is contraindicated and should be avoided due to risk of occluding arterial blood supply to a major portion of the spinal cord.

As illustrated here, the application of embolic therapy for the treatment of pain in metastatic lesions is rapidly expanding. New agents and techniques continue to be developed in an attempt to alleviate the pain and suffering of these previously unrelieved patients. By decreasing the vascularity and blood supply feeding these tumors, physicians are seeing a dramatic relief of pain and morbidity, both directly and indirectly. Hopefully, the decreases in tumor size and associated complications such as intraoperative blood loss are just the beginning of the benefits experienced by these patients secondary to embolic therapy.

REFERENCES

1. Randall RL. Tumors in Orthopedics. Current Diagnosis and Treatment in Orthopedics – 3rd Ed. Lange/McGraw-Hill: online edition, 2003. http://utdol.statref.com/document.aspx?fxid=46&docid=186

2. Sartor OA, DiBiase SJ, Management of Bone Metastases in Advanced Prostate Cancer. UpToDate Online 13.3, 2005. http:// utdol.com/application/topic/print.asp?file=prost_ca/7518.

3. Guise TA, Mundy GR. Cancer and bone. Endocr Rev 1998;19:18.

4. Nelson JB, Nabulsi AA, Vogelzang NJ, et al. Suppression of prostate cancer induced bone remodeling by endothelin receptor A antagonist atrasentan. J Urol 2003; 169:1143.

5. Hatrick NC, Lucas JD, Timothy AR, et al. The surgical treatment of metastatic disease of the spine. Radiother Oncol 2000;56:335–9.

6. Fornasier VL, Horne JG. Metastases to the vertebral column. Cancer 1975;36: 590–594.

7. Cleveland CS, Gonin R, Hatfield AK, et al. Pain and its treatment in outpatients with metastatic cancer. N Engl J Med 1994;330:592.

8. Twycross RG, Fairfield S. Pain in far-advanced cancer. Pain 1982;14:303.

9. Foley KM. Pain syndromes in patients with cancer. In: Advances in Pain Research and Therapy, Bonica JJ, Ventafridda B (Eds), Raven Press, New York, 1979, p. 59.

10. Portenoy RK. Cancer pain: epidemiology and syndromes. Cancer 1989;63:2298.

11. Bajwa ZH, Warfield CA. Cancer Pain and Cancer Pain Syndromes. UpToDate Online 13.3, 2005. www.uptodate.com

12. Honore P, Luger NM, Sabino MA, et al. Osteoprotegerin blocks bone cancer-induced skeletal destruction, skeletal pain and pain-related neurochemical reorganization of the spinal cord. Nat Med 2000;6:521.

13. Hu S, Zhu J. Sympathetic facilitation of sustained discharges of polymodal nociceptors. Pain 1989;38:85.

14. Devor M. Neuropathic pain and injured nerve: peripheral mechanisms. Br Med Bull 1991;47:619.

15. Burchiel KJ. Abnormal impulse generation in focally demyelinated trigeminal roots. J Neurosurg 1980;53:674.

16. Deyo RA, Diehl AK. Cancer as a cause of back pain: frequency, clinical presentation, and diagnostic strategies. J Gen Intern Med 1988;3:230.

17. Valji K. Vascular and Interventional Radiology. Saunders, Philadelphia, 1999, pp. 31–34.

18. Kaufman JA, Lee, MJ. The Requisites, Vascular and Interventional Radiology. Elsevier, Philadelphia, 2004, pp. 105–13.

19. Lepoire J, Montaut J, Picard L, Heppner H, Masingue M, Arnould G. Embolization preparatory to excision of spinal hemangioma. Neurochirurgie (France) 1973 Mar–Apr; 173–81.

20. Gottfried ON, Schloesser PE, Schmidt MH, Stevens EA. Embolization of metastatic spinal tumors. Neurosurg Clin N Am 2004;15:391–9.

21. Chuang VP, Wallace S, Swanson D, et al. Arterial occlusion in the management of pain from metastatic renal carcinoma. Radiology 1979;133(3 Part 1):611–14.

22. Varma J, Huben RP, Wajsman Z, Pontes JE. Therapeutic embolization of pelvic metastases of renal cell carcinoma. J Urol 1984;131:647–9.

23. Barton PP, Waneck RE, Reinhart E, et al. Embolization of bone metastases. JVIR7 1996;(1) Jan–Feb: 81–8.

24. Bendszus M, Klein R, Burger R, Warmuth-Metz M, Hofmann E, Solymosi L. Efficacy of Trisacryl gelatin microspheres versus polyvinyl alcohol particles in the preoperative embolization of meningiomas. Am J Neuroradiol Feb 2000;21:255–61.

25. Smit JW, Vielvoye GL, Goslings BM. Embolization of solitary spinal metastases for renal cell carcinoma: alternative therapy for spinal cord or nerve root compression. Surg Neurol 1989;31(4):268–71.

26. Coutheoux P, Alachkar F, Casasco A, et al. Arterial occlusion in the management of lumbar spine metastases. A preliminary study. J Neuroradiol 1985;12(2):151–2.

27. keuther TA, Nesbit GM, Barnwell SL. Embolization as treatment for spinal compression from renal cell carcinoma: case report. Surg Neurol 1989;31(4):268–71.

28. Coldwell DM, Stokes KR, Yakes WF. Embolotherapy: agents, clinical applications, and techniques. Radiographics 1994;14:623–43.

29. Kakinuma H, Sato K, Miura K, Sasaki S, Kato T. Chemoembolization with mitomycin-C microcapsules (MMC-mc) in the treatment of bone metastases from prostatic and renal cancer. Nippon Hinyokika Gakkai Zasshi 1994 Jul;85(7):1116–23.

30. Bowers TA, Murray, Charnsangavej C, Soo CS, Chuang VP, Wallace S. Bone metastases from renal carcinoma: the preoperative use of transcatheter arterial occlusion. J Bone Joint Surg 1982;64:749–54.

31. Roscoe MW, McBroom RJ, St. Louis E, Grossman H, Perrin R. Preoperative embolization in the treatment of osseous metastases from renal cell carcinoma. Clin Orthop Relat Res 1989 Jan;(238):302–7.

32. Gellad FR, Sadato N, Numaguchi Y, Levine AM. Vascular metastatic lesions of the spine: preoperative embolization. Radiology 1990;176:683–6.

33. Breslau J, Eskridge JM. Preoperative embolization of spinal tumors. J Vasc Interv Radiol 1995; Nov–Dec;6:871–5.

34. Smith TP, Gray L, Weinstein JN, Richardson WJ, Payne CS. Preoperative transarterial embolization of spinal neoplasms. J Vasc Interv Radiol 1995 Nov–Dec;6:863–9.

35. Hess T, Kramann B, Schmidt E, Rupp S. Use of preoperative vascular embolization in spinal metastasis resection. Arch Orthop Trauma Surg. 1997;116(5):279–82.

36. Manke C, Bretschneider T, Lenhart M, Strotzer M, Meumann C, Gmeinwieser J, Feuerbach S. Spinal metastases from renal cell carcinoma: effect of preoperative particle embolization on intraoperative blood loss. Am J Neuroradiol 2001; 22:997–1003.

37. Wirbel RJ, Roth R, Schulte M, Kramann B, Mutschler W. Preoperative embolization in spinal and pelvic metastases. J Orthop Sci 2005;10:253–7.

38. Guzman R, Dubah-Schwier S, Heini P, Lovblad KO, Kalbermatten D, Schroth G, Remonda L. Preoperative transarterial embolization of vertebral metastases. Eur Spine J 2005 Apr;14(3):263–8.
39. Bhojraj SY, Dandawate AV, Ramakantan R. Preoperative embolization, transpedicular decompression and posterior stabilization for metastatic disease of the thoracic spine causing paraplegia. Paraplegia 1992;30(4):292–9.
40. Berkefeld J, Scale D, Kirchner J, Heinrich T, Kollath J. Hypervascular spinal tumors: influence of the embolization technique on perioperative hemorrhage. Am J Neuroradiol 1999;20:757–63.
41. Rossi C, Ricci S, Boriani S, et al. Percutaneous transcatheter arterial embolization of bone and soft tissue tumors. Skeletal Radiol 1990;19:555–60.
42. Olerud C, Jonson H Jr., Lofberg AM, Lorelius LE, Sjostrom L. Embolization of spinal metastases reduces perioperative blood loss: 21 patients operated on for renal cell carcinoma. Acta Orthop Scand 1993;64:9–12.

Image-Guided Ablation of Painful Osteolyses

David T. Wang and Charles E. Ray, Jr.

INTRODUCTION

In the past, strategies for the mitigation of tumor pain have been limited to surgery, radiotherapy, or pharmacotherapy. Unfortunately, in many cases, these strategies fail because of increased morbidity, poor patient tolerability, or incomplete pain palliation. Though often curative, surgical excision is limited to the few who are adequate surgical candidates. In addition, surgery for tumors involving or adjacent to critical neurovascular structures, such as the spine, can be associated with significant morbidity.

Radiotherapy is considered by some to be the standard of care for patients with localized bone pain; however, the maximum benefit of radiotherapy may not be realized until 12–20 weeks later, with 50% having no benefit within four weeks (1). Furthermore, some tumors are insensitive to radiation therapy, and as a result 20–30% of patients who receive radiation therapy fail to respond (2). Moreover, the risk of irradiating normal tissue prevents repeated cycles of radiation therapy from becoming an effective long-term treatment option.

Pharmacotherapy may reduce pain in some patients; however, side effects from both opioid and nonopioid analgesics can be intolerable. Likewise, toxicity and/or poor therapeutic response limit the effectiveness of chemotherapy.

More options are becoming available in the management of cancer pain. In particular, interventional radiology has much to offer with regard to percutaneous or minimally invasive techniques. Any means by which percutaneous, controlled tissue necrosis of targeted tissue can be achieved has potential application. In practice, the main percutaneous strategies employ thermal ablation (burning or freezing) or chemical ablation (dehydration). Both strategies can provide either cure by direct tumor destruction or palliation by destruction of nerves compromised by the tumor.

THERMAL ABLATION

Thermal ablation can be accomplished in many ways. The most widely utilized thermal modality is radiofrequency ablation with other modalities such as laser ablation, extracorporeal high-intensity focused ultrasound (HIFU), and microwave ablation gaining popularity. Cryoablation, another popular ablative method, is categorized as a special case within the armamentarium of thermal therapies since it has its effect by freezing rather than heating tissue. Regardless of the modality, the goal of thermal ablation is to achieve controlled destruction of target tissue by exposing it to temperatures over 46°C or below −5°C, temperatures certain to produce coagulation necrosis (3).

Indications

Tumors involving bone are particularly painful. Although the pathophysiology is not clearly understood, stimulation of endosteal and periosteal nerve fibers by inflammatory agents resulting from bone destruction and direct stretching of nerve fibers from tumor expansion are probably the main mechanisms leading to pain (4).

Whether benign or malignant, the prototypical bone lesion best suited to thermal ablation is going to be small (less than 4 cm) (5), well marginated, easily localized with imaging, and situated away from critical neurovascular structures.

Osteoid osteoma typically meets these criteria and, therefore, is the most common bone lesion treated with thermal ablation. Considered benign, osteoid osteoma classically presents in the pediatric population. Frequently within the cortex of long bones, osteoid osteoma has a characteristic radiolucent nidus that is a meshwork of bone trabeculae with fibrous, vascular, and nervous tissue components (6). Classically, this lesion is more painful at night, often relieved with salicylates, and surprisingly painful despite its small size (typically less than 1.5 cm). Although the natural history of this lesion is spontaneous regression over years, the severity of pain can prompt treatment. Traditional treatment options included oral analgesics and surgical excision. However, for many patients, side effects from prolonged ingestion of nonsteroidal anti-inflammatory agents and complications from surgery make percutaneous thermal ablation attractive.

In addition to osteoid osteoma, palliation of pain from other primary bone tumors or metastases is another common indication for thermal ablation. When other strategies such as radiotherapy, surgery, and chemotherapy have failed or are contraindicated, thermal ablation of bone metastases may eliminate pain, improve quality of life, and decrease oral narcotic usage.

Contraindications to thermal ablation include bone lesions involving neurovascular bundles that, if compromised, could lead to paralysis or hemorrhage; spinal and sacral lesions are typical lesions that fall into this category. Bone lesions adjacent to a hollow viscus also present strategic challenges because thermal ablative techniques could cause perforation.

Radiofrequency Ablation

Radiofrequency ablation (RFA) for the treatment of malignant disease was first described in 1990 by McGahan et al., when his group used it to treat hepatic tumors (7). Since then, RFA has been used to treat renal, adrenal, breast, pulmonary, cerebral, prostatic, thyroid, parathyroid, and musculoskeletal neoplasms. In 1992, Rosenthal et al. used RFA in the treatment of osteoid osteoma, which lead to its subsequent application in the treatment of other painful bone lesions including chondroblastomas, hemangiomas, epithelioid hemangioendotheliomas, and metastases (8).

The efficacy of RFA in osteoid osteoma is well established. Rosenthal et al. reported complete pain relief two years post-RFA (the accepted time period to declare cure in the orthopedic literature) in 89% of the 126 procedures his group performed. In those patients who received RFA as their initial treatment, the success rate was 91% (9). Relief of pain from RFA of osteoid osteoma occurs within 24–48 hours (10).

The efficacy of RFA in osteolytic metastases has been demonstrated. Callstrom et al. and Goetz et al. reported similar results showing significant decreases in Brief Pain Index "worst pain in a 24-hour period" score that were sustained through 24 weeks (the mean survival time in patients with bone metastases) (2,11). Ninety-five percent of patients in the study by Goetz et al. experienced a greater than two-point drop in worst pain score in a 24-hour period (2). Furthermore, the mean worst pain score continued to decline through the 24th week post-RFA with an overall 69% decrease in mean worst pain score from before RFA. Other endpoints such as narcotic analgesic use also had decreasing trends by the 12th week post-RFA. Opioid use did increase at the 24th week, but this was attributed to pain from other locations (2).

EQUIPMENT

In RFA, a high-frequency alternating current (450–500 kHz) is used to emit radio waves from the tip of an electrode or needle inserted into targeted tissue. This alternating current is transmitted from the electrode to the tissue, causing vibration of local ions, thereby producing controlled frictional heat and a predictable zone of coagulation necrosis. The electrode is powered by an RF generator for which grounding pads must be used to complete the circuit.

The earliest RF electrodes were designed to produce focused tissue destruction for delicate ablation of cerebral seizure foci or aberrant cardiac conduction circuits and, therefore, were small. The utility of these small monopolar electrodes to produce necrosis was limited to a 1.6-cm diameter (12). Attempts to overcome this size limitation has led to the development of the multitined expandable electrode (umbrella RF electrode), the bipolar array, the cluster electrode, the perfusion electrode, and the internally cooled electrode (13), all of which have unique advantages and disadvantages beyond the scope of this chapter. These newer electrodes are capable of producing coagulation necrosis as large as 7 cm.

IMAGING

Whether confirming diagnosis or planning percutaneous access, preprocedural imaging is important for all ablative strategies. Preprocedural imaging may include conventional radiography, computed tomography (CT), magnetic resonance (MR) imaging, radionuclide bone scanning, fluoroscopy, or ultrasound. In fact, most patients with osteolyses will present to the interventionalist with multiple studies as part of their initial evaluation.

Intraprocedural imaging is the backbone of interventional radiology and indispensable with regard to percutaneous ablation. CT guidance is probably the most popular imaging modality; however, ultrasound and MR offer reasonable alternatives. Advantages of CT guidance include near-real-time monitoring of the zone of coagulation necrosis and, with regard to osteoid osteoma, CT offers superior nidus conspicuity. Ultrasound is more commonly used to guide ablation of soft tissue tumors, that is, liver or kidney lesions, but can also be used to image bone. Limitations of ultrasound result from the hyperechogenicity and gas produced by RFA that obscure accurate placement of additional electrodes (13). MR provides near-real-time imaging of coagulation necrosis similar to CT, and discrimination of ablated tissue can be followed by monitoring changes in the T1 signal (13). Caution should be exercised when using real-time imaging to declare treatment efficacy, particularly in malignant disease, because microscopic disease excluded from ablation may be inconspicuous at the time but later develops as tumor recurrence. Furthermore, as some chemotherapeutic agents can potentiate coagulation necrosis several days following ablation, the region of coagulation necrosis may be underestimated (13).

Postprocedural imaging is necessary to ensure adequate tumor ablation. Ideally, to ensure the greatest probability for successful retreatment repeat ablation should occur when residual or recurrent tumor is at the smallest detectable size. Although no strict guidelines exist, some authors recommend follow-up imaging in four weeks, whereas others recommend follow-up imaging should occur at approximately one year (13). Contrast-enhanced imaging will probably offer the best discrimination between recurrence and ablated tissue, and contrast-enhanced CT and MR are the most commonly used. Ultrasound with microbubble contrast may also be helpful. Finally, positron emission tomography may emerge as a useful follow-up imaging modality; however, it has challenges discriminating between residual tumor and the hypermetabolic inflammatory rim surrounding ablated tissue.

METHOD

Using the imaging modality of preference (CT, MR, fluoroscopy, or ultrasound), the bone lesion (primary or metastatic) is localized. Grounding pads are placed on the patient at equidistant sites from the RF source, and the patient skin is prepared using aseptic precautions. With or without periprocedural antibiotic prophylaxis, the patient is then anesthetized or consciously sedated.

Access to the bone lesion is sought through the shortest possible route unless prohibited by adjacent neurovascular structures that could be compromised. Ensuring adequate infiltration of local anesthetic, a skin incision large enough to accommodate the RF probe is made. The lesion is accessed with a bone-cutting biopsy needle of appropriate size (11–16 gauge); on occasion, a drill may be required to penetrate cortical bone. At this point, if the diagnosis is in doubt, as with an equivocal case of osteoid osteoma, biopsies may be obtained.

An appropriate RF electrode for the particular size lesion is introduced under image guidance. In the case of osteoid osteoma, the electrode is placed directly into the nidus. This maneuver should be done under general anesthesia because of intense pain that could cause patient movement jeopardizing electrode position (14). The RF generator is activated and the temperature allowed to rise to 100°C. At this target temperature, Callstrom et al. continue RF treatment for a minimum of five minutes, with a goal of 5–15 minutes (11). However, this time will vary with lesion size and the number and type of RF electrodes used. Upon successful ablation, the electrode is removed with or without tract cauterization, and local anesthetic may be injected into the surrounding soft tissues prior to wound dressing.

Some authors advocate cementoplasty for those patients where compromised bone integrity may lead to fracture. Following RFA of osteoid osteoma, most patients may bear weight immediately and return to normal activity and recreation. (14), although some authors caution against prolonged distance running (9).

COMPLICATIONS

In addition to the usual complications of bleeding and infection, the most common, and probably the most preventable, complication of RFA is a skin burn. Commonly, burns can occur at the probe entry site. Burns can also occur when metal instruments on the skin become heated by RF energy or when grounding pads are improperly placed. An incision at the RF probe entry point allowing for skin retraction can minimize skin surface burns. Another strategy to prevent skin burns is to wrap the probe with gauze moistened with chilled sterile water.

Less common than burns, neuropathy is serious problem that can occur when RF energy affects adjacent neurovascular structures, such as with spinal or pelvic lesions. Goetz et al. reported transient urinary incontinence in one patient who had treatment of a previously irradiated sacral metastasis (2). Nakatsuka et al. reported incomplete hemiplegia and radiculopathy in patients with spinal osteolyses (15).

Other possible complications include fractures, muscular hematomas, paresthesias, and osteomyelitis. Treatment failure, of course, is another possible adverse outcome.

MICROWAVE ABLATION

One of the newest thermal ablative techniques, microwave ablation uses electromagnetic energy with a frequency near 900 MHz to excite water molecules, producing friction and heat, and thereby inducing cell death by coagulation necrosis. Microwave ablation was first reported by Seki et al. in 1994 in the treatment of small hepatocellular carcinomas (16). Since then, microwave ablation has found experimental application in primary and metastatic tumors of liver, lung, kidney, adrenal gland, and bone.

In 1996, Fan et al. reported using intraoperative direct microwave thermal ablation in 62 patients with different bone tumors (17). After isolating tumor from adjacent normal tissue, the tumor was heated with a microwave antenna array while cooling the adjacent tissue with circulating water. Local tumor control was obtained in 57 of 62 patients (17).

In 2006, Simon and Dupuy reported a case of severe pain from a metastatic bladder cancer to the acetabulum of a 70-year-old male who failed radiation therapy (18). The patient was consciously sedated, and under CT fluoroscopic guidance, a 14.5-gauge microwave antenna was inserted into the lesion. The lesion was ablated for 10 minutes at a power level of 45 W, achieving temperatures between 63°C and 67°C. A postablation CT scan revealed complete thermocoagulation of the lesion. On follow-up two months later, the patient was pain free and CT scan showed decreased tumor size (18).

METHOD

Although literature regarding percutaneous microwave ablation of bone lesions is sparse, experience from RFA can be helpful in guiding microwave bone ablation. As with all ablative techniques, microwave ablation is performed with the patient under conscious sedation or general anesthesia. Likewise, standard surgical preparation and local anesthesia are employed. Under the operators imaging modality of preference (CT, ultrasound, or MR), the tumor is localized. Once the optimal approach is determined, the antenna is inserted in the tumor; drilling a cortical hole beforehand might be necessary. The antenna is attached to a microwave generator and activated, without need for grounding pads. The lesion is heated to a target temperature for a few minutes. Intraprocedural imaging can be used as a rough guide of tumor ablation extent. Following ablation, the antenna array is removed and the wound dressed.

MICROWAVE ABLATION: ADVANTAGES OVER RFA

Advantages of microwave ablation over RFA include higher intratumoral temperatures, larger zones of necrosis, shorter ablation times, and an improved convection profile (19). Also, multiple microwave antennae can be used to produce synergistic zones of coagulation necrosis to accommodate larger asymmetric tumors (18). Finally, because microwave thermal ablation does not require a grounding pad to complete an electrical circuit, surface burns do not occur. Complications of microwave ablation otherwise will be similar to RFA, including fractures and neurovascular compromise.

Extracorporeal High-Intensity Focused Ultrasound

The effect of HIFU on tissue has been known since the 1940s. Early clinical utility of HIFU was described in 1950s by producing deep brain lesions in cats and monkeys (20). Over the next half century, HIFU was used to treat various neurological conditions and in 1956 was suggested as a modality in the treatment of malignancy (20). Today, HIFU offers the greatest potential for a completely noninvasive modality for cancer treatment, and has been applied in the treatment of prostate, liver, breast, kidney, musculoskeletal, and uterine tumors.

Although diagnostic ultrasound employs electromagnetic energy in the frequency range of 1–20 MHz, typical frequencies used in HIFU range from 0.8 to 3.5 MHz. Despite lower frequencies than those used in diagnostic ultrasound, the amount of energy within the HIFU beam dwarfs the energy in diagnostic ultrasound beams by several orders of magnitude. Further, the energy in HIFU can be magnified, focused at any point, and precisely delivered to a small volume of tissue without collateral damage (21).

HIFU produces coagulation necrosis through the conversion of mechanical energy into heat and cavitation. Whereas other thermal ablative modalities rely on raising local tissue temperatures (typically above 43°C) for several minutes to produce coagulation necrosis, HIFU is capable of producing coagulation necrosis by way of a rapid temperature elevation over seconds (above 56°C for one second) (20).

HIFU in the treatment of bone tumors is relatively new and much of the experience has come from China. In 2005, Chen et al. report treating 96 cases of bone tumors with HIFU, including chondrosarcoma, malignant giant cell tumor, metastatic breast osteolyses, and osteosarcoma (22). In their first series of eight patients, four with primary stage II malignant bone tumors and four with metastatic breast osteolyses, no local recurrence was found in any of the cases at an average follow-up of 23 months (22). Furthermore, there is some preliminary data to suggest that HIFU ablation may enhance host antitumor immunity by increasing CD4 (+) lymphocyte counts (22).

METHOD

Although two general types of HIFU devices have been developed, extracorporeal and endocavitary, skeletal lesions are treated using an extracorporeal transducer under ultrasound, CT, or MRI guidance (21). Various transducers have been developed capable of frequencies ranging from 1.5 to 3.5 MHz.

Because ultrasonic waves pass harmlessly through normal tissue to the target lesion, access does not require local anesthetic, skin incision, or bone drilling. The procedure, however, is performed under general anesthesia or conscious sedation because the ablation can be painful.

Following lesion localization with ultrasound, CT, or MRI, a focused ultrasound transducer, powered by a generator, is placed on the skin over the target bone lesion. Gel is used to optimize contact and transmission. If ultrasound is the image guidance modality, color Doppler can be used for real-time imaging of HIFU thermal ablation. Taking into account the transducer characteristics, lesion depth, vascularity, and size, the target is then exposed to focused ultrasound energy for a short burst, on the order of milliseconds (up to one second), during which time the lesion experiences a rapid rise in temperature (20). The resulting zone of ablation is typically a 1–3 mm wide by 8- to 15-mm long cigar-shaped slice along the beam axis. The transducer is then translated on the patient's skin along the target lesion in a series of sequential ablations to produce a volume of coagulation necrosis.

COMPLICATIONS

Because energy deposition outside of the focal region is maximal at the interface between tissues of differing acoustic impedance, skin burns are a common complication. Burns are usually subcentimeter and superficial. Mild to moderate pain following ablation is typical, but usually controlled with analgesics. As with other ablative modalities, bone fracture can occur.

Laser Ablation

Lasers have been used for tumor ablation since the early 1980s and since then have found application in the ablation of esophageal, gastric, colonic, bronchial, hepatic, pancreatic, prostatic, cerebral, lymphatic, and osseous tumors. What makes laser ablation an ideal percutaneous therapy is the ability to direct laser energy precisely to target tissue through an optical fiber and produce a predictable volume of coagulation necrosis. A near-infrared wavelength laser, [neodymium yttrium aluminum garnet (Nd:YAG) diode laser (800- to 1100-nm wavelength)] is used. Laser ablation is capable of creating a spherical zone of coagulation necrosis approximately 10–16 mm in diameter, depending on the power used. Adjacent tissue is not affected. Because thermal rise during laser treatment is uncontrolled and not monitored, peak temperatures can reach between 100°C and 240°C (14).

For the most part, the indications of laser ablation in painful osteolyses are similar to those of RFA. However, because of its limited ablation size, laser ablation is better suited to smaller tumors, that is, osteoid osteoma, or those tumors that cannot be ablated by any other means (5).

The efficacy of laser ablation has been demonstrated repeatedly. In 83 patients with osteoid osteoma, Gangi et al. reported successful laser ablation achieving pain relief in the majority of patients within one day and nearly all patients within one week (23). Overall, his group attained a 92% cure rate with a recurrence rate of 7%. In a separate study, Witt et al. achieved a decrease in mean pain score from 7.5 to 0.95 (15 months after laser ablation of osteoid osteoma in 23 patients) (24).

Laser ablation has also been successful in ablation of spinal metastases. Groenemeyer et al. demonstrated pain relief in three patients with painful spinal osteolytic metastases refractive to chemotherapy and radiation, with persistent effect at three months (25).

METHOD

Laser ablation is performed similar to RFA or microwave ablation. Using general anesthesia or conscious sedation, the lesion is prepared using sterile technique and the overlying skin infiltrated with local anesthetic. Under CT, MR, fluoroscopy, or ultrasound guidance, a coaxial bone cutting biopsy needle is inserted into the lesion by hand; bone drilling can be performed if necessary. For osteoid osteoma, the nidus is the target for needle insertion. Some authors prefer using smaller needles, such as an 18-gauge spinal needle (23,24). Once the lesion is accessed, a bare-tipped 400-μm optical fiber connected to a laser generator is inserted through the needle into the lesion under imaging guidance. Some authors describe precharring (carbonization) the fiber tip by coagulating the patient's own blood before insertion into the lesion, in order to increase the size of and make predictable the zone of coagulation (23). The lesion is exposed to laser energy (800–1100 nm) using a continuous wave mode at a power of 2 W for 200–500 seconds, depending on lesion size (23,24). For larger lesions, additional fibers can be inserted using additional access points.

COMPLICATIONS

The complications of laser ablation will be similar to those of other thermal ablation techniques. Careful attention should be paid to adjacent neurovascular structures. Gangi et al. reported no intraprocedural complications during laser ablation but did report one case of postprocedural mild reflex sympathetic dystrophy of the wrist that resolved with conservative therapy (23).

One advantage of laser ablation over RFA is the smaller caliber of the optical fiber that allows for smaller access needles to be introduced. At the same time, smaller access can be somewhat limiting with regard to biopsy if histological verification is required. Also, the optical fiber is compatible with MR guidance.

Percutaneous Cryoablation

Although the use of freezing to treat disease has been known since the 1850s, the first reported cryotherapeutic treatment of a metastatic bone lesion was by Marcove et al. in 1964 when complete relief of pain was achieved following treatment of a painful metastatic humerus lesion refractive to radiation therapy (26,27). Since then, cryoablation has also been applied in the treatment of liver metastases and genitourinary malignancies (28,29).

The goal of cryoablation is to induce tissue necrosis by exposing targeted bone and/or tumor to temperatures below $-5°C$ (3). With subsequent thawing, cell membrane disruption, osmotic fluid shift, and protein denaturation ensue, ultimately leading to tissue necrosis. Marcove et al. showed that three freeze-thaw cycles using an open liquid nitrogen system, that is, "direct pour" of liquid nitrogen funneled into the curetted cavity of a giant cell tumor, produced necrosis within 1 inch of the cavity margin (26). Furthermore, work in 1984 by Malawer et al. using dog models demonstrated a predictable 7- to 12-mm rim of bone necrosis (30). These findings emphasized the usefulness of cryotherapy as an adjunct to surgical curettage and offered an alternative to invasive *en bloc* excisions. However, surgical exposure was still required to address these lesions because of the large size of the cryogen delivery systems. This problem lead to development of closed liquid nitrogen systems allowing smaller surgical exposure and improved control of freezing.

With the development of argon-based miniature cryoprobes (less than 3-mm diameter) that can be placed percutaneously, temperatures reaching $-100°C$ can be reached within seconds percutaneously (31,32). Furthermore, the ability to use multiple probes at once combined with the utility of varying probe sizes, some as small as 1.7-mm diameter, allow cryoablation to be tailored to almost any tumor shape.

INDICATIONS AND CONTRAINDICATIONS

Marcove has reported success using cryotherapy as an intraoperative adjunct to surgical curettage for the treatment of intraosseous lesions including unicameral bone cysts, aneurysmal bone cysts, giant cell tumors, chondroblastomas, fibromyxomas, fibrous dysplasias, eosinophilic granulomas, bone hemangiomas (vertebral), large enchondromas, low-grade fibrosarcomas, malignant fibrous histiocytomas, low- and medium-grade chondrosarcomas, focal myeloma, and osteogenic sarcomas, many of which were for cure (33). Furthermore, cryoablation as an intraoperative adjunct may be particularly useful for the treatment of patients with radioresistant disease and in those with pathological fracture (34).

With regard to percutaneous cryoablation, Callstrom et al. report preliminary data from an ongoing prospective trial as well as preliminary data by Sewell et al. suggesting success in the percutaneous treatment of painful primary and secondary bone neoplasms, both in terms of quality of life and pain relief (35,36). Data regarding the limitations of cryotherapy with respect to lesion size are few, however. Beland et al. reported producing a freeze zone of $8 \times 12 \times 6$ cm for a $13 \times 15 \times 17$–cm pubic ramus and pubic symphysis mass by using seven cryoprobes (37).

As for lesions unsuitable for cryoablation, some authors assert that malignant tumors with significant soft tissue extension such as high-grade bone sarcomas are not ideal lesions for cryotherapy because of the increased risk of damage to adjacent muscles and neurovascular bundles (27).

METHOD

The method for cryoablation mirrors that of other percutaneous ablative treatments. The bone lesion is localized with conventional radiography, fluoroscopy, CT, or MRI. After determining a direct access route and taking special note of critical neurovascular bundles, the patient is placed under conscious sedation or general anesthesia. Access to the lesion is then obtained under imaging guidance by first utilizing an 18-gauge bone-cutting biopsy needle to remove a core of overlying bone, or by using a drill bit to create a tract through cortical bone into the lesion of interest. Once access is gained, an argon-based cryoprobe (2- or 2.4-mm tip) is inserted into the lesion. Care is taken to protect overlying skin by utilizing a probe insulation sheath and placing warm saline gauze at the probe entry site to minimize surface freezing. Tissue sealant and skin-bonding agents placed near skin adjacent to the cryoprobes can also be used to limit inadvertent damage from freezing.

The cryoprobe is activated and the lesion subjected to at least two freeze-thaw cycles. The duration of freeze-thaw cycles vary widely among authors, but cycles consisting of an 8- to a 10-minute freeze, followed by a 5- to 10-minute thaw are common. Thawing can be induced either actively by flushing the argon system with helium or passively by allowing time for the thaw to occur. Imaging using MRI, CT, and ultrasound may be used to follow iceball formation to determine adequacy of lesion freezing and ensure satisfactory margins. Multiple cryoprobes may be required to produce larger iceballs in order to encompass larger lesions. Larger and highly vascular lesions are more likely to require additional freeze-thaw cycles. Following successful ablation, the probe is removed and the wound dressed.

COMPLICATIONS

As with other ablative treatments, unintended damage to adjacent structures is a primary concern. Freezing of neurovascular bundles can produce transient nerve palsies (26). Freezing of the skin can lead to blistering and skin necrosis, and predispose to infection.

Weakening of bone from tumor, resection, or cryosurgery predisposes to fracture (34,38). Prior to the use of polymethylmethacrylate cement, Marcove reported a postcryosurgery fracture rate of 25% (39). Therefore, some operators advocate subsequent cementoplasty one day after cryoablation, as a preventive measure (40).

Fat embolism has been reported as a rare complication of closed miniature cryoprobes, probably the result of increased intramedullary pressure from the spreading ice front (41).

Some complications of cryoablation are unique to open cryogen delivery, that is, the direct injection of liquid nitrogen can produce nitrogen gas embolism (34).

CRYOABLATION VERSUS RADIOFREQUENCY ABLATION

Cryoablation offers distinct advantages over RFA. First, the formation of an iceball, a reliable marker of the zone of cryoablation, can be monitored with CT, MRI, or sonography in real time. On CT, ice formation is demarcated by hypodense tissue attenuation. On ultrasound, the iceball reflects virtually all acoustic energy producing a hyperechoic rim beyond which no signal registers; this can be problematic if imaging beyond the ice rim interface is required. On MRI, ice formation is very distinct because the T1 and T2 relaxation times for ice differ from water, resulting in a markedly hypointense ball of ice on both T1 and T2. Gadolinium may also be helpful in distinguishing regions of blood flow occlusion (42).

In contrast to RFA, cryoablation may be performed using multiple probes simultaneously, facilitating larger zones of freezing and accommodating asymmetric tumors. Also, tissue displacement devices, such as balloons that allow ablation of lesions adjacent to bowel, are compatible with cryoablation and not with RFA.

Finally, cryoablation has been reported to produce a long-lasting analgesic effect extending from initial treatment into the posttreatment period. The concept of cryoanalgesia was reported by Lloyd et al. in 1976 using a probe with temperatures near 60°C to treat 64 patients with intractable pain (43). More recent work done in 2003 by Zhou et al. demonstrated a loss of somatosensory evoked potentials in rabbit sciatic nerves exposed to temperatures low as $-180°C$. These effects were temporary and returned after 40 days (44).

CHEMICAL ABLATION

Chemical ablative treatments have been described as early as 1909, and a myriad of chemical agents including phenol, acetic acid, and ethanol have been employed (45). Ethanol, the most common ablative chemical, has been described extensively in the treatment of benign and malignant hepatic tumors (46) and also has applications in the treatment of benign and malignant bone tumors (47), thyroid carcinoma (48), hypertrophic cardiomyopathy (49), and benign prostatic hypertrophy (45). Our focus will be its use in the treatment of painful bone lesions.

Indications for Ethanol Ablation

As a strategy for the control of pain in osseous tumors, ethanol ablation, also termed "alcoholization" or "percutaneous ethanol injection," has proven useful where other treatments, such as radiation, chemotherapy, and surgery have failed or are contraindicated (50). Furthermore, ethanol ablation can also be used as an adjunct to radiation, chemotherapy, or surgery in order to decrease pain in anticipation of definitive therapy or to debulk tumor.

Like other ablative treatments, the goal of ethanol ablation is to produce direct coagulation necrosis by causing dehydration of the cytoplasm, denaturation of proteins, small artery thrombosis, and, ultimately, fibrosis (51,52). Through this mechanism, direct ablation of the tumor and affected periosteal and endosteal nerves results in immediate pain relief, often within 24 hours (53).

Data regarding the outcomes of ethanol ablation in the ablation of painful bone tumors are rare. Gangi et al., in a series involving 64 patients with bone metastases in multiple locations, reported a 73% reduction in opiate usage and a reduction in tumor size of 28% after one injection (53,54). Duration of pain control varied from 2 to 7 months, with all patients succumbing to disease by seven months. El-Mowafi et al., in small series of 15 patients with osteoid osteomas, reported pain relief in all patients within 48 hours and a return to normal daily activities within two weeks (55).

METHOD

First, the bone lesion is characterized with unenhanced and contrast-enhanced contiguous CT scan imaging with particular attention to lesion size, location, adjacent neurovascular structures, and regions of necrosis (54). The patient is then consciously sedated.

After the overlying skin is anesthetized with 1% lidocaine, a small hand drill is used to introduce a 2-mm guide wire into the lesion. Next, a small incision large enough to accept a small cannulated drill bit (less than 5 mm) is made in the skin overlying the lesion. A sheath is inserted over the guide wire into the lesion and the guide wire removed. The drill bit is passed through the sheath into the lesion, creating a tract through which ethanol can be injected. Alternatively, access can be gained by inserting a 22-gauge needle directly into the lesion, particularly for superficial lesions.

Once the lesion has been accessed, a mixture of contrast (25% iohexol 240) and lidocaine is injected under fluoroscopy. This mixture is important for two reasons: the lidocaine mitigates any pain the injectate may stimulate and the contrast provides an estimate of bolus diffusion within the lesion.

Confident that the intended injection of ethanol will remain in the lesion without diffusing into nearby neurovascular structures, the operator injects a small amount of 95% ethanol into the lesion. Depending on the lesion size, the amount injected may vary from 1 to 30 ml. Additional injections can be performed depending upon sufficient distribution of ethanol within the lesion (evidenced by subsequent hypoattenuation of initial contrast injectate). The procedure is terminated if adjacent neurovascular structures become threatened by ethanol infiltration. With known inadvertent injections, immediate dilution with isotonic saline may help to minimize damage. Following successful ablation, the needle is removed and the wound dressed.

Acetic Acid

Injection of acetic acid, like ethanol ablation, has been more extensively described in the ablation of hepatic tumors than in the treatment of painful osteolyses. Because acetic acid and ethanol demonstrate identical cytotoxic characteristics, the method described above for ethanol injection can be extrapolated to acetic acid ablation. Some operators believe that acetic acid may be a more ideal ablative agent because of its ability to penetrate the tumor capsule and septa, a feature particularly importantly in relatively avascular tumors such as desmoids (47).

COMPLICATIONS

The most common complication of ethanol ablation involves inadvertent injection or diffusion of ethanol into adjacent innocent structures. If this occurs within a nerve sheath, neurolysis with subsequent neuralgia and/or paraparesis is possible.

CONCLUSIONS

New technologies like HIFU, laser ablation, and microwave ablation in the treatment of bone tumors are still in their infancy, whereas RFA and cryoablation are well established. Whether curative or palliative, image-guided ablation of tumors using either thermal or chemical means offers a minimally invasive and safe approach to the treatment of primary bone tumors and metastases. Furthermore, these techniques have been proven to provide durable pain relief. Finally, being familiar with the entire range of procedures is suggested, where one technique may be contraindicated, other techniques or combination of techniques may be helpful.

REFERENCES

1. Janjan NA. Radiation for bone metastases: conventional techniques and the role of systemic radiopharmaceuticals. Cancer 1997;80:1628–45.
2. Goetz MP, Callstrom MR, Charboneau JW, et al. Percutaneous image-guided radiofrequency ablation of painful metastases involving bone: a multicenter study. J Clin Oncol 2004;22:300–6.
3. Coldwell DM, Sewell PE. The expanding role of interventional radiology in the supportive care of the oncology patient: from diagnosis to therapy. Semin Oncol 2005;32:169–73.
4. Gangi A, Dietemann JL, Schultz A, Mortazavi R, Jeung MY, Roy C. Interventional radiologic procedures with CT guidance in cancer pain management. Radiographics 1996;16:1289–304.
5. Gangi A, Guth S, Imbert JP, Marin H, Wong LLS. Percutaneous bone tumor management. Semin Int Radiol 2002;19:279–86.
6. Pinto CH, Taminiau AHM, Vancershueren GM, Hogendoorn PCW, Bloem JL, Obermann WR. Technical consideration in CT-guided radiofrequency thermal ablation of osteoid osteoma: tricks of the trade. AJR Am J Roentgenol 2002;179:1633–42.
7. McGahan JP, Browning PD, Brock JM, Tesluk H. Hepatic ablation using radiofrequency electrocautery. Invest Radiol 1990;25:267–70.
8. Rosenthal DI, Alexander A, Rosenberg AE, Springfield D. Ablation of osteoid osteomas with a percutaneously placed electrode: a new procedure. Radiology 1992; 183:29–33.
9. Rosenthal DI, Hornicek FJ, Torriani M, Gebhardt MC, Mankin HJ. Osteoid osteoma: percutaneous treatment with radiofrequency energy. Radiology 2003;229:171–5.
10. Dupuy DE, Goldberg SN. Image-guided radiofrequency tumor ablation: challenges and opportunities – part II. J Vasc Interv Radiol 2001;12:1135–48.
11. Callstrom MR, Charboneau JW, Goetz MP. Painful metastases involving bone: feasibility of percutaneous CT- and US- guided radio-frequency ablation. Radiology 2002;224:87–97.
12. Goldberg SN, Gazelle GS, Dawson SL, Mueller PR, Rosenthal DI, Rittman W. Tissue ablation with RF: effect of probe size, ablation duration, and temperature on lesion volume. Acad Radiol 1995;2:399–404.

13. Goldberg SN, Dupuy DE. Image-guided radiofrequency tumor ablation: challenges and opportunities – part I. J Vasc Interv Radiol 2001;12:1021–32.
14. Papagelopoulos PJ, Mavrogenis AF, Galanis EC, et al. Minimally invasive techniques in orthopedic oncology: radiofrequency and laser thermal ablation. Orthopedics 2005;28:563–8.
15. Nakatsuka A, Yamakado K, Maeda M, et al. Radiofrequency ablation combined with bone cement injection for the treatment of bone malignancies. J Vasc Interv Radiol 2004;15:707–12.
16. Seki T, Wakabayashi M, Nakagawa T, et al. Ultrasonically guided percutaneous microwave coagulation therapy for small hepatocellular carcinoma. Cancer 1994;74: 817–25.
17. Fan QY, Ma B, Qiu X, Li Y. Preliminary report on treatment of bone tumors with microwave-induced hyperthermia. Bioelectromagnetics 1996;17:218–22.
18. Simon CJ, Dupuy DE. Percutaenous minimally invasive therapies in the treatment of bone tumors: thermal ablation. Semin Musculoskeletal Radiol 2006;10:137–44.
19. Simon CJ, Dupuy DE. Microwave ablation: principles and applications. Radiographics 2005;25:S69–83.
20. Kennedy JE, Ter Haar GR, Cranston D. High intensity focused ultrasound: surgery of the future? Br J Radiol 2003;76:590–9.
21. Kennedy JE. High-intensity focused ultrasound in the treatment of solid tumours. Nat Rev Cancer 2005;5:321–7.
22. Chen W, Zhou K. High-intensity focused ultrasound ablation: a new strategy to manage primary bone tumors. Curr Opin Orthop 2005;16:494–500.
23. Gangi A, Dietemann JL, Gasser B, et al. Interstitial laser photocoagulation of osteoid osteomas with use of CT guidance. Radiology 1997;203:843–8.
24. Witt JD, Hall-Craggs MA, Ripley P, et al. Interstitial laser photocoagulation for the treatment of osteoid osteoma. J Bone Joint Surg Br 2000;82:1125–8.
25. Groenemeyer DHW, Schirp S, Gevargez A. Image-guided percutaneous thermal ablation of bone tumors. Acad Radiol 2002;9:467–77.
26. Marcove RC, Miller TR. Treatment of primary and metastatic bone tumors by cryosurgery, JAMA 1969;207:1890–4.
27. Bickels J, Meller I, Shmookler BM, Malawer MM. The role and biology of cryosurgery in the treatment of bone tumors. A review. Acta Orthop Scand 1999;70:308–15.
28. Weaver ML, Atkinson D, Zemel R. Hepatic cryosurgery in treating colorectal metastases. Cancer 1996;76:210–14.
29. Wong WS, Chinn DO, Chinn M, Chinn J, Tom WL. Cryosurgery as a treatment for prostate carcinoma: results and complications. Cancer 1997;79:963–74.
30. Malawer MM, Marks MR, McChesney D, Piasio M, Gunther SF, Schmookler BM. The effect of cryosurgery and polymethylmethacrylate in dogs with experimental bone defects comparable to tumor defects. Clin Orthop Relat Res 1988;226:299–310.
31. Callstrom MR, Charboneau JW. Percutaneous ablation: safe, effective treatment of bone tumors. Oncology (Williston Park) 2005;19(Suppl 4):22–6.
32. Hebert JJ, Davis KW, Choi JJ, Blankenbaker DG, Tuite MJ, Lee FT. Cryoablation in the musculoskeletal system. Poster Presentation, Radiologic Society of North America Annual Meeting, November 2005, Chicago, IL.
33. Marcove RC. A 17-year review of cryosurgery in the treatment of bone tumors. Clin Orthop Relat Res 1982;163:231–4.
34. Veth R, Schreuder B, van Beem H, Pruszczynski M, de Rooy J. Cryosurgery in aggressive, benign, and low-grade malignant bone tumours. Lancet Oncol 2005;6: 25–34.
35. Callstrom MR, Charboneau JW, Goetz MP, et al. Image-guided ablation of painful metastatic bone tumors: a new and effective approach to a difficult problem. Skeletal Radiol 2006 Jan;35(1):1–15.
36. Sewell PE, Jackson MS, Dhillon GS. Percutaneous MRI-guided cryosurgery of bone tumors. Radiology 2002;225(S):514.

37. Beland MD, Dupuy DE, Mayo-Smith WW. Percutaneous cryoablation of sympto-
    matic extraabdominal metastatic disease: preliminary results. AJR Am J Roentgenol
    2005;184:926–30.
38. Dabak N, Tomak Y, Piskin A, Gulman B, Ozcan H. Early results of a modified
    technique of cryosurgery. Int Orthop 2003;27(4):249–53.
39. Marcove RC, Weis LD, Vaghaiwalla MR, Pearson R, Huvos AG. Cryosurgery in the
    treatment of giant cell tumors of bone. A report of 52 consecutive cases. Cancer
    1978;41:957–69.
40. Callstrom MR, Charboneau JW. (2005, October 1) Percutaneous ablation treats bone
    tumors safely, effectively – image-guided tumor destruction using radiofrequency,
    cryo techniques offers well-tolerated treatment with long duration of pain relief.
    Diagnostic Imaging. Retrieved May 16, 2006, from http://www.diagnosticimaging.
    com/showArticle.jhtml?articleID=171201841
41. Popken F, Meschede P, Erberich H, et al. Complications after cryosurgery with new
    miniature cryoprobes in long hollow bones: an animal trial. BMC Surg 2005;5:17.
42. Rubinsky B. Cryosurgery. Annu Rev Biomed Eng 2000;2:157–87.
43. Lloyd JW, Barnard JD, Glynn CJ. Cryoanalgesia. A new approach to pain relief.
    Lancet 1976;2:932–4.
44. Zhou L, Shao Z, Ou S. Cryoanalgesia: electrophysiology at different temperatures.
    Cryobiology 2003;46:26–32.
45. Plante MK, Folsom JB, Zvara P. Prostatic tissue ablation by injection: a literature
    review. J Urol 2004;172:20–6.
46. Lee MJ, Mueller PR, Dawson SL, et al. Percutaneous ethanol injection for the treat-
    ment of hepatic tumors: indications, mechanism of action, technique and efficacy.
    AJR Am J Roentgenol 1995;164:215–20.
47. Clark TW. Percutaneous chemical ablation of desmoid tumors. J Vasc Interv Radiol
    2003 May;14:629–34.
48. Nakada K, Kasai K, Watanabe Y, et al. Treatment of radioiodine-negative bone meta-
    stasis from papillary thyroid carcinoma with percutaneous ethanol injection therapy.
    Ann Nucl Med 1996;10:441–4.
49. Holmes DR Jr., Valeti US, Nishimura RA. Alcohol septal ablation for hypertrophic
    cardiomyopathy: indications and technique. Catheter Cardiovasc Interv 2005;66:
    375–89.
50. Cotten A, Demondion X, Boutry N, et al. Therapeutic percutaneous injections in the
    treatment of malignant acetabular osteolyses. Radiographics 1999;19:647–53.
51. Goldberg SN, Ahmed M. Minimally invasive image-guided therapies for hepatocel-
    lular carcinoma. J Clin Gastroenterol 2002;35:S115–29.
52. Sabharwal T, Salter R, Adam A, Gangi A. Image-guided therapies in orthopedic
    oncology. Orthop Clin North Am 2006;37:105–12.
53. Gangi A, Kastler B, Klinkert A, Dietemann JL. Injection of alcohol into bone meta-
    stases under CT guidance. J Comput Assist Tomogr 1994;18:932–5.
54. Gangi A, Dietemann JL, Schultz A, Mortazavi R, Jeung MY, Roy C. Interventional
    radiologic procedures with CT guidance in cancer pain management. Radiographics
    1996;16:1289–1304.
55. el-Mowafi H, Refaat H, Kotb S. Percutaneous destruction and alcoholisation for the
    management of osteoid osteoma. Acta Orthop Belg 2003;69:447–51.

Chronic Pelvic Pain in Women

Derek L. West

Chronic pelvic pain (CPP) can be defined as nonmenstrual pain of three or more months' duration that localizes to the anatomic pelvis and is severe enough to cause functional disability and require medical or surgical treatment (1). Chronic dysmenorrhea or menstrual pain of six or more months' duration that causes functional disability and requires medical or surgical treatment is also appropriately included in the definition. This condition can have a strong influence on the patient's quality of life, being associated with years of disability and suffering, loss of employment, and marital discord. In treating CPP, the primary aim is to improve the quality of life (Table 1) (2,3).

EPIDEMIOLOGY

CPP in women is a common gynecological problem with an estimated prevalence of 38 per 1,000 women (3.8%), which is higher than that of migraine headaches (2.1%) and is similar to that of asthma (3.7%) or back pain (4.1%) (4). Women with pelvic pain account for up to 40% of patients attending gynecological outpatient clinics and is estimated to occur in 15% of all women between the ages of 18 and 50 years (5). Such patients use three times more medication, have four times more nongynecological operations, and are five times more likely to have hysterectomy (6). In fact, 15% of all hysterectomies and 35% of diagnostic laparoscopies are performed because of chronic pelvic pain (1), and it is estimated that $881.5 million dollars are spent each year on its outpatient management in the United States (4).

ETIOLOGY AND PATHOGENESIS

CPP may originate from one or more organ systems or pathologies, and may have multiple contributing factors. The presence of pelvic pathology, history of abuse, and coexistent psychological morbidity all have a very high correlation with the presence of CPP.

Other risk factors are often associated with specific presenting symptomatology. Risks factors for dysmenorrheal (pain with menses) include young age

Table 1. Quality-of-Life Effect in Patients with CPP

Inability to exercise

Difficulty sleeping

Lack of enjoyment of leisure

Interference with socialization

Interference with sexuality

Source: Steege (3).

Table 2. Common Findings in CPP Syndrome

Duration of pain >6 months

Impaired function

Signs of depression

Pain out of proportion to pathology

Unresponsive to medical therapy or lifestyle changes

Altered family roles

Source: Steege (3).

(older than 30 years), thin body habitus (body mass index <20), smoking, and longer menstrual cycles. Risk factors for dyspareunia (pain with intercourse) include women who have been "circumcised," peri- or postmenopausal women, or those with pelvic inflammatory disease. Noncyclical pelvic pain is associated with endometriosis, pelvic adhesions, or history of sexual abuse (4).

By one definition, CPP is defined as pelvic pain of at least six months, duration (Table 2) (2,3). As one might expect from such a nonspecific definition, there is a broad spectrum of diseases that can be associated with CPP. Gynecological etiologies such as endometriosis, pelvic congestion syndrome, and leiomyomata are commonly associated with CPP. Alternatively, urological, gastrointestinal, and musculoskeletal etiologies must also be considered (Table 3) (2). In the majority of women, there are multiple etiologies of CPP, whereas in others, the etiology is not discernible (2).

Pain in CPP has been difficult to understand, especially in patients in whom "definitive" treatment has failed or no etiology could be elicited. Traditional pain models propose a direct relationship between tissue damage, stimulation of nociceptors, and pain (8). Nociceptive pain can be divided into somatic and visceral. Somatic pain originates from skin, muscle, bones, and joints, and is transmitted to the sensory cortex by peripheral sensory nerves. It is perceived as localized, sharp, or dull pain. Visceral pain originates from

Table 3. Some Gynecological Disease States That May Be Associated with CPP in Women

Gynecologic

Uterine	Extrauterine
Adenomyosis	Adhesions
Atypical dysmenorrhea	Adnexal cysts
Cervical stenosis	Chronic ectopic pregnancy
Endometrial polyps	Chlamydial infection
Intrauterine contraceptive device	Endometriosis
Symptomatic pelvic relaxation	Neoplasia of the genital tract
Uterine fibroids	Ovulatory pain
	Pelvic congestion

Extragynecologic

Bladder

Gastrointestinal

Musculoskeletal

Psychiatric

Source: Howard (2).

Table 4. Predisposing Psychosocial Variables in Psychosocial Pain Model

Familial pain models
Mood/anxiety state
Marital adjustment
Spouse responses
Abuse history
Somatization

bowel, is transmitted to the brain by the sympathetic nervous system, and is perceived as poorly localized, dull, or crampy, and is associated with autonomic phenomena (9,10). In addition to nociceptive pain, traditional pain models also take into account neurogenic pain, which is nonnociceptive. Neurogenic pain originates from injury to the central or peripheral nervous system and is perceived as burning pain or parasthesias. These traditional pain theories are adequate for most patients who have a discernible physical injury. This theory fails, however, for CPP patients without such findings, leaving many health care providers to oversimplify the pain as "not real" (8).

Newer pain theories are based on biopsychosocial models. In these models, a second type of non-nociceptive pain is identified: this type of pain is termed "psychogenic." These theories recognize the important role that emotional, environmental, and cognitive factors play in pain perception (Table 4) (8).

Mood, general health status, anxiety, family support, and employment status have been shown to have predictive value in nonpelvic chronic pain, such as back pain or arthritis. Based on these findings, biopsychosocial models combine sensory (nociceptive) stimuli, psychological factors, and socioenvironmental factors (psychogenic) in the assessment of chronic pain (8,10,11).

HISTORY AND PHYSICAL EVALUATION OF THE PATIENT WITH CPP

Given the numerous etiologies of CPP, a proper history and physical examination are crucial in diagnosing the causes of CPP in each individual patient. The quality and character of the pain, including alleviating or exacerbating factors, should be elicited. An obstetric and menstrual history is important, particularly as it pertains to the onset of symptoms. Given the psychogenic component of pain in these patients, an appropriate psychological history must be performed. This is particularly important as depression is both a positive predictor of pain severity and an indicator of responsiveness to treatment. Suicide, sexual abuse, and substance abuse are also found more frequently in these patients. An evaluation of social history for stressors must be performed, and a comprehensive review of systems should be performed. The International Pelvic Pain Society (www.pelvicpain.org) has a comprehensive questionnaire form that can help to guide history taking in CPP patients.

Physical examinations in CPP patients are beyond the scope of this chapter and are usually performed by gynecologists. However, a few key points will be emphasized. First, the physical exam should be performed in four different positions: standing, sitting, supine, and lithotomy. This is of particular importance when evaluating for the presence of varices. Second, from the lithotomy position, a digital and bimanual exam should be performed. If tolerated, a speculum exam should be performed as well.

Imaging plays a significant role in the evaluation of CPP patients. Ultrasound can diagnose an endometrioma, while magnetic resonance (MR) imaging can define endometrial implants in other organs. MR imaging has a high degree of specificity and sensitivity for adenomyosis and uterine fibroids. As will be discussed later, venograms, particularly using a tilt table, are the gold standard for pelvic congestion syndrome (PCS) (12).

PELVIC CONGESTION SYNDROME
Etiology and Pathophysiology

PCS is a form of CPP due to ovarian and pelvic varices. This clinical syndrome was first described by Taylor in 1949 (13). In 1958, Topolanski-Sierra described an association between ovarian and pelvic varices and chronic pelvic pain (14). Seen commonly in the reproductive years, there is a high prevalence of PCS among multiparous women. Hormonal changes in pregnancy and congenital absence of valves in the ovarian veins have been identified as risks factors for the formation of varices. Varices tend to occur more frequently on the left as a result of drainage of the ovarian vein into the left renal vein, as opposed to the right ovarian vein that drains directly into the inferior vena cava.

One specific cause of PCS is "nutcracker syndrome." This syndrome, typically seen in thin women, is caused by compression of the left renal vein between the superior mesenteric artery and the aorta. As a result, left renal venous hypertension develops, with gradients across the stenosis as high as 3 mm Hg. This pressure causes collateral venous drainage to develop around the renal pelvis via the gonadal vein. Often, the collateral venous drainage forms direct communications between the collateral vessels and the renal collecting system, leading to hematuria. Although treatment in the past was limited to surgical correction, intravascular stent placement across the left renal vein has been shown to be an attractive option. Long-term results are uncertain (15).

Clinical History

PCS is difficult to diagnose clinically. Patients present with shifting location of pain, dyspareunia, and postcoital pain. One clinical clue to the diagnosis is the exacerbation of pain while standing, likely due to the variceal distension. Physical exam may reveal associated varices in the thighs, buttocks, perineum, vulva, or vagina. Symptoms also often worsen in the postpartum period.

Imaging

As discussed earlier, cross-sectional imaging is primarily used to exclude other sources of chronic pelvic pain. On computed tomography (CT) or MR imaging, pelvic varices can be visualized as dilated, tortuous, contrast-enhancing parauterine tubular structures, isodense to other venous structures. Coakley et al. suggest that in order to diagnose pelvic varices, at least four ipsilateral tortuous parauterine veins of varying caliber (at least one of which measures over 4 mm in maximum diameter) or an ovarian vein diameter of greater than 8 mm should be visualized (16). One must be cautious when using cross-sectional imaging in diagnosis as most of these exams are performed in the supine position, which can collapse the varices and underestimate the degree of variceal dilation.

Ultrasound has been used extensively to evaluate patients with chronic pelvic pain. One report compared transvaginal and transabdominal ultrasonographic findings between patients with PCS and normal patients (17). Patients with PCS were found to have dilated left ovarian veins with reversal of flow (caudal), presence of varicocele, dilated arcuate veins crossing the uterine myometrium, polycystic changes of the ovary, and variable duplex wave forms during Valsalva maneuver. One specific benefit of ultrasound is that it can be performed in the upright or standing position, making the varices easier to detect (17).

In spite of these advances in cross-sectional imaging, selective retrograde venography of the ovarian veins remains the diagnostic gold standard. Because the supine position may cause collapse of the ovarian varices, this procedure should be performed on a tilt table. Findings suggestive of PCS include minimum ovarian vein diameter greater than 10 mm, uterine venous engorgement, congestion of the ovarian plexus, filling of ovarian veins across the midline, or filling vulvovaginal or thigh varices (18).

Treatment Options

MEDICAL AND SURGICAL

Medical treatment options for patients diagnosed with PCS are limited. Nonsteroidal anti-inflammatory drugs may provide short-term relief of symptoms. Addressing psychogenic factors such as stress and social issues may also be helpful in decreasing the likelihood of recurrence of symptoms. Medroxyprogesterone acetate and gonadotropin-releasing hormone agonists have also shown some benefit. However, medical management in PCS is often suboptimal and other forms of treatment are frequently needed.

Surgical options for PSC are limited to ovarian vein ligation or hysterectomy and bilateral oophorectomy. However, clinical outcome in these patients has been disappointing, with many patients not experiencing postsurgical relief of their symptoms (19).

ENDOVASCULAR

Endovascular ovarian vein embolization is becoming the primary treatment method for PCS (20–23). The procedure is typically performed from a transfemoral approach. A 7F guiding catheter or sheath is guided to the left renal vein. From this location, an initial left renal venogram is performed. A 4F angled glide catheter is guided into the left ovarian vein, where a second venogram is obtained. In cases where varices are not visualized, having the patient perform a Valsalva maneuver and/or tilting the table upright can be helpful. Embolization of the left ovarian vein is then performed using coils and/or gelfoam. If possible, the right ovarian vein is embolized in a similar manner. Several authors have also suggested improvements in outcomes when bilateral internal iliac embolization is performed, usually four to six weeks after the initial ovarian vein embolization (20). Although medical and surgical therapy for PCS has limited success, endovascular therapy has shown significant positive results, with a 73–78% symptomatic improvement rate (21). Further, in a 2006 long-term study, 83% of embolized patients had clinical improvement at two years postprocedure (20).

SUMMARY

CPP is a complex syndrome that encompasses many different etiologies. In these patients, the biopsychosocial model of pain is useful in increasing the efficacy of treatments. Although in many cases an underlying pathology may not be uncovered, cross-sectional imaging is often helpful in diagnosis. Further, several disease entities, including PCS and uterine leiomyomata (not discussed here) are amenable to endovascular therapy as a definitive treatment.

REFERENCES

1. APGO Educational Series on Women's Health Issues: Chronic Pelvic Pain: An Integrated Approach. Crofton, MD: APGO, 2000.
2. Howard FM. Chronic pelvic pain. Obstet Gynecol. 2003;101(3):594–611.
3. Steege JF. Scope of the problem. In: Chronic Pelvic Pain: An Integrated Approach. Steege JF, Metzger DM, Levy BS, eds. Philadelphia: W.B. Saunder's; 1999; p. 9.

4. Pallavi L, Luciano M, Gray R Hills R, Khan K. Factors predisposing women to chronic pelvic pain: systematic review. BMJ. 2006;332(7544):749–55.

5. Harris RD, Holtzman SR, Poppe AM. Clinical outcome in female patients with pelvic pain and normal pelvic ultrasound findings. Radiology. 2000;216:440–3.

6. Reiter RC, Gambone JC. Demographics and historic variables in women with idiopathic chronic pelvic pain. Obstet Gynecol. 1990;75(3 Pt 1):428–32.

7. Davies L, Ganger K, Drummond M, Saunders D, Beard R. The economic burden of intractable gynecological pain. J Obstet Gynecol. 1992;12:46–54.

8. Reiter RC. Evidence based management of chronic pelvic pain. Clin Obstet Gynecol. 1998;41(2):422–35.

9. Gunter J. Chronic pelvic pain an integrated approach to diagnosis and treatment. Obstet Gynecol Survey. 2003;58:615–23.

10. Raj PP, Abrams BM, Benson HT, et al. eds. Practical Management of Pain, 3rd Edition. St. Louis: Mosby, Inc.; 2000.

11. Turk DC, Rudy TE. Toward a comprehensive assessment of chronic pelvic pain patients. Behav Res Ther 1987;25:237–49.

12. Kuligowska E, Deeds L, Lu K. Pelvic pain: overlooked and underdiagnosed gynecologic conditions. Radiographics. 2005;25:3–20.

13. Taylor HC. Vascular congestion and hyperaemia: Part 1. Physiologic basis and history of the concept. Am J Obstet Gynecol. 1949;57:211–30.

14. Topolanski-Sierra R. Pelvic phlebography. Am J Obstet Gynecol. 1958;76:44–5.

15. Ahmed K, Sampath R, Khan MS. Current trends in the diagnosis and management of renal nutcracker syndrome: a review. Eur J Endovascular Surg. 2006;31:410–6.

16. Coakley FV, Varghese SL, Hricak H. CT and MRI of pelvic varices in women. J Comput Tomogr. 1999;23(3):429–34.

17. Seong JP, Joo WL, Young TK, Dong HL, Yup Y, Joo HO, Hae KL, Chu YH. Diagnosis of pelvic congestion syndrome using transabdominal and transvaginal sonography. Am J Roentgenol. 2004;182:683–8.

18. Maleux G, Stockx L, Wilms G, Marchal G. Ovarian vein embolization for the treatment of pelvic congestion syndrome: long term technical and clinical results. J Vasc Interv Radiol. 2000;11(7):859–64.

19. Beard RW, Kennedy RG, Gangar KF, et al. Bilateral oophorectomy and hysterectomy in the treatment of intractable pelvic pain associated with pelvic congestion. Br J Obstet Gynecol. 1991;98:988–92.

20. Kim HS, Malhotra AD, Rowe PC, et al. Embolotherapy for pelvic congestion syndrome: long-term results. J Vasc Interv Radiol. 2006;17(2 Pt 1):289–97.

21. Machan L: Embolization in the female pelvis. In: Textbook of Endovascular Procedures. Dyet JD, Ettles D, Nicholson AA, eds. Philadelphia: Churchill-Livingstone; 2000; p. 367.

22. Venbrux AC, Chang AH, Kim HS, et al. Pelvic congestion syndrome (pelvic venous incompetence): impact on ovarian and internal iliac vein embolotherapy on mentrual cycle and chronic pelvic pain. J Vasc Interv Radiol. 2002:17;171–8.

23. Sichlau MJ, Yao JS, Vogelzang RL. Transcatheter embolotherapy for the treatment of pelvic congestion syndrome. J Obstet Gynecol. 1994;83(5 Pt 2):892–6.

PART II

Systemic Pain Control

Sedation and Analgesia Medications

George Behrens, Hector Ferral, and Nilesh H. Patel

INTRODUCTION

The performance of minimally invasive interventional radiology procedures has increased in a significant fashion over the past 20 years. The trend in modern medicine has definitely moved toward solving medical problems with minimally invasive techniques. This trend toward minimally invasive techniques has made it extremely important for the interventionalist to be able to provide adequate sedation and analgesia during interventional procedures. Providing effective and safe sedation and analgesia has become part of the standards of care for any interventional radiology practice.

Selected patients undergoing very simple procedures may not require any sedation or analgesia; however, most of the therapeutic procedures currently performed in interventional radiology suites require the patient to be under moderate sedation and analgesia, which is also known as "conscious sedation" or, more appropriately, "sedation and analgesia."

The purpose of this chapter is to provide an overview of the most important components of sedation that an interventional radiologist should know about sedation and analgesia. The chapter will address the use of medications, mechanisms of action, doses, and antagonists, as well as the appropriate ways to monitor the patient.

DEFINITIONS

The terms sedation and analgesia refer to a fluctuant state of conscious depression induced by pharmacological agents (1). In 2002, the American Society of Anesthesiologists (ASA) published well-defined guidelines for sedation and analgesia by nonanesthesiologists. The document specifies the spectrum of sedation/analgesia and provides qualitative parameters for the classification of stages of sedation (Table 1). These sedation stages are defined by the patients' level of consciousness, airway maintenance, spontaneous ventilation, and cardiovascular

Table 1. Classification of Stages of Sedation

	Responsiveness	Airway	Spontaneous ventilation	Cardiovascular function
Anxiolysis	Normal	Unaffected	Unaffected	Unaffected
Conscious sedation	Good response to verbal or tactile stimulation	No intervention required	Usually maintained	Adequate
Deep sedation	Good response after repeated or painful stimulation	Intervention may be required	Usually maintained	May be inadequate
General Anesthesia	Unarousable, even with painful stimulus	Intervention often required	May be impaired	Frequently inadequate

function (1,2). The stages range from anxiolysis to general anesthesia, with defined criteria at each level.

Anxiolysis is a drug-induced state during which patients respond normally to verbal commands, and both respiratory and cardiovascular functions are intact (1).

Conscious sedation is a conscious depression during which patients respond purposefully, alone or accompanied by light tactile stimulation, to verbal commands. The ventilation is spontaneous and adequate, and cardiovascular function is maintained (1).

Deep sedation is the depression of consciousness during which patients cannot be easily aroused but respond purposefully following repeated or painful stimuli. Patients may require assistance in maintaining a patent airway and spontaneous ventilation. Cardiovascular function is usually maintained (1).

General anesthesia is the point at which consciousness is lost and the patient is not arousable. The patient requires respiratory assistance and cardiovascular function is often impaired (1).

A sedative drug decreases activity, moderates excitement, and calms the patient, whereas a hypnotic drug produces drowsiness and facilitates the onset and maintenance of a state that resembles natural sleep. The benzodiazepines share both sedative and hypnotic properties and contribute to muscle relaxation as well. The main effect of the benzodiazepines results from action of these drugs on the central nervous system (CNS), increasing the levels of inhibitory neurotransmission pathway. Opiates are drugs derived from opium including morphine, codeine, and a wide variety of semisynthetic drugs. The term opioid is more inclusive, applying to all agonists and antagonists with morphine-like activity. Anti-inflammatory drugs, such as the commonly used nonsteroidal anti-inflammatory drugs (NSAIDs), are a heterogeneous group of compounds, often chemically unrelated, which share certain therapeutic actions and side effects, basically by inhibition of cyclooxygenase (COX) enzyme.

PREPROCEDURAL EVALUATION

All patients undergoing sedation and analgesia require medical evaluation before the procedure to stratify the risk and to manage any problems related to preexisting medical conditions. Patient evaluation before sedation and analgesia should include a short questionnaire regarding medical history, a focused physical examination, and compiling a list of current medications and drug allergies. The patient risk should be assessed based on the ASA classification and specified in the patient's chart or preprocedural paperwork. The patient medical record must have documentation that appropriate informed consent has been obtained for the procedure and for sedation and analgesia. If the patient is a minor or is incapable of signing an informed consent, then the consent must be obtained from the parent or legal guardian of the patient. The practitioner must provide verbal and written instructions to the patient or responsible person. This information will include the drugs being administered to the patient, both during and after sedation. The side effects and all precautions need to be discussed. Successful sedation requires planning and knowledge. Knowledge of the comorbidities and drug actions during drug administration will be extremely helpful to decide what to do in case of complications. Most of the known complications during sedation and analgesia can be prevented by a good preprocedural evaluation.

Patient Selection

The ASA physical status is not a risk stratification system. Rather, it is intended to give practitioners a common language in referring to the severity of systemic disease in various patients. Each patient should be given the proper ASA classification as part of the routine preprocedure screening (Table 2). In most instances, patients who are ASA classification I or II are considered appropriate candidates for sedation and analgesia. In certain cases, patients with ASA classification III might be considered appropriate for sedation and analgesia. The presence of an anesthesiologist is strongly recommended during procedures performed for ASA IV and V patients.

Preprocedural fasting

The relationship between preprocedural fasting time and incidence of adverse events has not been definitively defined (2–4). However, the ASA guidelines recommend fasting for procedures that require sedation and analgesia (Table 3). The recommended fasting times before sedation and analgesia are as follows: fast for two hours after clear liquids (water, nonpulp fruit juice, tea, or black coffee). Milk is similar to solids in gastric emptying time. A four-hour fast is recommended after "breast milk" or more complex juices. A six-hour fasting is recommended after a light meal (toast and clear liquids) before receiving sedation. Meals that include meat, or fried or fatty foods may prolong gastric emptying time. Both the amount and type of foods ingested must be considered when determining an appropriate fasting period. No specific fasting-time guidelines are offered for emergency procedures, and the sedation needs to be modified to anxiolysis level. The ASA also states that "the literature does not provide sufficient data to test the hypothesis that preprocedural fasting results in a decreased incidence of adverse outcomes"(5).

Table 2. ASA Physical Status Classification System	
Physical Status	
ASA-1	A normal healthy patient
ASA-2	A patient with mild systemic disease that results in no functional limitations
	Examples: hypertension, diabetes mellitus, chronic bronchitis, morbid obesity, extremes of age
ASA-3	A patient with severe systemic which results in functional limitations
	Examples: poorly controlled diabetes mellitus with vascular complications, angina pectoris, prior myocardial infarction, pulmonary disease that limits activity
ASA-4	A patient with severe systemic disease that is a constant threat to life
	Examples: unstable angina pectoris, advanced pulmonary, renal or hepatic dysfunction
ASA-5	A moribund patient who is not expected to survive without the operation
	Examples: ruptured abdominal aortic aneurysm, pulmonary embolus, head injury with increased intracranial pressure
ASA-6	A declared brain-dead patient whose organs are being removed for donation

Table 3. ASA Guidelines for Preprocedural Fasting	
Fast	
Two hours	Clear liquids
Four hours	Complex liquids
Six hours	Light meal
More than eight hours	Fatty foods

Patient Monitoring

All patients undergoing to IR procedures must have continuous monitoring before, during, and after the administration of sedatives. Monitoring may detect early signs of patient distress, such as changes in pulse, blood pressure, ventilatory status, cardiac electrical activity, and clinical and neurological status, before clinically significant compromise occurs. A baseline set of vital signs must be obtained before the administration of sedative agents; this information should be documented in the patient's chart. Standard monitoring of sedated patients includes recording the heart rate, blood pressure, respiratory rate, and oxygen saturation. Although electronic monitoring equipment often facilitates assessment of patient status, it does not replace a well-trained and vigilant assistant. When given during procedures, supplemental oxygen administration has been shown to reduce the magnitude of oxygen desaturation (6). Continuous electrocardiogram (EKG) monitoring is reasonable in high-risk patients, although the necessity for such monitoring has not been shown conclusively in controlled trials. Patients who may benefit from EKG monitoring include those who have a history of significant cardiac or pulmonary disease, elderly patients, and those in whom prolonged procedures are anticipated.

In our practice, we monitor all patients undergoing either diagnostic or therapeutic procedures. Parameters that should be monitored are (a) level of consciousness, which serves as a guide to the depth of sedation and to the potential need for cardiopulmonary support; (b) ventilatory function, by observation or auscultation during lighter stages of sedation; (c) oxygenation using pulse oximetry; and (d) hemodynamics with continuous electrocardiography and noninvasive blood pressure monitoring a minimum of every five minutes.

PHARMACOLOGICAL AGENTS

The ideal sedative/analgesic should optimize performance of the procedure by minimizing patient's movement, maximizing comfort for the patient, and having no side effects. Specifically, it should provide a sedative/hypnotic effect (a dose-dependent depression of consciousness), analgesia (if necessary for supplementing local anesthesia), and amnesia, ideally with minimal cardiovascular and respiratory effects. Rapid-onset and short-acting or reversible agents would allow optimal control over these effects. Unfortunately, no single drug accomplishes all of these goals. With some basic understanding of the pharmacology of some of the more commonly used sedatives, combinations of these drugs can achieve the desired effect. The use of specific medications for sedation and analgesia is individual to the practitioner.

Benzodiazepines

Benzodiazepines act primarily by potentiation of a major inhibitory neurotransmitter, γ-aminobutyric acid (GABA), throughout the CNS but especially in the basal ganglia, hippocampus, cerebellum, hypothalamus, and spinal cord (7). The interaction of GABA with the receptor facilitates the aperture of chloride ion channels, allowing influx of chloride into the neuronal cell, thus hyperpolarizing the membrane potential and limiting the cell's response to excitatory stimuli. Pharmacological properties include relief of anxiety, sedation, and anterograde amnesia, with a minimum of cardiovascular and respiratory depression. Benzodiazepines are not analgesics, and for this reason they are typically combined with opioids such as fentanyl, producing a synergistic response in both sedative qualities and respiratory depressive effects. Careful titration should be taken to prevent severe hypoventilation and apnea episodes, especially when given concomitantly with opioids in elderly patients. The duration of action can be increased secondary to decreased metabolic clearance, making the patient more susceptible to respiratory depression or paradoxical agitation.

MIDAZOLAM
Midazolam is the most commonly used parenteral benzodiazepine. It is frequently combined with fentanyl as the most accepted "cocktail" used for sedation and analgesia in interventional radiology. This popularity can be attributed to a rapid onset of action (1–5 minutes) and a short duration of action (30–60 minutes). This duration of action compares favorably with other

Midazolam			
Ingredients	Midazolam HCl	Dose	0.5–2.5 mg
Brand Name	Versed	Supplemental Dose	0.25–1 mg
Cost	$1.06/vial	Onset Action	1–5 minutes
FDA Approval	1985	Duration of Effect	60–90 minutes
		Contraindication	Hypersensitivity or narrow-angle glaucoma
		Comment	Reduce dose 30–50% in elderly or when used with narcotics

benzodiazepines, such as diazepam (21–37 hours) or lorazepam (10–20 hours) (8). If a sedation level is achieved, repeat doses can be given every five minutes to maintain the patient at the same level of sedation. The time of onset is affected by the total dose administered, the concurrent administration of narcotic, and drugs used for premedication. Midazolam also has superior amnestic properties when compared with the other benzodiazepines. The typical intravenous dose for sedation is 0.03–0.1 mg/kg, with special considerations in the elderly and in patients with hepatic failure due to an increase in the plasma half-life (2-fold and 2.5-fold, respectively). It is important to consider reducing the dose with the concomitant use of narcotics. Sedative effects are variable among patients, and in some cases, the recovery can be prolonged and accompanied by delayed recovery of superior function (9).

The drug is metabolized in the liver by hydroxylation and conjugation, and then it is excreted in the urine (10). The side effects of midazolam are dose dependent, and include hypoventilation and hypoxemia (11). These side effects are more prominent when midazolam is combined with other CNS depressants such as narcotics, barbiturates, or anesthetics. Hypotension also can occur with high doses. Midazolam is contraindicated in patients with a known hypersensitivity to the drug or in patients with acute narrow-angle glaucoma. Benzodiazepines can be used in patients with open-angle glaucoma only if they are receiving appropriate therapy.

Our common dosing regimen for the adult population is 1 mg of midazolam with 50 mcg of fentanyl before the procedure (with the patient on the table). A second round is given just before starting the procedure and once the desired level of sedation is obtained, we continue with full rounds or half rounds every 10–15 minutes depending on the level of patient arousal.

DIAZEPAM

Diazepam is a long-acting benzodiazepine used for the short-term management of anxiety disorders, acute alcohol withdrawal, and as a skeletal muscle relaxant. Diazepam can be administered orally, rectally, and parenterally. Diazepam is the most rapidly absorbed benzodiazepine following an oral dose. The absorption following an intramuscular (IM) injection is slow and erratic.

Diazepam

Ingredients	Diazepam	Dose	2.5–5 mg
Brand Name	Valium	Supplemental Dose	2.5–20 mg
Cost	$2.54/vial	Onset Action	1–5 minutes
FDA Approval	1981	Duration of Effect	12–60 hours
		Comment	Long-acting benzodiazepine. Do not mix or dilute

Anticonvulsant, skeletal muscle relaxant, and anxiolytic effects are usually evident after the first dose. The onset of action after an intravenous dose is 1–5 minutes. The duration for some clinical effects (e.g., sedation, anticonvulsant activity) is much shorter than would be expected considering the very long half-life for diazepam (30–60 hours). The typical intravenous dose can be low as 2.5 to 5 mg before the procedure, and then supplemental doses titrated from 2.5 to up to 20 mg intravenously (IV), depending on response and patient tolerability. The oral dose is 10 mg given 45–60 minutes before the procedure.

Diazepam is primarily metabolized in the liver with the production of long-half-life active metabolites. These metabolites are subsequently glucuronidated and excreted in the urine.

Benzodiazepine Antagonist

FLUMAZENIL

Flumazenil or Romazicon® is a competitive benzodiazepine antagonist in the central nervous system and is used to reverse the sedation effect, ventilatory depression, and psychomotor impairment caused by benzodiazepines. It has a one hour half-life. Because the half-life of flumazenil is so short, a resedation effect by long-acting benzodiazepines may occur in 3–9% of the patients, requiring a second dose of the antagonist in some cases. The usual dose is 0.1–0.2 mg intravenously every minute until reversal of benzodiazepine overdose signs is observed. The onset of reversal is usually evident within 1–2 minutes after injection. Eighty percent response will be reached within three minutes, with the peak

Flumazenil

Ingredients	Flumazenil	Dose	0.1–0.2 mg
Brand Name	Romazicon	Supplemental Dose	Same at 1 minute
Cost	$82.86/vial	Onset Action	0.5–1 minute
FDA Approval	1991	Duration of Effect	60 minutes
		Comment	Increased risk of seizure in patients with long-term benzodiazepine therapy

effect occurring at 6–10 minutes. The pharmacokinetics is not significantly altered by age, gender, or renal function. Adverse effects are infrequent in patients who receive 1 mg or less, although injection site pain, agitation, and anxiety may occur. Flumazenil is known to precipitate withdrawal seizures in patients who are physically dependent on benzodiazepines, even if such dependence was established in a few days of high-dose sedation. Flumazenil is contraindicated in patients with a known hypersensitivity to the drug or in patients who have been given a benzodiazepine for control of a potentially life-threatening condition (e.g., control of elevated intracranial pressure or status epilepticus).

Opioids

Opioids bind to specific receptors located throughout the central nervous system including the spinal cord and other tissues. Four major types of opioid receptors have been identified: mu (μ), kappa (κ), delta (δ), and sigma (σ). Of those receptors, μ receptors (with subtypes μ-1 and μ-2) are the most clinically relevant. Stimulation of μ-1 receptors produces supraspinal analgesia, and μ-2 activation produces respiratory depression, miosis, decreased gastrointestinal motility, and euphoria. Kappa-receptor stimulation also produces some degree of analgesia, miosis, and respiratory depression. Respiratory depression is caused by the direct action of an opiate on respiratory centers in the brain stem. Opiate agonists increase smooth muscle tone in the stomach, small intestine, large intestine, and biliary and gastrointestinal sphincters. Opiate agonists also decrease secretions from the stomach, pancreas, and biliary tract. The combination of effects of opiate agonists on the gastrointestinal tract results in constipation and delayed digestion. Urinary smooth muscle tone is also increased by opiate agonists. The tone of the bladder detrusor muscle, ureters, and vesical sphincter is increased, which sometimes causes urinary retention. Other significant clinical side effects include cough suppression, hypotension, nausea, and vomiting. The antitussive effects of opiate agonists are mediated through direct action on receptors in the cough center of the medulla, and cough suppression can be achieved at lower doses than those required to produce analgesia. Hypotension is possibly due to an increase in histamine release and/or depression of the vasomotor center in the medulla. Induction of nausea and vomiting possibly occurs from direct stimulation of the vestibular system and/or the chemoreceptor trigger zone. Opioids can produce drug dependence; psychic dependence, physical dependence, and tolerance may develop upon repeated administration of opioids and therefore should be prescribed and administered with caution. All opioids are regulated by federal narcotic laws.

FENTANYL

Fentanyl is a synthetic opioid that binds with relative specificity to μ-receptors (μ-1/μ-2). It is 80–100 times more potent than morphine and 750 times more potent than meperidine. The onset of action of fentanyl is almost immediate when the drug is given intravenously, making it relatively easy to titrate; however, the maximal analgesic and respiratory depressant effect may not be noted for several minutes. The usual duration of action of the

Fentanyl			
Ingredients	Fentanyl Citrate	Dose	25–75 µg
Brand Name	Sublimaze	Supplemental Dose	25–50 µg
Cost	$1.40/vial	Onset Action	0–5 minutes
FDA Approval	1968	Duration of Effect	30–60 minutes
		Comments	Hepatic impairment prolongs the effect

analgesic effect is 30–60 minutes after a single IV dose of up to 100 µg. Fentanyl is typically given IV at a dose of 0.5 to 2 µg/kg every 1–2 minutes. It is prudent not to administrate at intervals shorter than 2 minutes.

Larger doses of fentanyl may produce apnea. As with most medications used in procedural sedation and analgesia, lower doses should be used in the elderly population. Fentanyl appears to have fewer emetic side effects than either morphine or meperidine. Additional benefits include preserving cardiac stability, and the drug does not cause histamine release as does morphine. As a result, the incidence of hypotension and skin manifestations (flushing and rash) is minimal. Fentanyl has minimal amnestic effects and is not typically used as a single agent. Therefore, it is commonly combined with amnestics and anxiolytics such as midazolam.

As with other opioids, the most common serious adverse reactions reported to occur with fentanyl are respiratory depression, apnea, rigidity, and bradycardia. If these remain untreated, respiratory arrest, circulatory depression, or cardiac arrest could occur. An advantage over other narcotics is that fentanyl seems to have minimal cardiovascular effects; therefore, it is less likely to cause hypotension. Fentanyl is contraindicated in patients with known hypersensitivity to the drug or other opioid agonist.

MORPHINE

Morphine is a pure opiate agonist with relative selectivity for the µ-receptor, although at higher doses it can interact with other opiate receptors. The principal therapeutic action of morphine is analgesia. Other therapeutic effects of morphine include anxiolysis, euphoria, and a relaxed feeling. Morphine is still

Morphine			
Ingredients	Morphine Sulfate	Dose	2.5–10 mg
Brand Name		Supplemental Dose	0.8–10 mg/hour
Cost	$23.80/vial	Onset Action	1–5 minutes
FDA Approval	1984	Duration of Effect	4–6 hours
		Comment	Contraindicated in patients with hepatic and/or renal insufficiency

a widely used opioid in the management of acute and chronic pain. The onset of action after intravenous injection is around 3–5 minutes, but IM or subcutaneous administration results in slower absorption, which can range between 15 and 20 minutes. Peak analgesia is obtained about 20 minutes after intravenous injection, and 50–90 minutes after subcutaneous and IM injections. Morphine is rapidly and widely distributed and crosses the blood brain barrier. At therapeutic doses, plasma protein binding is only 20–35%. The primary site of metabolism is the liver and excretion is via the kidneys; the dose should therefore be reduced in patients with liver disease. There is no predictable relationship between morphine serum concentrations and analgesic response; however, there is a minimum effective analgesia plasma concentration for any given patient, which varies from patient to patient. Also, there is no relationship between morphine concentrations and incidence of adverse events, although higher concentrations are associated with more adverse events than lower concentrations. Several factors may affect a patient's response to a given opiate agonist including age, prior opiate therapy, medical condition, and emotions.

As with all drugs in the opiate class, morphine can cause respiratory depression, cough depression, and nausea, and vomiting. These may occur in part due to a direct effect on the brainstem and medulla. Antitussive effects may occur with doses lower than those usually required for analgesia. In the gastrointestinal tract, morphine decreases the gastric, biliary, and pancreatic secretions; causes a reduction in bowel motility; and causes a marked increase in biliary tract pressure as a result of spasm of the sphincter of Oddi. Morphine may also cause spasms of the sphincter of the urinary bladder. In therapeutic doses, morphine does not usually cause major effects on the cardiovascular system. Morphine, like other opiates, produces peripheral vasodilatation that may result in orthostatic hypotension and fainting. Release of histamine can occur, which may play a role in opiate-induced hypotension. Manifestations of histamine release and/or peripheral vasodilatation may include pruritus, flushing, red eyes, and sweating.

Morphine clearance is decreased in the elderly and in cirrhotic patients; drug administration in these patients should be performed with caution. Morphine sulfate is contraindicated in patients with respiratory depression, acute or severe bronchial asthma, and upper airway obstruction. It is also contraindicated in any patient who has or is suspected of having paralytic ileus, suspected or known head injury, or increased intracranial pressure. Morphine sulfate may cause vasodilatation that may exacerbate hypotension and hypoperfusion and, therefore, is contraindicated in patients with circulatory shock.

Morphine has several pharmacological disadvantages when considered as a drug for sedation and analgesia for interventional procedures. The onset of action is slower in comparison with fentanyl, and despite shorter half-life, morphine's clinical effects are longer than those of fentanyl. For this reason, morphine is popular as a postoperative analgesic when pain is expected for a prolonged period of time. The main side effects are related to histamine release causing flushing, hives, and rash. The incidence of nausea and untoward central nervous system effects are greater as well. Morphine does not fit the model of a rapid-onset, short-acting, low-side-effect agent as well as fentanyl.

In our practice, we use morphine for pain control after certain procedures including chemoembolization, uterine fibroid embolization, and sclerotherapy of vascular malformations. We use intravenous morphine via pump; our standard regimens are (a) 0.5 mg every six minutes, with a maximum dose of 20 mg in a four-hour period, and (b) 1 mg every eight minutes, with a maximum dose of 30 mg in a four-hour period.

We usually employ an antiemetic drug to reduce the nausea and vomiting related to both the procedure and the morphine effect. We find that these regimens work extremely well in controlling pain for these patients.

MEPERIDINE

Meperidine is a synthetic narcotic with a weak analgesic property. Meperidine is primarily a κ-opiate receptor agonist, and due to its chemical structure, it also has local anesthetic effects. Meperidine is recommended for relief of moderate to severe acute pain. It is one-tenth as potent as morphine with side effects unlike those of other opioids. There is some evidence, which suggests that meperidine may produce less smooth muscle spasm, constipation, and depression of the cough reflex than equianalgesic doses of morphine. Some patients exhibit an increase in heart rate probably caused by chemical structural similarity to atropine. The onset of action is slightly more rapid than with morphine, and the duration of action is slightly shorter. Following intravenous administration, onset of analgesia occurs within one minute and the time to peak effect is 5–7 minutes. When given via the intramuscular or subcutaneous route, the onset of action is noted within 10–15 minutes and the peak of effect occurs within one hour. The duration of analgesia is around 2–4 hours but decreases with chronic use. Dosage should be adjusted according to necessity, severity of the pain, and response of the patient. IM administration is preferred when repeated doses are required. If intravenous administration is required, the dosage should be decreased and the drug should be injected very slowly, preferably utilizing a diluted solution. Rapid intravenous injection increases the incidence of serious adverse reactions, such as severe respiratory depression, apnea, hypotension, peripheral circulatory collapse, and cardiac arrest. The usual dosage is 50–150 mg intramuscularly or subcutaneously every three or four hours as necessary. In children, the dosage is 1–1.5 mg/kg intramuscularly or subcutaneously up to the adult dose, every three or four hours as necessary.

Meperidine is metabolized to normeperidine in the liver, a metabolite capable of inducing seizures and delirium. These toxic reactions to this

Meperidine			
Ingredients	Meperidine HCl	Dose	50–150 mg
Brand Name	Demerol	Supplemental Dose	25–100 mg
Cost	$19.20/vial	Onset Action	1–7 minutes
FDA Approval	1942	Duration of Effect	2–4 hours
		Comment	Use with caution in patients with renal and/or hepatic insufficiency. Do not used concurrently with MAO inhibitors

compound may be greater in patients with impaired hepatic or renal function. In elderly patients, the drug should be given at the lower end of the dose range and the patient observed closely because these patients are more likely to have decreased renal function. Meperidine is contraindicated in patients who are receiving monoamine oxidase (MAO) inhibitors or those who have recently received such agents. There are reports of severe and occasionally fatal reactions after meperidine administration in patients who have received MAO inhibitors within 14 days. The mechanism of these reactions is unclear but may be related to a preexisting hyperphenylalaninemia. Meperidine is also contraindicated in patients with respiratory depression, acute or severe bronchial asthma, upper airway obstruction, who have or are suspected of having paralytic ileus, head injury, or increased intracranial pressure. The respiratory depressant effects of meperidine can cause CO_2 retention with subsequent elevation of cerebrospinal fluid pressure; this effect may be markedly exaggerated in the presence of head injury, other intracranial lesions, or a preexisting increase in intracranial pressure.

REMIFENTANIL

Remifentanil is a μ-receptor agonist with rapid onset and peak effect and an ultrashort duration of action. The effects of remifentanil have a direct correlation between dose, blood levels, and response. The peak effect occurs within 3–5 minutes after a single dose of remifentanil, which effectively subsides within 5–10 minutes after discontinuation of therapy. Good grades of analgesia are reached with infusions of 0.05–0.1 μg/kg/minute, with blood concentrations of 1–3 ng/ml. As a practical rule, every 0.1 μg/kg/minute change in the IV infusion rate will lead to a corresponding 2.5 ng/ml change in remifentanil blood concentration, with a necessity of delay of around 5–10 minutes to reach the steady state. At doses larger than 5 ng/ml or greater than 0.2 μg/kg/minute, remifentanil can cause hypotension, bradycardia, and respiratory depression. Skeletal muscle rigidity is related directly to dose and speed of administration. Unlike other opioids, remifentanil is rapidly metabolized by blood and tissue esterases. The pharmacokinetics of remifentanil are unaffected by the presence of renal or hepatic impairment. The rapid elimination of remifentanil permits the titration of infusion rate without concern for prolonged duration of action. The μ-receptor activity of remifentanil can be reversed by opioid antagonists such as naloxone. Only personnel specifically trained in the use of intravenous and general anesthetics should administer remifentanil.

Remifentanil			
Ingredients	Remifentanil HCl	Dose	0.05–0.1 μg/kg/minute
Brand Name	Ultiva	Supplemental Dose	0.05 μg/kg/minute
Cost	$70.70/vial	Onset Action	0–1 minute
FDA Approval	1996	Duration of Effect	3–10 minutes
		Comments	Should be used by trained personnel

Naloxone			
Ingredients	Naloxone HCl	Dose	0.4–0.8 mg
Brand Name	Narcan	Supplemental Dose	0.1–0.2 mg up to 10 mg
Cost	$1.75/vial	Onset Action	1–2 minutes
FDA Approval	1971	Duration of Effect	1–2 hours
		Comment	Do not use in Patients who are suspected to be physically dependent on opioids

Opioid Antagonist

NALOXONE

Naloxone is a pure opiate-receptor antagonist with little or no agonistic activity. Classically, it is used to reverse the clinical effects of opiate analgesics overdose. Naloxone is thought to antagonize µ-, kappa-, and delta-receptors. This antagonism is competitive and short lived. Thus, repeat doses of naloxone may be required when long-acting opiates are involved.

The onset of action is 1–2 minutes after IV administration and 2–5 minutes after subcutaneous or IM administration. Onset of action can be delayed in hypotensive patients. The plasma half-life ranges from 60 to 90 minutes. The usual dose is 0.4–0.8 mg IV, IM, or SC, up to a total dose of 10 mg; the doses can be repeated every 2–3 minutes to attain the desired response. Naloxone is metabolized in the liver and excreted by the kidney (12). Naloxone itself produces no physical or psychological dependence and will not worsen respiratory depression if administered for nonopiate overdose. It should be used with discretion when considering administering it to patients who are sedated from opiates but who do not exhibit respiratory depression. In patients who have not recently received opioid drugs, naloxone shows no pharmacological effects, even at high doses.

Other Drugs

PROPOFOL

Propofol is an intravenous, nonbarbiturate anesthetic that is structurally unrelated to other intravenous anesthetic agents. The mechanism of action of propofol appears to be related to inhibition of a specific subtype of glutamate receptors and agonistic activity at the GABA receptor. The popularity of propofol as a sedative and induction agent is related to its rapid onset and short duration of action, producing rapid awakening and recovery in most patients (13). The onset of action is as rapid as 40 seconds, with a typical duration of action of 3–5 minutes (14). The usual dose is 100–150 µg/kg/minute injected over a period of 3–5 minutes, trying to titrate to desired clinical effect while closely monitoring respiratory function. For maintenance infusions in most

Propofol			
Ingredients	Propofol	Dose	100–150 µg/kg/minute during 3–5 minute
Brand Name	Diprivan	Supplemental Dose	25–50 µg/kg/minute adjusted to clinical response
Cost	$7.09/vial	Onset Action	<1–2 minutes
FDA Approval	1989	Duration of Effect	3–5 minutes
		Comments	Should be used by trained personnel

patients, an IV infusion of 25–75 µg/kg/minute is given during the first 10–15 minutes, followed by 25–50 µg/kg/minute adjusted to clinical response. Doses of 150–200 µg/kg/minute usually produce deep sedation or general anesthesia. When used at subhypnotic doses, propofol provides an easily titratable level of sedation, with anxiolysis and amnesia similar to those of midazolam (15). When propofol is administered slowly, most patients will be adequately sedated and the peak drug effect can be achieved while minimizing undesirable cardio-respiratory effects.

Controversy exists concerning the safe use of propofol by practitioners who are not anesthesiologists. Gastroenterologists in particular have pursued the use of propofol for sedation during endoscopic procedures. Several large randomized controlled studies have been published demonstrating its safe use by gastroenterologists, often with nurses administering the drug (16,17). Propofol is metabolized in the liver where it rapidly is converted to inactive metabolites that are excreted by the kidney. The pharmacokinetics of propofol do not appear to be affected by chronic hepatic or renal disease.

Unlike many other general anesthetics, propofol possesses antiemetic activity (18). Pain during the injection occurs in 28–90% of patients. The concomitant use of a low dose of IV lidocaine can prevent the pain resulting from propofol injection (19).

Nonsteroidal Anti-imflammatory Drugs

NSAIDs are used as first-line agents for the symptomatic relief of inflammatory and pain conditions, and fever relief. NSAIDs constitute one of the most widely used groups of drugs in the USA (20), with 70 million prescriptions and more than 30 billion over-the-counter tablets sold annually (21). NSAIDs are a chemically varied class of compounds with common therapeutic effects. NSAIDs mediate inflammation through inhibition of the COX enzyme, which is responsible for the production of prostaglandins from arachidonic acid (22,23). NSAIDs also work as antipyretics through inhibition of production of prostaglandin E2 in the hypothalamus. Analgesic properties appear to be due to attenuation of the prostaglandin-mediated effect on nociceptors that are activated by chemical mediators of pain, such as bradykinin, histamine, nitric oxide (24).

There are two general types of COX inhibitors: nonselective and selective. The majority of NSAIDs are nonselective, leading to inhibition of both COX-1 and COX-2. The inhibition of COX-1 is responsible for many of the unwanted gastrointestinal side effects of NSAIDs. The new selective compounds do not appear to be more effective mediators of inflammation or analgesics, but they do appear to cause fewer gastrointestinal side effects due to the lack of COX-1 effects (Table 4).

Variability in response to NSAIDs is described among patients, although the exact cause is not fully understood. Several pharmacological factors such as dose response, plasma half-life, and urinary excretion, as well heterogeneity in gene expression are the most accepted explanations (25–27). NSAIDs are available in a variety of preparations, including sustained release, slow release, and suppository. Most NSAIDs are totally absorbed from gastrointestinal tract, bound to plasmatic proteins by more than 90%, and metabolized principally through the liver with production of inactive metabolites that are excreted in the bile and urine. Most NSAIDs undergo partial metabolism in the liver with elimination in the urine or feces. Plasma half-lives of NSAIDs range from 2 hours for ibuprofen to longer than 80 hours for piroxicam.

NSAIDs are relatively safe drugs that have a number of well-documented side effects at therapeutic doses. Important toxicities occur in the gastrointestinal tract, kidney, platelets, and other organ systems. Effects on platelets are also recognized. The adverse gastrointestinal effects occur in at least 10–20% of patients, resulting in increase of NSAID-associated morbidity and mortality (28). The mortality rate among patients hospitalized for NSAID-induced upper gastrointestinal bleeding is 5–10% (29), and certain groups of patients are at greater risk for developing peptic ulcer complications. In these cases, consideration should be given to use a gastroprotective therapies in order to reduce the risk of adverse gastrointestinal events. The available strategies include the use of COX-2-specific NSAIDs, replacement of gastric prostanoids with misoprostol, synthetic analog of prostaglandin E1 (30,31), or coadministration of a proton pump inhibitor (30,32). However, misoprostol is often poorly tolerated due to diarrhea or abdominal pain (33). Unfortunately, despite the number of

Table 4. Risk Factors for Gastrointestinal Complications of NSAIDs
Advancing age
High dose of NSAID
History of peptic ulcer
Anticoagulation or aspirin therapy
Corticosteroid therapy
Alcohol
Cigarette smoking
Source: Wolfe et al. (29).

Table 5. Nonsteroidal Anti-inflammatory Drugs

Drug	Brand Name	Cost/Day ($)	Presentation (mg)	Maximal Dose (mg/day)	Tmax (hour)	T (hour)	Comments
Celecoxib[a]	Celebrex	3.8	100, 200, 400	400 (800 mg in FAP)	3	11	Contraindicated with sulfonamide allergy
Diclofenac	Voltaren	4.2	25, 50, 75 100 (ER)	225	1–2	2	More incidence of elevation of transaminase
Etodolac	Lodine	5.2	200, 300, 400, 500, 600	1200	1–2	6–7	
Fenoprofen	Nalfon	2.74	200, 300, 600	3200	1–2	2–3	More risk of idiosyncratic nephropathy
Flurbiprofen	Ansaid	3.6	50, 100	300	1.5–2	3–4	
Ibuprofen	Motrin, Advil	0.3	200 (OTC), 300, 400, 600, 800	3200	1–2	2	Contraindicated in severe liver disease
Indomethacin	Indocin	2.4	25, 50, 75 (SR)	200	1–4	2–13	
Ketoprofen	Orudis	3.7	12.5 (OTC), 25, 50, 75100, 150,200 (SR)	300	0.5–2	2–4	Adjust dose is required in severe renal disease, hepatic disease, and elderly
Ketorolac	Toradol	5.3	PO:10 IM/IV: 15, 30	120 IV/IM 40 mg PO	0.3–1	4–6	Adjust dose in renal failure and elderly
Meloxicam	Mobic	3.3	7.5	15	5–6	20	
Nabumetone	Relafen	2.6	500, 750	2000	3–6	24	Reduce dose in renal disease; avoid in severe liver disease
Naproxen	Aleve	0.4	125 (OTC), 250, 375, 500	1500	2–4	12–15	Decrease dose in renal disease, liver disease, and the elderly
Oxaprozin	Daypro	3.2	600	1800 or 26 mg/kg/day	3–6	49–60	Adjust dose in renal failure
Piroxicam	Feldene	3.7	10, 20	20	2–5	3–86	Reduce dose in liver disease and elderly
Sulindac	Clinoril	2.5	150, 200	400	2–4	16	Decrease dose in renal disease, liver disease, and the elderly
Valdecoxib[a]	Bextra	3.5	10, 20	20	1–3	8–11	Contraindicated in patients with sulfa allergy; caution in severe renal and liver disease

[a]COX-2 specific.
Source: Harris et al. (37).

strategies available for risk reduction, there is a high failure rate to adequately protect patients using NSAIDs.

Non-gastrointestinal-related side effects of NSAIDS are also well documented. NSAIDs inhibit platelet aggregation, but except for aspirin, this inhibition is reversible and depends on the concentration of drug in the platelet. The antiaggregation effect of aspirin can last for up to 4–6 days, until the bone marrow can form new platelets (34). Prostaglandins play a vital role in solute and renovascular homeostasis (35). Prostaglandins are known to regulate renal sodium resorption by their ability to inhibit active transport of sodium in both the thick ascending limb and the collecting duct of the kidney, and to increase renal water excretion by blunting the actions of vasopressin (36). Decreased sodium excretion in NSAID-treated patients can lead to weight gain and peripheral edema. This effect may be sufficient to cause clinically important exacerbations of congestive heart failure. At the current time, there is no documented difference between COX-2-specific and nonspecific NSAIDs with regard to renal effects (35). In addition to sodium retention, NSAIDs may cause altered blood pressure or acute renal failure (uncommon and most of the time reversible). Another adverse renal effect resulting from NSAIDs involves an idiosyncratic reaction accompanied by massive proteinuria and acute interstitial nephritis.

A wide variety of cutaneous reactions have been associated with NSAIDs. Almost all the NSAIDs have been associated with cutaneous vasculitis, erythema multiforme, Stevens-Johnson syndrome, or toxic epidermal necrolysis. NSAIDs are also associated with urticaria, angioedema, anaphylactoid, or anaphylactic reaction. Up to 10–20% of the general asthmatic population, especially those with the triad of vasomotor rhinitis, nasal polyposis, and asthma, are hypersensitive to aspirin. In these patients, ingestion of aspirin and nonspecific NSAIDs leads to severe exacerbations of asthma with naso-ocular reactions.

CONCLUSIONS

A wide range of medications are available for use both during and following interventional procedures. Choosing an appropriate regimen is vital to maximize the desired effect of any given regimen while minimizing its adverse effect. In order to achieve this desired effect, the interventionalist must take an active role in being familiar with commonly used medications.

REFERENCES

1. Gross JB, Bailey PL, Connis RT, et al. American Society of Anesthesiologists Task Force on Sedation and Analgesia by Non-Anesthesiologists. Practice guidelines for sedation and analgesia by non-anesthesiologists. Anesthesiology 2002;**96**:1004–17.
2. Practice guidelines for preoperative fasting and the use of pharmacologic agents to reduce the risk of pulmonary aspiration: application to healthy patients undergoing elective procedures: a report by the American Society of Anesthesiologist Task Force on Preoperative Fasting. Anesthesiology 1999;**90**:896–905.

3. Hoffman GM, Nowakski R, Troshynski TJ, Bereas RJ, Weisman SJ. Risk reduction in pediatric procedural sedation by application of an American Academy of Pediatrics/ American Society of Anesthesiologists process model. Pediatrics 2002;**109**:236–43.

4. Agrawal D, Manzi SF, Gupta R, Krauss B. Preprocedural fasting state and adverse events in children undergoing procedural sedation and analgesia in a pediatric emergency department. Ann Emerg Med 2003;**42**:636–46.

5. American College of Emergency Physicians. Clinical policy for procedural sedation and analgesia in the emergency department. Ann Emerg Med 1998;**31**:663–77.

6. Bailey PL, Pace NL, Ashburn MA, Moll JW, East KA, Stanley TH. Frequent hypoxemia and apnea after sedation with midazolam and fentanyl. Anesthesiology 1990;**73**:826–30.

7. Goodchild CS. GABA receptors and benzodiazepines. Br J Anaesth 1993;**71**:127–33.

8. Buhrer M, Maitre PO, Crevoisier C, Stanski DR. Electroencephalographic effects of benzodiazepines. II. Pharmacodynamic modeling of the electroencephalographic effects of midazolam and diazepam. Clin Pharmacol Ther 1990;**48**:555–67.

9. Kanto J, Aaltonen L, Himberg JJ, Houi-Viander M. Midazolam as an intravenous induction agent in the elderly: a clinical and pharmacokinetic study. Anesth Analg 1986;**65**:15–20.

10. Oldenhof H, deJong M, Steenhoek A, Janknegt R. Clinical pharmacokinetics of midazolam in intensive care patients, a wide interpatient variability? Clin Pharmacol Ther 1988;**43**:263–9.

11. Meyer BR. Benzodiazepines in the elderly. Med Clin North Am 1982;**66**:1017–35.

12. Handal KA, Schauben JL, Salamone FR. Naloxone. Ann Emerg Med 1983;**12**: 438–45.

13. Wilder-Smith OH. Borgeat A. Propofol and pharmacokinetic modeling. Anesth Analg 1992;**74**:316–7.

14. Schnider TW, Minto CF, Shafer SL, et al. The influence of age on propofol pharmacodynamics. Anesthesiology 1999;**90**:1502–16.

15. Veselis RA, Reinsel RA, Feshchenko Va, Wronski M. The comparative amnestic effects of midazolam, propofol, thiopental, and fentanyl at equisedative concentrations. Anesthesiology 1997;**87**:749–64.

16. Vargo JJ, Zuccaro G Jr, Dumot JA, et al. Gastroenterologist-administered propofol versus meperidine and midazolam for advanced upper endoscopy: a prospective, randomized trial. Gastroenterology 2002;**123**:8–16.

17. Rex DK, Overley C, Kinser K, et al. Safety of propofol administered by registered nurses with gastroenterologist supervision in 2000 endoscopic cases. Am J Gastroenterol 2002;**97**:1159–63.

18. Borgeat A, Wilder-Smith OH, Saiah M, Rifat K. Subhypnotic doses of propofol possess direct antiemetic properties. Anesth Analg 1992;**74**:539–41.

19. Gehan G, Karoubi P, Quiret F, Leroy A, Rathat C, Pourriat JL. Optimal dose of lignocaine for preventing pain on injection of propofol. Br J Anaesth 1991;**66**:324–6.

20. Paakkari H. Epidemiological and financial aspects of the use of non-steroidal anti-inflammatory analgesics. Pharmacol Toxicol 1994;**75**(2):56–9.

21. Lichtenstein DR, Syngal S, Wolfe MM. Nonsteroidal antiinflammatory drugs and the gastrointestinal tract. The double-edged sword. Arthritis Rheum 1995;**38**:5–18.

22. DeWitt DL, Meade EA, Smith WL. PGH synthase isoenzyme selectivity: the potential for safer nonsteroidal antiinflammatory drugs. Am J Med 1993;**95**:40S–4S.

23. Marnett LJ, Rowlinson SW, Goodwin DC, Kalgutkar AS, Lanzo CA. Arachidonic acid oxygenation by COX-1 and COX-2. Mechanisms of catalysis and inhibition. J Biol Chem 1999;**274**:22903–6.

24. Ito S, Okuda-Ashitaka E, Minami T. Central and peripheral roles of prostaglandins in pain and their interactions with novel neuropeptides nociceptin and nocistatin. Neurosci Res 2001;**41**:299–332.

25. Vane JR, Botting RM. Mechanism of action of anti-inflammatory drugs. Adv Exp Med Biol 1997;**433**:131–8.

26. Rodnan GP, Benedek TG. The early history of antirheumatic drugs. Arthritis Rheum 1970;**13**:145–65.

27. Lee YS, Kim H, Wu TX, Wang KM, Dionne RA. Genetically mediated interindividual variation in analgesic responses to cyclooxygenase inhibitory drugs. Clin Pharmacol Ther 2006;**79**:407–18.

28. Cryer B. A COX-2-specific inhibitor plus a proton-pump inhibitor: is this a reasonable approach to reduction in NSAIDs' GI toxicity? Am J Gastroenterol 2006;**101**:711–3.

29. Wolfe MM, Lichenstein DR, Singh G. Gastrointestinal toxicity of nonsteroidal anti-inflammatory drugs. N Engl J Med 1999;**340**:1888–99.

30. Scheiman JM. Pathogenesis of gastroduodenal injury due to nonsteroidal antiinflammatory drugs: implications for prevention and therapy. Semin Arthritis Rheum 1992; **21**:201–10.

31. Graham DY, Agrawal NM, Roth SH. Prevention of NSAID-induced gastric ulcer with misoprostol: multicentre, double-blind, placebo-controlled trial. Lancet 1988;**2**(8623):1277–80.

32. Chan FK, Huang LC, Suen BY, et al. Celecoxib versus diclofenac and omeprazole in reducing the risk of recurrent ulcer bleeding in patients with arthritis. N Engl J Med 2002;**347**:2104–10.

33. Silverstein FE, Grahan DY, Senior JR, et al. Misoprostol reduces serious gastrointestinal complications in patients with rheumatoid arthritis receiving nonsteroidal anti-inflammatory drugs. A randomized, double-blind, placebo-controlled trial. Ann Intern Med 1995;**123**:241–9.

34. Antithrombotic Trialists' Collaboration. Collaborative meta-analysis of randomised trials of antiplatelet therapy for prevention of death, myocardial infarction, and stroke in high risk patients. BMJ 2002;**324**:71–86.

35. Brater DC. Anti-inflammatory agents and renal function. Semin Arthritis Rheum, 2002;**32**:33–42.

36. Brater DC, Harris C, Redfern JS, Gertz BJ. Renal effects of COX-2-selective inhibitors. Am J Nephrol 2001;**21**:1–15.

37. Harris ED Jr., Budd RC, Firestein GS, et al. (eds). Kelley's Textbook of Rheumatology, 7th Edition – Text with Continually Updated Online Reference, 2-Volume Set. Philadelphia: WB Saunders, 2005, pp. 845–6.

Guidelines for Sedation Administered by Nonanesthesiologists

Iftikhar Ahmad

The purpose of sedation during interventional procedures is to alleviate pain and anxiety. Administration of sedation makes performance of interventional procedures possible in young children and uncooperative adults. Anesthesiologists are trained to administer and monitor all levels of sedation. However, it is a common practice for nonanesthesiologists to administer sedation in a variety of hospital and office settings.

Sedation is a continuum of decreasing levels of consciousness ranging from anxiolysis to general anesthesia. During anxiolysis, also known as minimal sedation, the patient's level of anxiety is decreased; they are responsive to all external stimuli and maintain all protective reflexes. These patients may have some impairment of their cognitive functions. Moderate sedation is a medically controlled state of depressed consciousness in which patients respond purposefully to verbal and tactile stimuli and maintain all protective refluxes. In deep sedation, the level of consciousness is further depressed where patients only respond to painful stimuli. These patients generally maintain their respiratory drive and cardiovascular functions but their gag reflex may be depressed intermittently. General anesthesia involves medically induced complete loss of consciousness from which patients cannot be aroused by any form of external stimuli. These patients lose all protective refluxes and their respiratory and cardiovascular functions are depressed. In most clinical settings, nonanesthesiologists administer and monitor moderate sedation (where not otherwise specified, the word sedation implies moderate sedation in this chapter).

Safe administration of sedation by nonanesthesiologists is governed by guidelines generated by the American Society of Anesthesiologists (ASA) and the Joint Commission for Accreditation of Healthcare Organizations (JCAHO).

The *American Society of Anesthesia* formed a 10-member task force comprising anesthesiologists in academic and private practices as well as nonanesthesiologists who routinely administered sedation in their practices. The participants of the task force were chosen from all parts of the United States. This task force reviewed published literature and conducted surveys relating to safety and efficacy of various methods of administering sedation. Based on literature review and survey results, the task force formulated draft recommendations and held open forums during two major national meetings to solicit input on these draft recommendations. ASA guidelines for sedation administered by nonanesthesiologists were first published in *Anesthesiology* in 1996 (1) and the revision was published in *Anesthesiology* in 2002 (2).

Based on the strength of published data in support of a given recommendation, the task force graded the recommendation as supportive, suggestive, equivocal, inconclusive, or insufficient. Similarly, the survey responses from the consultants were graded from one through five ranging from strongly disagree to strongly agree.

These guidelines are only intended for administration of moderate sedation by nonanesthesiologists during interventional and diagnostic procedures. These guidelines do not address minimal or deep sedation. Because of the differences in the level of sedation and patient monitoring, administration of moderate sedation outside the settings of interventional or diagnostic procedures, such as premedication and postoperative analgesia, are also not covered by these guidelines.

The guidelines recommended by the ASA are intended to assist the health care provider in administering sedation in a safe and effective fashion. These guidelines are broad in scope and general in application. The guidelines are only recommendations and are not binding. They can be adapted, altered, or altogether ignored by the health care professional administering sedation.

JCAHO is an agency whose mission is to improve the safety and quality of patient care though accreditation of health care facilities and to provide related services to support and improve performance of health care organizations. To this goal, JCAHO employs many tools including the conduction of surveys, site visits, and inspection of various health care organizations for the purpose of accreditation. JCAHO also establishes organizational standards to be implemented by health care organizations. These standards of practice are published in a compressive accreditation manual that can be accessed online at the JCAHO official Web site (3). JCAHO standards for sedation apply in all hospital or office settings where the administration of sedation, irrespective of its intent, is reasonably expected to suppress the patients protective reflexes.

ASA guidelines address all aspects of sedation from consent to medications and recovery. JCAHO guidelines, in contrast, are more operational in nature and discuss staffing, equipment, and documentation.

AMERICAN SOCIETY OF ANESTHESIA GUIDELINES

Preprocedure Patient Evaluation

The clinician administering sedation should obtain the patient's medical history including previous reactions to sedation, allergies to drug and other substances, time of last oral intake, and history of alcohol, tobacco, or substance abuse. The patient should also undergo a focused physical examination. Vital signs should be obtained and the heart, lungs, and airways should be evaluated. Only those laboratory tests that will be helpful in the decision-making process during administration of sedation should be ordered.

The published literature provides insufficient evidence of any relationship between preprocedure patient evaluation and the outcome of administering sedation. There is, however, some evidence that preexisting medical conditions may adversely affect the outcome of sedation. The consultants strongly agree that a history should be taken, and a focused physical examination should be performed on all patients receiving sedation.

Consent

The patient or their legal guardians should be properly counseled about the risks, benefits, limitations, and alternatives of administering sedation.

There is insufficient literature regarding benefits of obtaining informed consent for sedation. The consultants agree in the case of moderate sedation and strongly agree in the case of deep sedation that an informed consent for administering sedation should be obtained in all patients.

Oral Intake Status

The guidelines recommend six hours of fasting after ingestion of a solid meal and four hours after liquids. After ingestion of clear liquids, patients can receive sedation after two hours. Clear liquids for this purpose are defined as transparent or semitransparent liquids of any color.

There is insufficient literature in support of better outcomes of sedation in patients who were fasting before the procedure. Sedation does, however, suppress airway reflexes. The consultants agree in the case of moderate sedation and strongly agree in the case of deep sedation that for elective interventional procedures, enough time should be allowed for gastric emptying so as to prevent aspiration during the procedure. In emergent situations, consultants suggest altering the target level of sedation, delaying the procedure if possible, or protecting the airway by endotracheal intubation.

Monitoring Level of Consciousness

The patient's level of consciousness should be monitored by assessing their response to verbal commands. Spoken responses from the patients also assure that they are breathing adequately.

Published literature is noncontributory as to whether monitoring the patient's level of consciousness either reduces risk or improves outcome. However, the consultants strongly agree for both moderate and deep sedation that monitoring the patient's responsiveness reduces the risk and improves outcome.

Monitoring Pulmonary Ventilation

Drug-induced respiratory depression is the main cause of morbidity and mortality related to sedation. During administration of sedation, ventilatory function should be monitored by observation and auscultation. Although related to ventilation, monitoring blood oxygen levels by pulse oximetry is an independent physiological process and does not substitute for monitoring of ventilation directly.

There is insufficient literature in support of monitoring pulmonary ventilation during administration of sedation. Consultants strongly agree that monitoring ventilation during sedation improves outcome. Consultants also agree that monitoring capnography decreases risk during deep sedation but are equivocal of its role during moderate sedation. In circumstances where patients are physically separated from the health care provider monitoring their sedation, consultants agree that an automated apnea monitor can reduce the risk of adverse outcome.

Monitoring Pulse Oximetry

Guidelines recommend that pulse oximetry should be continuously monitored in all patients during sedation, preferably with an audible alarm set to alert of decreasing oxygenation.

Published literature suggests that pulse oximetry can detect oxygen desaturation in patients receiving sedation. Consultants strongly agree that early detection of oxygen desaturation reduces the risk of adverse outcome during sedation. Consultants also agree that pulse oximetry detects cardiovascular depression earlier than clinical observation alone.

Monitoring the Patient's Hemodynamic Status

The level of sedation is inversely related to the patient's ability to respond adequately to changing hemodynamic stresses. Lower level of sedation, in contrast, leads to stress-related hypertension and tachycardia. Early detection of changes in patient's heart rate and blood pressure are therefore essential in maintaining a balance between the patient's comfort and the adequate level of consciousness. Blood pressure should be automatically recorded every 5–15 minutes throughout the procedure, and response to verbal and tactile stimuli should be assessed at routine intervals.

There is insufficient published data to reach a conclusion regarding the effects of agents used for sedation on patient's hemodynamic status. The consultants agree that sedative and analgesic agents blunt the autonomic homeostatic responses. Consultants strongly agree that monitoring patient's vital signs on a short regular interval reduces the likelihood of adverse outcome.

Consultants also strongly agree that continuous electrocardiography during deep sedation reduces the likelihood of adverse outcome; for patients receiving moderate sedation, consultants are equivocal in their recommendation. Consultants are of the opinion that patients with other cardiovascular comorbidities should be monitored with continuous electrocardiography irrespective of their level of sedation.

Personnel Monitoring the Patient

The task of administering sedation and the performance of diagnostic or invasive procedures should not be assigned to the same health care provider. The provider administering deep sedation should have no other responsibilities other than monitoring the patient. For moderate sedation, however, the provider can be assigned other minor tasks once the patient reaches a stable level of sedation.

No published data are available on this issue. For moderate sedation the consultants agree, and for deep sedation the consultants strongly agree, that the person responsible for administering and monitoring sedation should be independent of the person performing the procedure so that the caregiver responsible for monitoring the patient can concentrate solely on the patient monitoring.

Personnel Training

A health care provider trained in basic life support should be present in the procedure room and a provider trained in advanced cardiac life support should be available and able to respond within five minutes. Because sedation is a continuum of decreasing levels of consciousness, and because each patient responds differently to medications, the personnel responsible for administering and monitoring sedation should be able to recover patients from sedation levels deeper than intended for any given case.

There are no published data addressing the training of the personnel monitoring sedation. The consultants agree that the personnel monitoring the patients should receive special training in recognizing early signs of respiratory and cardiovascular depression.

Emergency Equipment

A crash cart with all emergency equipment should be readily available in case of an emergency. The crash cart should stock all relevant pharmacological antagonists and age-appropriate equipment to maintain an airway, obtain blood pressure measurements, maintain intravenous access, and provide supplemental oxygen. A defibrillator should be readily available.

The literature is noncontributory on the availability of emergency equipment during the administration of sedation. Consultants agree that availability of emergency equipment may reduce the risk of a poor outcome associated with sedation.

Supplemental Oxygen

Supplemental oxygen with appropriately sized delivery equipment to administer oxygen should be available in the procedure room.

Published literature supports, and the consultants agree, that the use of supplemental oxygen reduces the risk of a poor outcome during moderate and deep sedation.

Analgesic and Sedative Agents

It is the consensus of the task force that the combination of sedatives and analgesics is effective in administering sedation, and that a fixed combination of these agents may not allow the individual agents to be titrated according to the patient's specific needs. It is also the recommendation of the task force that each sedative or analgesic agent be administered individually and tailored to the patient's needs, keeping in mind the patient's respiratory and cardiovascular status.

There is insufficient literature concerning the safety of a single dose of analgesic and sedative agent based on patient's age, height, and weight, against incremental small doses titrated to achieve the desired effect. The consultants strongly agree that sedative and analgesic agents should be administered in small incremental doses to achieve the desired effect. Health care providers should allow sufficient time to lapse between each dose to assess its effect before administering the subsequent doses. The literature suggests that the combination of sedative and analgesic agents is effective in producing sedation. However, the literature is equivocal as to whether or not the combination of these agents is more effective than a single agent alone. The published literature also suggests that a combination of analgesics and sedatives increases the likelihood of ventilatory and cardiovascular depression.

Reversal Agents

Specific antagonists to opioids (naloxone) and benzodiazepines (flumazenil) should be readily available to reverse respiratory depression caused by the sedative and analgesic agents. Health care providers should be careful that sudden reversal of sedation can cause severe pain and hypertension. This effect may be especially true in the case of patients who are on chronic benzodiazepine or narcotic therapy. Patients who suffer from hypoxia or apnea during sedation should be encouraged to breathe deeply, be given supplemental oxygen, and receive positive-pressure ventilation if spontaneous ventilation is inadequate. It is also important to realize that the pharmacological effect of the reversal agents is short, and patients need to be monitored after apparent recovery because of continued effects of sedative and analgesics that can outlast the reversal agents.

The literature supports the availability of pharmacological reversal agents to sedatives and analgesics, and the consultants strongly agree that availability of these agents reduces poor outcome of sedation.

Recovery Care

Patients receiving sedation continue to be at risk of respiratory and cardiovascular depression after the procedure. Because of variation in the elimination of agents based on patient's metabolic processes, agents used for administering sedation have variable residual effects that may continue after the completion of the procedure.

There is insufficient literature supporting postprocedure patient care. The consultants strongly agree that patients should be observed in a well-staffed area until they reach the predetermined discharge criteria.

Special Situations

Patients with other severe comorbid conditions, extremes of age, and those with a history of drug or alcohol abuse are at increased risk of poor outcome. Consultants agree that preprocedural consults from appropriate medical specialists decreases the risk of sedation. Consultants are equivocal regarding the benefit of consulting anesthesiologists on the outcome of sedation for patients with sedation-related risk factors like morbid obesity, sleep apnea, difficult airways, and uncooperative tendencies. The task force is of the opinion that whenever possible, the relevant medical specialist should be consulted.

JOINT COMMISSION FOR ACCREDITATION OF HEALTH CARE ORGANIZATIONS

Staff

JCAHO guidelines mandate that only qualified health care providers should administer sedation. Qualified health care providers include physicians and dentists with current clinical competency in administering sedation. Current clinical competency constitutes a current BLS certification and biennial review of sedation educational material with successful completion of written sedation examination. Anesthesiologists, emergency care physicians, critical care physicians, and pulmonologists by virtue of their training are exempt from the above requirements. Qualified nurses should have a current BLS certification and should be current in their competency in medication administration, nursing care, and patient monitoring.

Administration of sedation in the clinical setting mandates that there should be enough staff members available to evaluate the patient prior to the procedure, administer sedation, perform the procedure, monitor the patient, recover the patient safely from sedation, and discharge them when stable. There is no specific minimum number of staff required to be available during the procedure. The staff should have a minimum competency-based education, training, and experience to safely assess the patient prior to the procedure and administer sedation in a safe manner.

Equipment

The health care facility where the sedation is being administered should have appropriate equipment to safely administer and monitor sedation. Oxygen should be readily available within the procedure room from either a permanent or portable source. Age-appropriate airway maintenance and oxygen delivery equipment, suction equipment, emergency cart, and monitoring equipment including pulse oximetry, blood pressure, and electrocardiogram monitoring devices should be available. Appropriate pharmacological reversal agents should be readily available.

Documentation

An informed consent should be obtained from all patients receiving sedation. The health care provider obtaining the consent should counsel the patient or their health care proxy about the risk and benefits of sedation.

Sedation assessment should be documented in the patient's medical record. The assessment should address the following:

- History of snoring or sleep apnea. All patients undergoing sedation require assessment of their airway including the ability to hyperextend their neck and documentation of any loose teeth or dentures.
- History of allergic reactions to medications, particularly the ones used for administering sedation.
- Neurological examination with respect to level of consciousness.
- Time and nature of last oral intake.
- Vital signs.
- Physical examination of cardiovascular and respiratory systems.
- Patient's risk stratification and documentation of their ASA physical status classification.
- Plan for sedation.

ASA physical status classification is as follows:

- Class I: Healthy patient
- Class II: Mild-to-moderate well-controlled systemic disorder
- Class III: Severe systemic disorder that limits normal activities
- Class IV: Severe life-threatening illness
- Class V: Moribund, poor chance of survival

Just prior to starting the procedure, a "procedural pause" (time-out) should be observed where the patient, the site of the procedure, and the procedure being performed should be positively identified with active verbal communication. The health care provider administering sedation needs to reevaluate the patient for their level of consciousness and to reassess the vital signs if indicated.

Patients with ASA Class III or higher may be considered for anesthesia consult. Patients with other comorbid conditions like obesity, pregnancy, mental incapacity, and extremes of age may also benefit from an anesthesia consult.

All complications related to sedation should be documented in the patient's medical record. Discharge orders should be properly written, documenting that the patient has returned to baseline physical and mental status, that sufficient time has lapsed to ensure that no delayed compromise of cardiorespiratory status can occur, and that the patient is being discharged into the care of a responsible adult with written information about the procedure and sedation.

REFERENCES

1. Practice guidelines for sedation and analgesia by non-anesthesiologists. A report by the American Society of Anesthesiologists Task Force on Sedation and Analgesia by Non-Anesthesiologists. Anesthesiology. 1996. 84(2):84 459–71.
2. Practice guidelines for sedation and analgesia by non-anesthesiologists. American Society of Anesthesiologists Task Force on, Sedation and Analgesia by, Non-Anesthesiologists. Anesthesiology. 2002 96(4):96 1004–17.
3. www.jcaho.org

Pediatric Sedation for Radiological Imaging Studies and Interventions

Keira P. Mason

Infants and children, who undergo radiological imaging studies, whether diagnostic or interventional, may require sedation. Sedation may be indicated in order to minimize motion artifact, facilitate successful completion of the procedure and, potentially, minimize risk to the patient (e.g., a sedation that would be required to achieve a cerebral angiogram in order to minimize risk of vascular damage related to the patient inadvertently moving during the study). There are a variety of sedatives available; most of the standard and most popular sedatives have been in existence for almost 100 years.

Triaging patients as being appropriate to receive sedation is the first important step in managing these children. Sedation may be administered by a variety of health care professionals that include a physician (radiologist, hospitalist, emergency medicine, pediatric, intensivist), nurse, or nurse practitioner. With the advent of new Current Procedural Terminology (CPT) billing codes in January 2006, there is now a billing code that enables a physician to bill for being physically present and responsible throughout the sedation. There are moderate sedation codes that reflect services provided by the same physician performing the diagnostic or therapeutic service that the sedation supports as well as codes for sedation services provided by a physician (other than an anesthesiologist) other than the health care professional performing the diagnostic or therapeutic service. As a consequence of these new billing codes, an increasing number of nonanesthesiologists are taking an active interest in delivering and setting up their own sedation services.

PATIENT SELECTION

A thorough medical history and review of systems should be completed prior to scheduling a patient. The surgical, sedative and anesthetic history is also reviewed and documented. All current medications and drug allergies are noted. Any potentially relevant clinical consults, and laboratory and clinical studies should be reviewed or ordered prior to triaging this patient. All children scheduled for nursing sedation should receive a prescreen telephone call from a radiology nurse the day before the scheduled study. A screening nurse is critical to this process. The nurse reviews the medical history, relays NPO instructions, and reminds the parents to administer the child's routine medications with a sip of clear fluid. All this patient information should be clearly documented and attached to a standard, hospital-approved sedation work-up form.

At our institution, there are clearly defined guidelines on which patient meets medical criteria to receive nurse-administered sedation. The patients scheduled for nursing sedation are typically American Society of Anesthesiologists (ASA) level 1 and level 2, but rarely level 3 (Table 1). A list of medical conditions that would immediately contraindicate nurse-administered sedation can help guide this triage process as well as ensure consistency of decision making (Table 2). In the event that there are questions regarding the medical status of a child, it is important to designate a "go-to" physician, usually an anesthesiologist, who will review the data and make the final decision regarding sedation appropriateness. In the event that the anesthesiologist requires additional information, consultations are arranged with appropriate specialty services (anesthesiology, otolaryngology, surgery, nephrology, or endocrinology). If the patient is deemed appropriate to receive sedation, then personal discussion between the consulting physician and the physician who will be supervising the sedation must ensue in order to ensure that there is agreement. The supervising physician must give final approval for sedation after reviewing the child's medical history and current medical status, prior to ordering the medications.

It is important for the practitioner responsible for sedation to also understand the procedure requested. For example, a patient may be medically appropriate to undergo sedation for an magnetic resonance imaging (MRI) scan but may be an inappropriate sedation candidate for sedation for a nephrostomy tube placed with the patient prone in interventional radiology. After determining that the patient meets the medical criteria for sedation, the technical nuances of the procedure must be reviewed. This may often require a collaborative discussion between the practitioner responsible for the sedation and the radiologist who will be performing the study. In the event that the procedure is deemed high risk (cerebral embolization), associated with significant pain (sclerotherapy with doxycycline), or long in duration, the collaborative decision may be that the patient should be referred to general anesthesia for management. Additional

---

Table 1. ASA Physical Status Classification

1	A normal healthy patient
2	A patient with mild systemic disease
3	A patient with severe systemic disease
4	A patient with severe systemic disease that is a constant threat to life
5	A moribund patient who is not expected to survive without the operation
6	A declared brain-dead patient whose organs are being removed for donor purposes

Source: http://www.asahq.org/clinical/physicalstatus.html

Table 2. "RED FLAGS" for sedation

---

1. Apnea

2. Full-term infant less than 1 month of age (unless an in-patient admitted to the hospital)

3. Respiratory compromised patients

4. Uncontrolled/unpredictable gastroesophageal reflux or vomiting that poses an aspiration risk

5. Craniofacial abnormality that may make it difficult to establish effective mask airway

6. Cyanotic cardiac disease or unstable cardiac status

7. Painful procedure that may be challenging to provide adequate analgesia without a general anesthetic

8. High-risk procedure that may require presence of an anesthesiologist for resuscitation

9. Procedure that requires absolute immobility only achievable with a general anesthetic

10. Procedure being performed in remote location that is so removed that immediate emergency back up assistance would be virtually impossible

11. Inadequate qualified personnel available to provide safe procedural sedation

---

considerations should be the physical layout of the procedure room and its geographical proximity to the operating rooms. In the event of an emergency and the need for backup assistance from the "code team" and anesthesiologists, the layout is important. If the radiological suites are physically isolated and distant from backup assistance, this may guide the practitioners to request anesthesia services.

PATIENT SEDATION GUIDELINES

To minimize the chance of drug delivery error or miscalculation, it is helpful to have preprinted order sheets that should be approved by the Hospital Sedation Committee as recommended by Joint Commission for Accreditation of Healthcare Organizations (JCAHO). The practice standards adopted by the American Society of Anesthesiologists in 1986 for basic intraoperative monitoring apply as well to extramural locations. Practice standards and guidelines promulgated by the American Academy of Pediatrics (1) are exceeded by established practice standards in anesthesiology (2). Significant variances may exist when nonanesthesiologists sedate (3). Practice Standards for Nonanesthetizing Locations were adopted by the ASA in 1994 (4). According to practice standards mentioned, sedated patients need to be monitored with pulse oximetry and noninvasive blood pressure monitoring.

A director of anesthesia services for this extramural radiology site can help to facilitate and coordinate anesthesia and sedation services. This director can also serve as a consultant for the nonanesthesia medical and nursing staff. By being available to answer questions, do on-site consults, examine patients, and provide back up support or emergency airway expertise, the anesthesiologist can also support a nurse-administered sedation program. Nurses who provide sedation under the supervision of the ordering extramural physician (gastrointestinal, radiology, dental) should be Pediatric Advanced Life Support (PALS)- and Basic Life Support (BLS)-certified. The JCAHO Anesthesia and Sedation Manual sets guidelines for credentialing of all personnel (physicians and nurses) who administer sedation (5).

MEDICATIONS

The selection of a sedation agents depends on the patient's underlying medical condition, age, drug tolerance, and anticipated procedure. Beware that parents and radiologists may have the unrealistic expectation that sedation will provide ideal conditions, complete analgesia, and guarantee successful completion of the procedure. Each medication has its own property that can include a hypnotic, anxiolytic, and/or analgesic. In order to appropriately make a sedation plan for each procedure, it is important to understand the properties of each medication and its potential synergistic actions with adjuvant medication.

Chloral Hydrate and Pentobarbital

Historically, chloral hydrate (Major Pharmaceuticals, Rosemont, IL) and pentobarbital (Nembutal; Abbott, North Chicago, IL) have been the hypnotics of choice for pediatric sedation (6–9). Both medications have no analgesic properties. They are useful for nonpainful procedures as a sole agent [MRI, computerized tomography (CT), nuclear medicine]. They can also be used with adjuvant analgesics in order to promote a hypnotic, sedative state for interventional procedures. Rates of successful sedation with chloral hydrate and pentobarbital range from 85% to 98% (10,11). Both pentobarbital and chloral hydrate are medications that each have almost 100 years of clinical experience. Because of their extended half-life (which approaches 24 hours), they have been associated with prolonged recovery times and sedation-related morbidity. Adverse events with these medications include oxygen desaturation, nausea, vomiting, hyperactivity, respiratory depression, and failure to adequately sedate (7,12).

Chloral hydrate is a medication that is predominantly given as an oral sedative. It does not exist in an intravenous form. Pentobarbital, in contrast, can be given by various routes. Most importantly, it may be given intravenously, intramuscularly, and orally. Children less than one year of age respond well to these two medications when given in the oral form. Pentobarbital, flavored with cherry syrup, is more palatable and equally effective as chloral hydrate (13). Comparing the two medications, oral pentobarbital has been associated with fewer respiratory events as compared to chloral. The incidence of a drop in oxygen saturation during sedation was over seven times higher in patients sedated with oral chloral hydrate compared to those sedated with pentobarbital (adjusted odds ratio = 7.3, 95% confidence interval: 2.0–36.5, likelihood ratio test = 8.1, p = .004) (14). Although some practitioners are reluctant to administer oral sedation to a child who will not have intravenous access during the examination, at least one study has shown that oral pentobarbital has similar efficacy and a lower rate of respiratory complications compared with intravenous pentobarbital in infants less than 12 months of age (15).

Consideration should be given to the use of oral pentobarbital in infants less than 12 months of age, regardless of the presence of an IV. Patients over one year of age receive intravenous sedation because it is more predictable and reliable. Pentobarbital is titrated up to 6 mg/kg intravenously to provide sedation and hypnosis. Patients who are on barbiturate therapy (for seizures) can be more tolerant to barbiturates and may receive up to 8 mg/kg.

Dexmedetomidine

Both pentobarbital and chloral hydrate, as hypnotics, have no analgesic properties. A recent addition to the sedative market is dexmedetomidine (Dex) (Precedex; Hospira, Lake Forest, IL). Only approved for use in intubated adults, Dex does not yet have approval by the Food and Drug Administration (FDA) for pediatric use. Rarely, Dex can cause potentially life-threatening cardiovascular complications in some adults and children (16–20). Regardless, it is being used for pediatric sedation in certain settings. These settings include diagnostic radiological imaging studies, the intensive care unit, and moderately painful procedures. Dex is a highly selective α2 adrenoceptor agonist that has sedative and analgesic effects and a short half-life of 1.5–3 hours after intravenous dosing (21–23) This is a significantly shorter half-life than that of pentobarbital and chloral hydrate. A short half-life could make Dex easier to titrate, quicker to recover from, and potentially associated with fewer prolonged sedation-related adverse events.

A significant advantage of Dex is that when administered to adults within clinical dosing guidelines, there are no accompanying changes in resting ventilation (21,24,25). Some feel that Dex actually mimics some aspects of natural sleep (21). It can produce dose-dependent decreases in blood pressure and heart rate as a result of its α2 agonist effect on the sympathetic ganglia with resulting sympatholytic effects (24,25). An additional advantage of Dex is that antagonists to α2 agonists exist and could potentially provide for a quick reversal of the hemodynamic or sedative effects (16).

There is limited prospective literature in children regarding Dex. The majority of publications are case reports and series describing Dex for sedation of children who are ventilated, detoxifying from opioids and benzodiazepines, failing traditional sedation techniques for MRI imaging, or undergoing an awake craniotomy (26,27). Digoxin is a contraindication to Dex administration because it has been associated with bradycardia and cardiac arrest (19). There are no other absolute contraindications to Dex usage. At our institution, Dex has replaced pentobarbital for all CT and nuclear medicine studies as well as some MRI scans.

Dex is administered as an initial loading dose of 2 mcg/kg IV Dex, and is administered over a 10-minute period. Patients are monitored initially with pulse oximetry. As the level of sedation increases, additional monitors are added in conjunction with the patient's tolerance. Typically, the child does not tolerate nasal prong capnography and insufflation of the noninvasive blood pressure cuff until there is a Ramsay Sedation Score of four (28). The imaging study is initiated as soon as the desired level of sedation has been achieved, sometimes even during the initial loading dose. Dex has a mean time to sedation of approximately 10 ± 2 minutes and a mean recovery time of only 32 ± 18 minutes (29). There have been no reported significant adverse events.

As an $\alpha2$ agonist, similar in property to clonidine, there is some literature to support that Dex has some analgesic properties (30–32). It may be useful for select interventional radiology procedures that require sedation and minimal analgesia. It can be particularly effective when supplemented with a local anesthetic during the procedure.

Ketorolac

For procedures that are unable to be achieved with hypnotics, sedatives, or infiltration with local anesthesia, analgesics are requisites. There are a variety of analgesics available. Analgesics can include ketorolac tromethamine (Toradol; Abbott Labs, N. Chicago, IL) administered intravenously every six hours with a maximum of 72 hours of administration. Ketorolac may be useful as a one-time administration to provide analgesia for simple, short procedures such as biopsies. As a nonsteroidal anti-inflammatory agent, ketorolac may inhibit platelet aggregation and prolong bleeding time, which may be an undesirable effect for some interventional procedures. Alternative analgesics could include narcotics or ketamine.

Narcotics

The choice of narcotic should depend on the duration of the procedure and the extent of analgesia required. Morphine (Baxter Healthcare Corp., Deerfield, IL) and fentanyl (Baxter) are the more popular narcotics. Morphine requires approximately 10 minutes for effect and has a duration of action of approximately two hours. Fentanyl works quicker, has 100 times the potency of morphine, and can produce analgesia in minutes. It generally needs to be redosed at least every 30–60 minutes depending on the procedure. Narcotics should be administered prior to (in anticipation of) the painful stimulus so that adequate analgesia is present at the time of the stimulus.

Ketamine

Ketamine, 2-(o-chlorophenyl)-2-(methylamino) cyclohexane, a phencyclidine and cyclohexamine derivative, was developed and introduced into clinical anesthesia practice in the 1960s. It may be administered via intravenous, intramuscular, oral, rectal, nasal, epidural, or intrathecal routes. The use of ketamine for pediatric sedation and analgesia has been described in various nonoperating room settings that include emergency departments (33), gastroenterology (34), oncology (35), dental (36), and radiology suites (37,38). A review of the literature reveals that despite the widespread use of ketamine by nonanesthesiologists, there is no consistent protocol for ketamine administration. Ketamine can produce the rapid onset of deep sedation and analgesia with minimal respiratory depression and cardiovascular side effects (39,40). Historically, ketamine has been a medication administered primarily by anesthesiologists, and subsequently emergency room physicians, for both operating room and outside-operating room procedures. Ketamine is unique because it provides deep sedation and profound analgesia while still maintaining airway muscle activity and upper airway patency (41).

Ketamine is an effective sedative and analgesic. It has potent analgesic properties and the advantage of preserving respiratory drive with a negligible risk of respiratory depression. Ketamine has the advantage of preserving respiratory status while producing more analgesia than would be achieved with a narcotic. When given in small bolus doses, it provides analgesia for an average of 30 minutes. As an infusion, ketamine can produce a continuous state of analgesia, which may be titrated up and down in response to (or in anticipation of) the painful stimulus. It is especially useful for patients who are going to undergo an exceptionally painful procedure (doxycycline sclerotherapy, chest tube) are on chronic opioids or have a high tolerance to opiates. Ketamine provides an effective alternative to narcotics in these patients.

Hallucinations, delusions, nightmares, and emergence delirium are phenomenon most commonly described as a potential side-effect of ketamine; these are more commonly noted in adults (42,43). The presence of these adverse events in the pediatric population is controversial (36,44). In adults, the concomitant administration of benzodiazepines (midazolam or diazepam) with ketamine has been shown to decrease the incidence of these events. Again, the utility of benzodiazepines in reducing these events in children is controversial (45–47). Some reports indicate that the addition of benzodiazepines leads to an increased incidence of oxygen desaturation events (48). Under age five, there is no definitive evidence that benzodiazepine administration will reduce the hallucinations, delusions, and excitatory behavior that can occur with ketamine. Children over age five may in fact benefit from concomitant benzodiazepine administration.

Most of the experience with ketamine in children is drawn from the emergency department.

A review of the emergency department literature demonstrates that intramuscular injection in children (12 months to 7 years) of a combination of ketamine (3 mg/kg), midazolam (0.05 mg/kg), and glycopyrrolate (0.005 mg/kg) provides reliable sedation within approximately six minutes, with no respiratory or cardiovascular complications (49). No emergence delirium or hallucinations were noted. In addition, respiratory drive and protective airway tone was intact with this combination. Additional literature evaluating 1,022 cases of ketamine intramuscular sedation in the pediatric emergency room reveals that at doses of 4 mg/kg, IM ketamine provides acceptable sedation in 98%, with a small risk (1.4%) of transient airway complications that included airway malalignment, laryngospasm, apnea, and respiratory depression. All were treated without intubation or sequela, and all patients maintained their airway reflexes. Only 1.6% demonstrated moderate-to-severe recovery agitation, and none demonstrated signs of hallucinations or delirium (49). There is no difference in time to discharge or adverse events when comparing 4–5 mg/kg IM ketamine. A separate investigation revealed that intravenous ketamine (1–2.0 mg/kg) provides sedation/anesthesia within two minutes with no deleterious cardiopulmonary or respiratory effects (47). It is important to realize, however, that large doses of ketamine can produce a state of general anesthesia.

In an effort to provide adequate analgesia and sedation for this patient population, the department of anesthesia can work closely with the department of radiology to develop a safe protocol for ketamine administration by credentialed radiology nurses under the supervision of radiologists. At our institution, ketamine is administered by either the intravenous or intramuscular route as 2.0 mg/kg bolus (in two divided doses over 10 minutes), followed by a ketamine infusion titrated between 50 and 125 mcg/kg/minute. The infusion is titrated to the same endpoint on each child: minimal response to painful stimulation elicited by deep nail bed pressure or ear lobe pinch.

Recovery time following ketamine administration averages 48 ± 40 minutes (50). In an evaluation of ketamine infusion at my institution, the average infusion rate was 76 ± 50 mcg/kg/minute. Multivariate analysis indicated that independent of gender, procedure, or ASA status, patients less than two years of age had a higher risk of sedation failure, oxygen desaturation, or need for resuscitation ($p < 0.05$) (50). Based on these findings, caution should be taken when selecting patients less than two years of age.

Because of the lack of clearly documented benefit of supplementing ketamine sedation with benzodiazepines and in order to reduce the risk of adverse events resultant from concomitant benzodiazepine administration, we reserve the use of ketamine plus benzodiazepines for those children over five years of age. Procedures include peripheral central intravenous catheters, chest tubes, G-tubes or nephrostomy tubes, percutaneous biopsies, sclerotherapy, drainage, and angiography.

Propofol

There has been an increasing interest by nonanesthesiologists in using propofol as a sedation agent. The anesthesia literature, however, supports propofol as an agent that, when administered for sedation purposes, requires dosing upward from 100 mcg/kg/minute (51). Even at this low dosing range, the cross-sectional area of the airway at the level of the tongue and epiglottis narrows and patients can manifest signs of obstruction (52,53). There are multiple reports in the nonanesthesiology literature claiming that propofol can be safely administered by gastroenterologists, pediatricians, nurse practitioners, and emergency room physicians. In fact, propofol is a recognized sedation agent by the American College of Gastroenterology. In 2003, The American Society for Gastrointestinal Endoscopy published their Standards of Practice, which included the administration of propofol for deep sedation by gastroenterologists credentialed in basic and advanced life support. Anesthesia assistance was necessary only in the event of prolonged procedures, presence of severe comorbidities, or anatomic risk of airway obstruction (54). Seven months following the publication of these gastrointestinal practice guidelines, the ASA issued a statement regarding propofol. Specifically, the statement claimed that propofol should only be administered by "persons trained in administration of general anesthesia ... (but) exempts intubated, ventilated" patients in critical care settings (55).

When being used for sedation purposes by nonanesthesiologists, propofol should be administered with caution. It can cause apnea and respiratory depression with little warning. Even in the hands of experienced anesthesiologists, propofol can have an unpredictable effect on respiration. To date, propofol is not being widely used by nonanesthesiologists (nurses, radiologists) for interventional radiological procedures.

PRACTICAL CONSIDERATIONS

At most institutions, the department of radiology encompasses the largest volume sedation area in the hospital. As recommended by the JCAHO, the Department of Anesthesia should oversee all sedation protocols and meet on a regular basis to review adverse events, policies, and procedures and to make recommendations for improvements. A computerized database can be helpful in order to maintain information on all sedations: patient demographics, medications (dosages and routes of administration), time required to sedate and to discharge home, ASA physical status classification, and adverse events and failed sedations. This database facilitates access to outcome statistics. JCAHO recommends that adverse sedation outcomes be reviewed regularly in order to review existing protocols, trial new protocols, and make changes if necessary.

For example, using a computerized database, a review of 16,467 sedations performed in a radiology department that uses pentobarbital, fentanyl, and versed revealed a total of only 70 (0.4%) pulmonary adverse events (56). These included 58 oxygen desaturations, 2 pulmonary aspirations, 10 airway resuscitations, and no (0%) cardiovascular events. There were no cardiac arrests and no need for intubations. Adverse events were compared between sedation regimens, and multiple logistic regression analysis was applied to identify predictors of an adverse event. Nearly 30% of the patients who had an adverse event had a medical history of serious respiratory illness (20 of 70 = 29%). Logistic regression indicated that age, weight, gender, and type of procedure were not associated with an increased risk for an adverse event. Single sedation agents were associated with a lower risk than the administration of multiple agents ($p < .001$) (56).

Caution should be used when administering multiple sedation agents. All sedation agents are synergistic, and one can unexpectedly precipitate respiratory depression. When administering a second or third medication, the practitioner should be conservative and modest in the dosage amounts. Adequate time should be allotted between dosages to ensure that the maximum effect has been achieved before adding more medication. Especially when adding a third sedative, the risk of significant morbidity and mortality increases dramatically (57,58).

Pediatric sedation is an evolving practice in which practitioners from different specialties utilize a variety of classes of medications and administer them via various routes. Some of these drugs are "historic" and have been utilized for almost 100 years, whereas others are relatively new. Many drugs administered to children have not even been approved by the FDA for pediatric usage. In fact, since 1995, midazolam (versed) is the only sedative that has been approved by the FDA for pediatric usage (1997). The paucity of approved medications for pediatric usage is attributed largely to the small retail need and generated income. Only 6.8% of all retail prescriptions are for children less than three years of age, and only 7% of marketed retail prescriptions are for children between the ages of 4 and 12. With such a small market for pediatric prescriptions, most drug companies are reluctant to spend the time and expense to pursing FDA approval. In 2003, Congress passed the Pediatric Research Equity Act in order to address the perceived unfairness of drug companies in pursuing drug testing for medications with potential pediatric utility. This act stipulated that the FDA may require the pharmaceutical company to test a new medication under the following conditions: the drug may be of potential benefit, is already being used for children, or in the absence of a pediatric label poses a potential risk (59).

Following the introduction of CPT billing codes specific for moderate sedation, pediatric sedation by nonanesthesiologists is becoming a potentially lucrative topic of interest and attention. To date, most of the sedatives available have been used for many decades with only a few recent additions. As the FDA mandates more pediatric drug testing under the Pediatric Research Equity Act, hopefully someday the pediatric patient will have a wider armamentarium available to safely and effectively provide sedation for a variety of different procedures.

REFERENCES

1. American Academy of Pediatrics Committee on Drugs. Guidelines for monitoring and management of pediatric patients during and after sedation for diagnostic and therapeutic procedures. Pediatrics 1992;89:1110–5.
2. American Academy of Pediatrics, Section on Anesthesiology. Guidelines for the pediatric perioperative anesthesia environment. Pediatrics 1999;103:512.
3. Keeter S, Benator RM, Weinberg SM, Hartenberg MA. Sedation in pediatric CT: national survey of current practice. Radiology 1990;175:745–52.
4. http://www.asahq.org/publicationsAndServices/standards/14.pdf. American Society of Anesthesia. Guidelines for nonoperating room anesthetizing locations (Approved by House of Delegates on October 19, 1994, and last amended in October 15, 2003).
5. Joint Commission on Accreditation of Healthcare Organization. 2001. Anesthesia and Sedation. Joint Commission Resources, Inc., Oakbrook Terrace, IL.
6. Ferrer-Brechner T, Winter J. Anesthetic considerations for cerebral computer tomography. Anesth Analg 1977;56:344–7.
7. Greenberg SB, Faerber EN, Aspinall CL, Adams RC. High-dose chloral hydrate sedation for children undergoing MR imaging: safety and efficacy in relation to age. AJR Am J Roentgenol 1993;161:639–41.
8. Greenberg SB, Faerber EN, Aspinall CL. High dose chloral hydrate sedation for children undergoing CT. J Comput Assist Tomogr 1991;15:467–9.
9. American Academy of Pediatrics Committee on Drugs and Committee on Environmental Health. Use of chloral hydrate for sedation in children. Pediatrics 1993;92:471–3.
10. Thompson JR, Schneider S, Ashwal S et al. The choice of sedation for computed tomography in children: a prospective evaluation. Radiology 1982;143:475–9.
11. Napoli KL, Ingall CG, Martin GR. Safety and efficacy of chloral hydrate sedation in children undergoing echocardiography. J Pediatr 1996;129:287–91.
12. Ronchera-Oms CL, Casillas C, Marti-Bonmati L et al. Oral chloral hydrate provides effective and safe sedation in paediatric magnetic resonance imaging. J Clin Pharm Ther 1994;19:239–43.

13. Chung T, Hoffer FA, Connor L et al. The use of oral pentobarbital sodium (Nembutal) versus oral chloral hydrate in infants undergoing CT and MR imaging – a pilot study. Pediatr Radiol 2000;30:332–5.

14. Mason KP, Sanborn P, Zurakowski D et al. Superiority of pentobarbital versus chloral hydrate for sedation in infants during imaging. Radiology 2004;230:537–42.

15. Mason KP, Zurakowski D, Connor L et al. Infant sedation for MR imaging and CT: oral versus intravenous pentobarbital. Radiology 2004;233:723–8.

16. Scheinin H, Aantaa R, Anttila M et al. Reversal of the sedative and sympatholytic effects of dexmedetomidine with a specific alpha2-adrenoceptor antagonist atipamezole: a pharmacodynamic and kinetic study in healthy volunteers. Anesthesiology 1998;89:574–84.

17. Belleville JP, Ward DS, Bloor BC, Maze M. Effects of intravenous dexmedetomidine in humans. I. Sedation, ventilation, and metabolic rate. Anesthesiology 1992;77:1125–33.

18. Ingersoll-Weng E, Manecke GR Jr., Thistlethwaite PA. Dexmedetomidine and cardiac arrest. Anesthesiology 2004;100:738–9.

19. Berkenbosch JW, Tobias JD. Development of bradycardia during sedation with dexmedetomidine in an infant concurrently receiving digoxin. Pediatr Crit Care Med 2003;4:203–5.

20. Venn RM, Bradshaw CJ, Spencer R et al. Preliminary UK experience of dexmedetomidine, a novel agent for postoperative sedation in the intensive care unit. Anaesthesia 1999;54:1136–42.

21. Hall JE, Uhrich TD, Barney JA et al. Sedative, amnestic, and analgesic properties of small-dose dexmedetomidine infusions. Anesth Analg 2000;90:699–705.

22. De Wolf AM, Fragen RJ, Avram MJ et al. The pharmacokinetics of dexmedetomidine in volunteers with severe renal impairment. Anesth Analg 2001;93:1205–9.

23. Dyck JB, Maze M, Haack C et al. The pharmacokinetics and hemodynamic effects of intravenous and intramuscular dexmedetomidine hydrochloride in adult human volunteers. Anesthesiology 1993;78:813–20.

24. Talke P, Lobo E, Brown R. Systemically administered alpha2-agonist-induced peripheral vasoconstriction in humans. Anesthesiology 2003;99:65–70.

25. Talke P, Richardson CA, Scheinin M, Fisher DM. Postoperative pharmacokinetics and sympatholytic effects of dexmedetomidine. Anesth Analg 1997;85:1136–42.

26. Tobias JD, Berkenbosch JW. Sedation during mechanical ventilation in infants and children: dexmedetomidine versus midazolam. South Med J 2004;97:451–5.

27. Finkel JC, Elrefai A. The use of dexmedetomidine to facilitate opioid and benzodiazepine detoxification in an infant. Anesth Analg 2004;98:1658–9, table of contents.

28. Ramsay MA, Savege TM, Simpson BR, Goodwin R. Controlled sedation with alphaxalone-alphadolone. Br Med J 1974;2:656–9.

29. Mason KP, Zgleszewski SE, Dearden JL. Dexmedetomidine for pediatric sedation for CT imaging studies. Anesth Analg, 2006;103(1):43–8.

30. Jackson KC, Wohlt P, Fine PG. Dexmedetomidine: a novel analgesic with palliative medicine potential. J Pain Palliat Care Pharmacother 2006;20:23–7.

31. Bamgbade OA. Dexmedetomidine for peri-operative sedation and analgesia in alcohol addiction. Anaesthesia 2006;61:299–300.

32. Rich JM. Dexmedetomidine as a sole sedating agent with local anesthesia in a high-risk patient for axillofemoral bypass graft: a case report. AANA J 2005;73:357–60.

33. Dachs RJ, Innes GM. Intravenous ketamine sedation of pediatric patients in the emergency department. Ann Emerg Med 1997;29:146–50.

34. Kirberg A, Sagredo R, Montalva G, Flores E. Ketamine for pediatric endoscopic procedures and as a sedation complement for adult patients. Gastrointest Endosc 2005;61:501–2.

35. Marx CM, Stein J, Tyler MK et al. Ketamine-midazolam versus meperidine-midazolam for painful procedures in pediatric oncology patients. J Clin Oncol 1997;15:94–102.

36. Roelofse JA, Joubert JJ, Roelofse PG. A double-blind randomized comparison of midazolam alone and midazolam combined with ketamine for sedation of pediatric dental patients. J Oral Maxillofac Surg 1996;54:838–44; discussion 45–6.

37. Bennett JA, Bullimore JA. The use of ketamine hydrochloride anaesthesia for radiotherapy in young children. Br J Anaesth 1973;45:197–201.

38. Cotsen MR, Donaldson JS, Uejima T, Morello FP. Efficacy of ketamine hydrochloride sedation in children for interventional radiologic procedures. AJR Am J Roentgenol 1997;169:1019–22.

39. White PF. Ketamine update: its clinical uses in anesthesia. Semin Anesthesia 1998;7:113–26.

40. Way WL, Trevor AJ. 1986 Pharmacology of Intravenous Nonnarcotic Anesthetics. 2nd ed.: Churchill Livingstone, NY.

41. Drummond GB. Comparison of sedation with midazolam and ketamine: effects on airway muscle activity. Br J Anaesth 1996;76:663–7.

42. Fine J, Finestone SC. Sensory disturbances following ketamine anesthesia: recurrent hallucinations. Anesth Analg 1973;52:428–30.

43. Meyers EF, Charles P. Prolonged adverse reactions to ketamine in children. Anesthesiology 1978;49:39–40.

44. Sherwin TS, Green SM, Khan A et al. Does adjunctive midazolam reduce recovery agitation after ketamine sedation for pediatric procedures? A randomized, double-blind, placebo-controlled trial. Ann Emerg Med 2000;35:229–38.

45. Wathen JE, Roback MG, Mackenzie T, Bothner JP . Does midazolam alter the clinical effects of intravenous ketamine sedation in children? A double-blind, randomized, controlled, emergency department trial. Ann Emerg Med 2000;36:579–88.

46. Hollister GR, Burn JM. Side effects of ketamine in pediatric anesthesia. Anesth Analg 1974;53:264–7.

47. Green SM, Johnson NE. Ketamine sedation for pediatric procedures: Part 2, review and implications. Ann Emerg Med 1990;19:1033–46.

48. Sussman DR. A comparative evaluation of ketamine anesthesia in children and adults. Anesthesiology 1974;40:459–64.

49. Green SM, Rothrock SG, Lynch EL et al. Intramuscular ketamine for pediatric sedation in the emergency department: safety profile in 1,022 cases. Ann Emerg Med 1998;31:688–97.

50. Mason KP, Michna E, DiNardo JA et al. Evolution of a protocol for ketamine-induced sedation as an alternative to general anesthesia for interventional radiologic procedures in pediatric patients. Radiology 2002;225:457–65.

51. Frankville DD, Spear RM, Dyck JB. The dose of propofol required to prevent children from moving during magnetic resonance imaging. Anesthesiology 1993;79:953–8.

52. Evans RG, Crawford MW, Noseworthy MD, Yoo SJ. Effect of increasing depth of propofol anesthesia on upper airway configuration in children. Anesthesiology 2003;99:596–602.

53. Reber A, Wetzel SG, Schnabel K et al. Effect of combined mouth closure and chin lift on upper airway dimensions during routine magnetic resonance imaging in pediatric patients sedated with propofol. Anesthesiology 1999;90:1617–23.

54. www.acg.gi.org/media/rcleases/mar82004.asp.

55. www.asahq.org/news/propofolstatement.htm.

56. Sanborn PA, Michna E, Zurakowski D et al. Adverse cardiovascular and respiratory events during sedation of pediatric patients for imaging examinations. Radiology 2005;237:288–94.

57. Cote CJ, Karl HW, Notterman DA et al. Adverse sedation events in pediatrics: analysis of medications used for sedation. Pediatrics 2000;106:633–44.

58. Cote CJ, Notterman DA, Karl HW et al. Adverse sedation events in pediatrics: a critical incident analysis of contributing factors. Pediatrics 2000;105:805–14.

59. www.fda.gov/opacom/laws/prea.html.

Nontraditional Pain Management in Interventional Radiology

Salomao Faintuch, Gloria Maria Martinez Salazar,
Felipe Birchal Collares, and Elvira V. Lang

INTRODUCTION

Appropriate pain management (or lack thereof) is gaining increasing attention. The California Board of Registration in Medicine now requires CME in pain management. Court cases address the "right to pain relief." A recent trend in judicial standard setting with regard to pain management is expressed in the opinion of Nowatske vs. Osterloh, Wisc 1996 (1): "Should customary medical practice fail to keep pace with developments and advances in medical science, adherence to custom might constitute a failure to exercise ordinary care." Another judgment went as far to declare that "it is entirely possible that what is the usual or customary procedure might itself be negligence" (1). Although this legal interpretation has been applied predominantly to end-of-life pain management, one can see how juries sympathetic to any kind of medical suffering may react to ensure that what is known to reduce pain be used judiciously. There is a well-known place for analgesics, narcotics, sedatives, and anesthetics in interventional radiology (2,3). However increasing number of reports support an evidence-based use of nonpharmacological adjuncts for invasive procedures, and an increasing number of patients request such services. This chapter is intended to provide an overview of such methods, with special emphasis in procedural pain and distress management as they relate to interventional radiology.

RATIONALE FOR USE OF NONPHARMACOLOGICAL ADJUNCTS

Mild and moderate pharmacological sedation during and after interventional radiological procedures is widely practiced and well established (2) but can have limited effectiveness and serious side effects (3–5). The anesthetic risk associated with the use of monitored anesthesia care, which is used for more invasive procedures, is comparable to that seen with use of general anesthesia (6). Nonpharmacological adjuncts for pain management are increasingly being utilized in different medical settings (7–11), including interventional radiology (12–14). The rationale for their use emphasizes procedural safety, as well as on the opportunity to address psychological factors (fear, anxiety, and tension) that patients may experience during medical procedures (15,16). The U.S. Public Health Service guidelines (Clinical Practice Guidelines for Acute Pain Management), published in 1992, recommended relaxation exercises and cognitive approaches without providing specifics or outcome data (17). Since then, outcome data from prospective trials have become available showing benefits of such modalities (12,18,19), further justifying their consideration (20).

OVERVIEW OF NONTRADITIONAL TECHNIQUES FOR PAIN MANAGEMENT DURING INVASIVE MEDICAL PROCEDURES

The management of pain with nonpharmacological adjuncts is being increasingly studied (20) and accepted by patients (21). Clinical trials of nonpharmacological pain management have been published in various settings and medical specialties, including lumbar punctures (22), vascular and renal interventions (12), cardiac interventions (23), bone marrow aspiration (24), breast biopsies (9), and skin laceration repair in the pediatric emergency department (11). Although heterogeneity of approaches complicates meta-analyses (25), large enough trials are now available, at least on hypnotic interventions (12,18), to justify their evidence-based status (20). An additional advantage of such interventions is their beneficial effect on anxiety (16,26), which is often prevalent in the patient population presenting for procedures.

The National Center for Complementary and Alternative Medicine, a branch of the National Institutes of Health, classifies nontraditional medical approaches into five categories: alternative medical systems (e.g., acupuncture, homeopathy), body-mind therapies (e.g., biofeedback, hypnosis, relaxation/meditation, imagery techniques, prayer, spiritual practice), biologically based therapies (e.g., herbal medicine, high-dose mega vitamins, special diets), energy therapies (e.g., transcutaneous electrical nerve stimulation, healing touch, Reiki), and manipulative- or body-based methods (e.g., massage therapy exercise/movement therapies, chiropractic) (27). Of these, alternative medical systems, mind-body therapies, and energy will likely be the easiest to be integrated into the interventional radiology practice, whereas biologically based or manipulative- or body-based methods during procedures would be more difficult to implement. We will therefore focus on the former and describe their principles, applications for acute management of pain and anxiety, and, if available, the experience of their use in interventional radiology or similar settings.

USE OF ALTERNATIVE MEDICAL SYSTEMS AND ENERGY THERAPIES IN ACUTE PAIN MANAGEMENT

Transcutaneous Electrical Nerve Stimulation

The main mechanism of action of transcutaneous electrical nerve stimulation (TENS) is the inhibition of nociceptive C-fibers through stimulating A-fibers, depending on the amplitude of stimulation at the segmental spinal cord level. Additional pathways include the effect of TENS in decreasing activity of dorsal horn neurons that transmit information to supraspinal levels and the release of endorphins. It is described as a simple technique without side effects that involves attachment of stimulating electrodes in a specific dermatomal area to be treated (28). Local application of TENS has been shown to be a rapid and effective treatment for analgesia in patients with renal colic (29), postthoracotomy pain (30), and following cardiac interventions (31). It has not been tested in interventional radiology but could conceivably be of use to address preexisting pain that interferes with immobilization on the table. However, studies are still needed to assess utility during invasive procedures.

Acupuncture

The theory of acupunture is based on the concept that specific patterns of continuous energy flow (Qi) through the body are vital to human health (32). This technique involves placement of intradermal metallic needles that are typically manipulated with the practitioners' hands, in specific anatomical points, to restore the essential patterns of flow in the body. The analgesic effect of acupuncture has been studied for postoperative pain management of patients undergoing abdominal surgery (33). Preoperative insertion of acupuncture needles, which remained in place during surgery, was shown to reduce postoperative pain, analgesic requirements, nausea and vomiting, as well as plasma cortisol and epinephrine levels. In a pilot trial with patients having thoracic surgery, preoperative acupuncture proved to be acceptable to patients and did not interfere with standard preoperative care (34). Whereas acupuncture was used for brain, head and neck, and chest surgical pain management in China (35), a recent review of the literature in the field of surgery did not support the use of acupuncture as an adjunct to standard anesthesia (36). To our knowledge, results about applications in interventional radiology have not been published.

USE OF MIND-BODY THERAPIES IN ACUTE PAIN MANAGEMENT

Mind-body therapies are described as a variety of techniques that enhance the mind's capacity to affect bodily functions and symptoms (27). Relaxation techniques, biofeedback, guided imagery, hypnosis, and prayer are encompassed by this category. Although these techniques are listed separately, they often overlap; most include some element of relaxation training and imagery, and even verbalization of prayer has communalities with hypnotic immersion and suggestions.

Relaxation Techniques and Relaxation Response

The term relaxation response was coined by Herbert Benson and describes elicitation of a psychophysiological state of relaxation and decreased sympathetic arousal (37). Initially used for femoral angiographies (14), these interventions have been described as an effective adjunct in reducing pain following intestinal operations (38) and during bone marrow transplantation (19). However, recent trials using these interventions to reduce perioperative stress in colorectal resections have not proven it to be of clinical relevance, despite patients' acceptance and positive responses (39).

The mechanism was described as "a set of coordinated physiologic changes that included decreased oxygen consumption, heart rate, and levels of arterial blood lactate; increased production of alpha, theta, and delta waves on the electroencephalogram; and psychological changes of decreased anxiety and hostility" (37). As such, the use of this technique in the management of patients' pain and anxiety during femoral angiographies was evaluated in a randomized study (14). Prior to angiography, patients were instructed to listen to audiotapes (relaxation response, music, and blank tapes) throughout the length of the procedure. At the completion, patients were asked to rate their experience regarding pain. The nurses also were asked to provide pain and anxiety ratings based on the observation of patients. The results showed that patients who listen to relaxation response tapes reported significantly less pain and anxiety during the procedure and requested a smaller amount of medications; their nurses also described them as having less pain and anxiety. The relaxation response was considered to be a simple, an inexpensive, an efficacious, and a practical method to reduce pain, anxiety, and medication usage.

Different investigators, however, have shown limited efficacy of relaxation in interventional radiology, with techniques that do not provide specific skills for patients to cope with their procedure-related distress (40). Bugbee et al. designed a randomized trial to compare relaxation techniques versus medication, aiming at anxiety reduction during breast core-needle biopsies. It showed significantly less anxiety for women in the medication group, as compared to the relaxation group. The authors suggested that more comprehensive relaxation resources, in addition to training patients before the procedure, could have resulted in a greater effectiveness for this treatment group, instead of the sole provision of audio-taped music and ocean sounds.

Unaddressed in the tape-based relaxation response treatments are issues that may result from startle reflexes in response to invasive stimuli or actions, and communications from health care providers in the room. Based on our experience, the provision of relaxation that includes a structured coping mechanism (hypnosis or guided imagery) is preferable to simple relaxation, as it empowers patients to deal with distress not only during the intervention but possibly also during recovery and in future medical procedures.

Biofeedback

Biofeedback provides real-time information from psychophysiological recordings (i.e., body temperature variations, muscle tension) about the levels at which physiological systems are functioning (41). These records are mostly measured from the surface of the skin, and the information is sent to a computer for processing and then displayed on monitors. This method requires the presence of a skilled therapist who can use the immediate feedback information while incorporating it into a specific technique (relaxation, breathing, and imagery/hypnosis exercises). Therefore, the provider can instruct patients to alter their physiological processes by using biofeedback as a guide.

Biofeedback is used in many different environments including schools (to improve concentration), sports (to enhance performance), and medicine. Research has shown the utility of biofeedback-guided treatment for diverse medical conditions including constipation, migraine headaches, and tension headaches (42,43). One of the most common applications is the management of pediatric migraines (42,44). Examples include patients suffering from tension headaches, who are managed with EMG (electromyography) feedback, or with migraines, controlled with thermal biofeedback.

The use of biofeedback techniques in interventional radiology may be limited due to the fact that multiple training sessions with a skilled coach are usually required. Therefore, this may likely be impractical for application in the management of acute procedural distress. Nonetheless, in patients with chronic medical conditions who require repeated interventions, this modality may have the potential of being helpful.

Guided Imagery

Guided imagery involves the generation (by oneself or guided by a practitioner) of different mental states through the ability of visualization and imagination. Individuals can evoke "images" with focus on any or all sensory experiences such as visual, auditory, sensory, gustatory, and olfactory elements. These images are elicited with the goal of attaining a psychophysiological state of relaxation; when a specific outcome is targeted, the process would usually be described as hypnosis. This attempt of distinction already indicates the overlap between various mind-body techniques such as hypnosis, relaxation training, and imagery. One may keep this in mind when assessing clinical studies that evaluate the use of these techniques. Terminology apart, the use of imagery has been shown to reduce pain in patients undergoing bone marrow transplantation (19) and in the postoperative period following tonsillectomies/adenoidectomies (45). However, the use of imagery in patients undergoing colorectal resections did not yielded significant clinical effect in reducing postoperative pain and analgesic requirements, despite patient's openness to this intervention (39).

Prayer

Prayer is considered one of the most ancient healing practices for sick individuals. Scientifically, it has been studied in different trials, in the form of off-site intercessory prayer with patients undergoing percutaneous coronary interventions for acute coronary syndrome (23,46–48). Off-site intercessory prayer involved the provision of patients' name, illness, and procedure to be performed by phone, e-mail, or Internet connection to different prayer groups (i.e., Catholic, Buddhist, Jewish). In the analysis of the effect of intercessory prayer in procedural distress related to percutaneous coronary intervention and its clinical outcomes, Krucoff et al. did not find significant clinical improvements with the use of this method in such patients in a pilot study (46), as well as in a randomized trial (48). Recently, Benson et al. evaluated the effect of receiving intercessory prayer or being certain of receiving such intervention in recovery of patients after coronary artery bypass graft (CABG) surgery (47). This randomized trial showed that intercessory prayer itself had no effect on complication-free recovery from CABG, but patients who were certain that intercessors would pray for them presented with a higher rate of complications than patients who were uncertain but did receive this intervention.

Hypnosis

Hypnosis can be defined as a form of focused concentration, similar to what happens when a person becomes absorbed in a book or movie. The patient is guided into a state of focused attention and physical relaxation that permits the subconscious mind to become open to receive beneficial suggestions. These suggestions can be constructed with the purpose of behavior modification, or to alter patients' thoughts and feelings.

The capacity to modulate the experience of pain is one of the most valuable applications of hypnosis (49). Therefore, its use as a pharmacological adjunct can provide substantial aid before (26) and during (12,50) medical procedures. Aside from being an adjunct, hypnosis has been effective as the sole means of analgesia during open surgery in selected patients (51–53).

The literature has shown that patients who offered hypnosis for different medical purposes experienced substantial benefits despite considerable variation in hypnotic techniques (54), indicating a potential for expansion of its use.

Preoperative hypnosis has proven to be a valuable method to reduce anxiety in patients undergoing ambulatory surgical procedures (26). In this context, patients were randomly assigned to receive one of three types of intervention prior to their operation: hypnosis (n = 26), attention-control (n = 26), and standard of care (n = 24). Their anxiety levels were assessed with the use of questionnaires and visual analog scale on a scale from 0 to 10, before and after the intervention, as well as during the surgical procedure. The authors found that patients in the hypnosis group were significantly less anxious after the intervention as compared to the other groups. In addition, while in the operating room, hypnosis patients reported a significant decrease from baseline anxiety levels (56%), in comparison to a 10% and 47% increase in the attention-control and standard of care groups, respectively.

Another study demonstrated the effectiveness of preoperative hypnosis in patients undergoing excisional breast biopsies, with significantly reduced post-surgical pain and distress (9).

A larger experience (20 studies) with the use of adjunct hypnosis in surgical patients was compiled in a meta-analysis conducted by Montgomery (55). The results indicated that 89% of patients in the included studies benefited from adjunctive hypnosis, in one or more of the following parameters: decreased anxiety/pain, decreased amount of medication used, faster treatment or recovery time.

In interventional radiology, adjunct hypnosis significantly reduced pain, anxiety, drug use, and complications during peripheral vascular and percutaneous renal interventions (12). In this study, 241 patients were randomized to receive: standard care treatment (n = 79), structured attention (n = 80), or self-hypnotic relaxation (n = 82). All patients had free access to IV sedative/narcotic in a patient-controlled analgesia model. Pain and anxiety levels were assessed through verbal scores reported on 0–10 scales, obtained before and every 15 minutes during the procedure. In this study, pain increased linearly with procedure time in the standard care group and, although to a lesser degree, in the attention control group, but did not increase in the hypnosis group. Anxiety decreased linearly from baseline with procedure duration in all three groups with the greatest decline in the hypnosis group. Analysis of drug administration during the procedure showed that patients in the standard care group requested and received significantly more drugs in a patient-controlled analgesia model (1.8 drug units requested, 1.9 drug units received; with 1 unit corresponding to either 1 mg versed or 50 µg fentanyl) than those in the attention group (0.8 units requested and received) and in the hypnosis group (0.9 units requested and received). Also, average procedure duration was significantly shorter in the hypnosis group than in the standard group (61 vs. 78 minutes). Procedure duration for the attention group was in between but not significantly different from that of the other two groups (mean = 67 minutes). Interestingly, adverse events were also less common in the hypnosis group.

While one could have expected a given improvement of hemodynamic stability in the empathy and hypnosis group merely based on a reduction of drug use, the significant reduction of hemodynamic instability in the hypnosis group suggests that hypnosis-specific effects were responsible for this clinically important outcome. This is supported by findings of an ongoing study with patients undergoing tumor embolization with our group (unpublished data).

The physiological responses to the use of hypnosis have also been investigated for percutaneous transluminal coronary angioplasty (PTCA). The selective influence of hypnosis on cardiac vegetative tone is well known, with an improved heart rate variability profile (56). Likewise, the downregulation of the sympathetic drive during PTCA through the selective influence of hypnosis was demonstrated in 2004 (57).

Decision-making processes employed during procedural analgesia require skilled practitioners and specific guidelines to ensure safety and proper management of pain, particularly for the pediatric population (58). As such, there is an expanding role of nonpharmacological techniques in alleviating pain and anxiety especially in children undergoing frequent invasive procedures (22), as well as in the emergency department (11). Hypnosis has been proposed as an attractive option for pain management in children because they are generally considered even more responsive to this type of intervention than adults (59). In the radiology setting, the use of hypnosis during voiding cystourethrography was evaluated in a randomized study with 44 patients (50). Children assigned to the hypnosis group demonstrated significantly lower distress levels during the procedure compared to the control group. Parents of the children also reported that the procedure was significantly less traumatic for their children, when compared to their previous cystourethrograms. Moreover, the medical staff reported less difficulty in performing the procedure in the hypnosis group, which resulted in shorter procedure duration, as compared to the control condition.

HYPNOSIS IN INTERVENTIONAL RADIOLOGY

Adequate anxiolysis and analgesia must be appropriately provided to patients in the interventional radiology suite. Unfortunately, patient comfort requirements are usually unknown by the time they arrive at the procedure room. Hence, there is an increasing concern regarding predictive factors for pain during and after interventional radiology procedures (5,16).

The patterns, incidence, and predictive factors for pain in this context were evaluated in patients after they underwent procedures, such as percutaneous biliary drainage, central venous access, gastrostomy tube insertion, and esophageal/duodenal stenting, and others (5). The authors concluded that although the pattern and severity of pain can be variable after these procedures, it is indeed a common problem that is often inadequately managed.

In a recent publication, assessment of the effect of patient's state baseline anxiety during vascular and renal interventions showed that baseline anxiety level is a predictor of trends in procedural pain and anxiety, need for medication, and duration of procedure (16). The authors concluded that nonpharmacological adjuncts provide a beneficial impact in patients with both low and high levels of anxiety, with the latter having the most to gain because they require more resources and are at a greater risk of being suboptimally assessed in a standard of care condition.

When preparing a patient for an upcoming procedure, one must consider time, cost, and the involvement of members of the patient's family (particularly in the pediatric population) (50). Individualized interventions that require repeated encounters with the hypnotherapist are less likely to be adopted in the interventional radiology setting and may not even be necessary for most patients.

Video and audiotapes can be employed as preparatory and procedural methods that do not demand excessive amounts of staff time, and have been reported to be useful in promoting relaxation and reducing drug use during dental surgery (60,61), gastrointestinal endoscopy (62), and femoral angiography (14). However, a 13% rejection rate was also described (63), and because of the lack of a therapist-patient relationship, videos and audiotapes may not be as powerful in preventing adverse events such as vomiting (61). In general, the presence of a "live therapist" is felt to be preferable (53). Very anxious patients may also require a process that addresses their worries specifically, before they will be able to relax and engage in hypnosis. This opportunity would be lost if only an electronic medium were used.

Given patient's awareness during medical procedures (53) and the fact that patients who come for a doctor's visit or a medical procedure are highly suggestible (64), the medical staff should be careful in their choice of words when interacting with a patient (65). Unfortunately, there is a strong belief in the medical community that announcing upcoming stimuli and events as painful and then expressing sympathy is a more "honest" approach and therefore beneficial to their patients. However, such statements tend to become self-fulfilling prophecies. Therapists, who prepare patients prior to procedures and are not in the procedure room with them, may want to be particularly conscious of these negative suggestions and include measures of "immunization" against such comments (such as the hypnotic suggestion "and use only the suggestions that are helpful for you"). In contrast, it is important to recognize the emotional investment of the procedure team in the patient's pain management, and it is crucial to acknowledge their experience and enlist their contribution and collaboration when designing hypnosis programs in medical settings.

In the conception of a validated model of hypnotic intervention for interventional radiology procedures, we demonstrated the safety and effectiveness of the use of hypnosis while in the procedure room (12,66,67). When the patient is lying on the procedure table, he or she is often exposed to the idea of having medical hypnosis for their first time. The main reason for this setup (i.e., no preprocedure preparation) is the lack of time and structure for a preparatory visit in a very busy interventional radiology clinic. We do not consider it as important to assess patients' hypnotizability prior to the procedure. Poor performance on a hypnotizability test could conversely introduce bias and sabotage later usage. Emphasis should rather be placed on rapid rapport techniques, in the form of structured attentive behavior to quickly establish a patient-provider relationship. Detailed descriptions of these standardized interventions have been published (13).

The structured attentive behavior includes the following components: (a) matching the patients' verbal communication pattern, (b) matching the patients' nonverbal communication pattern, (c) attentive listening, (d) provision of the perception of control ("Let us know at any time what we can do for you."), (e) swift response to patients' requests, (f) encouragement, (g) use of emotionally neutral descriptors (e.g., "What are you experiencing?," "Focus on a sensation of fullness, numbness, coolness, or warmth" – when painful stimuli are imminent), and (h) avoidance of negatively loaded suggestions (e.g., "How bad is your pain?," "You will feel a sting and burn now," "I know that you are sore").

For guidance to self-hypnotic relaxation, we typically use scripts, in part because much of our work occurs in a research context. Scripts also help providers learn and reinforce hypnotic vocabulary and permit exchange of personnel during the procedure when the choice of induction is known. We use one script that is relatively immune to interruptions by bystanders and permits patients to drift into and out of hypnosis as they wish (reprinted in the appendix).

The provision of structured attention and hypnosis by a provider is sometimes seen as impractical in the interventional radiology setting. In our experience, the clinical benefits of hypnosis can be extended to cost savings with reductions of up to $338 (US) per case, if every patient were offered hypnosis as compared to standard sedation (68,69). The cost advantage of adjunct hypnosis persists in a sensitivity analysis, even when a health care provider exclusively dedicated to performing hypnosis is added to the medical team, unless this person's hourly wage exceeded $330/hour ($633,600/year). Emphasis in the training of personnel in nonpharmacological interventions for analgesia and anxiolysis has led to the development of electronic teaching modules designed for radiology (70). The use of those materials is recommended as a supplement to traditional live courses, shortening the time required to be spent with instructors, for completion of biobehavioral skills training.

SAFETY CONSIDERATIONS WITH THE USE OF HYPNOSIS

Although the literature provides evidence confirming the safety of hypnosis as an adjunct to pharmacological pain control, it has been recommended that its use should be limited to licensed health care practitioners. Moreover, inadequate training in hypnosis has been suggested to be associated with a greater likelihood of occurrence of negative effects (71) (rarely, drowsiness, confusion, headaches, and, even less frequently, anxiety or panic described in case reports) (71–74). Thus, it is important that the person structuring hypnosis should be sufficiently capable and prepared to recognize the potential for adverse events and intervene accordingly.

There is theoretically a minor risk that psychotic patients could become worse when told to interact with their imagery during the self-hypnotic process. However, psychotic patients are typically not very hypnotizable and thus may not respond to hypnotic suggestion as well as others (75). It is conceivable that a patient may experience an "abreaction," which is a forceful reenactment of a past traumatic experience. We therefore do not regress patients to times in the past. Even "happy times" in a patient's life may have hidden painful aspects and the setting of the interventional radiology suite, where darkness, immobilization, and a position of less power can elicit comparisons to past abuse. Having anchored the patient in an imaginary place of safety upfront can then be very helpful in returning to a resourceful status.

In our clinical and research practice, we always review the patients' medical records prior to the use of adjunct hypnosis. If there is any clinical evidence or suspicion of psychosis or other major psychiatric disorder, hypnosis is not provided and a mental health care specialist is consulted.

CONCLUSIONS

The use of nontraditional techniques of pain control and anxiolysis can be successful, even in a busy interventional radiology practice. In such a clinical scenario, the use of empathic attentive skills, avoidance of negative suggestions, and provision of hypnosis can easily manage heightened patient fear and anxiety. This approach does not require additional involvement of time once these skills are learned, and hypnosis can contribute to improve patients' outcomes and the quality of medical care in this environment.

ACKNOWLEDGMENTS

This work was supported by the National Institutes of Health, National Center for Complementary and Alternative Medicine 1K24 AT 01074 and

RO1-AT-0002-07, and the U.S. Army Medical Research and Materiel Command DAMD17-01-01. The funding agencies were not involved in the writing of this manuscript. The content is solely the responsibility of the authors and does not necessarily reflect the official views of the funding agencies.

APPENDIX

Self-hypnotic Relaxation Script

We want you to help us to help you learn a concentration exercise to help you get through the procedure more smoothly. It can be a way to help your body be more comfortable through the procedure and also to deal with any discomfort that may come up during the procedure. It is just a form of concentration, like getting so caught up in a movie or a good book that you forget you're watching a movie or reading a book.

Now, what I want to do is to show you how you can use your imagination to enter a state of focused attention and physical relaxation. If you hear sounds or noises in the room, just use those to deepen your experience or allow them to drift away. You only have to have your mind respond to the suggestions that are helpful to you.

There are a lot of ways to relax but here's one simple way:

On one, I want you to do one thing, look up. On two, do two things,
    slowly close your eyes and take a deep breath in.
On three, do three things, breathe out, relax your eyes, and let your body float. That's good. Just imagine your whole body floating, floating through the table,

each breath deeper and easier. Right now, I want you to imagine that you are floating somewhere safe and comfortable, in a bath, a lake, a hot tub or just floating in space, each breath deeper and easier. Notice how with each breath you let a little more tension out of your body as your whole body floats, safe and comfortable, each breath deeper and easier.

Good, now with your eyes closed and remaining in this state of concentration please describe for me how your body is feeling right now. Where do you imagine yourself being, what is it like? Can you smell the air? Can you see what's around you? Good. Now this is your safe and pleasant place to be and you can use it in a sense to play a trick on the doctors. Your body has to be here but you don't. So just spend your time being somewhere else you would rather be.

Now, if there is some discomfort, and there may be some during the procedure, as they prepare you and insert the line, or as you feel the dye entering your body, there is no point in fighting it. You can admit it, but then transform the sensation. If you feel some discomfort, you might find it helpful to make that part of your body to feel warmer as if you were in a bath. Or cooler, if that is more comfortable, as if you had ice or snow on that part of your body. This warmth or coolness becomes a protective filter between you and the discomfort. If you have any discomfort right now imagine that you are applying a hot pack or you are putting snow or ice on it and see what it feels like. Develop the sense of warmth or cool tingling numbness to filter any hurt out of the discomfort. With each breath, breathe deeper and easier, your body is floating, filter the hurt out of the discomfort. Now again with your eyes closed and remaining in the state of concentration, describe what you are feeling right now.

1. **If they are in a safe and comfortable place, reinforce it:** What is it like now? What do you see around you? What are you doing?
2. **If they are in discomfort, say:** The discomfort is there but see if you can add coolness, more warmth, or make it lighter or heavier.

    If no longer in discomfort, say: Good, continue to focus on those sensations

    If still in discomfort, say: See if you can focus on another part of your body. Now rub your fingertips together and notice all the delicate sensations in your fingertips and see how much you can observe about what it feels like to rub you thumb and forefingers together. How do you feel now?

    If not in discomfort, say: Good, continue to focus on those sensations.

    If still in discomfort, say: Now imagine yourself being at . . . *(patient's safe place)* where you said you felt relaxed and comfortable. What is it like now? What is the temperature like? What do you see around you?
3. **If they state that they are worried, say:** OK, your main job right now is to help your body feel comfortable so we will talk about what's worrying you. But first, no matter what we discuss, concentrate on your body floating. So let's get the floating back into your body. Imagine that you arc in your favorite spot and when you're ready, let me know by nodding your head and then we will talk about what's worrying you. But remember no matter what we discuss, concentrate on your body floating, and feel safe and comfortable. So what's worrying you? (Discuss with patient)

How do you feel now?

If not worried, say: Continue to concentrate on your body floating and feel safe and comfortable in your favorite place.

If after discussing the patient has a persistent worry, say: OK. Picture in your mind a screen, like a movie screen, a TV screen or a piece of clear blue sky. First, picture a pleasant scene on it. Now, picture a large piece of blue screen divided in half. All right, now on the left half, picture what you are worrying about on the screen. Now, on the right half, picture what you will do about it. Or what you would recommend someone else to do about it. Keep your body floating, and if you are worrying about the outcome, OK admit it to yourself, but your body doesn't have to get uptight about it. You may, but your body does not have to.

Good. You know that whatever happens there is always something that you can do. But for now just concentrate on keeping your body floating and feeling safe and comfortable.

Sometime during the procedure, say: If you feel any sense of discomfort you are welcome to let me know about it. Use the filter to filter the hurt out of the discomfort, but by all means let me know and I will do what I can to help you with it too. Whatever you do just keep your body floating, and concentrate on being in the place where you feel safe and comfortable.

When finished, say: OK. The procedure is now over. We are going to leave formally this state of concentration by counting backwards from three to one. On three get ready, on two, with your eyes closed roll up your eyes, and on one let your eyes open and take a deep breath in and let it out. That will be the end of the formal exercise but when you come out of it you will still have the feeling of comfort that you felt during it and feel proud about having been able to help yourself so well through this procedure. Ready? Three, two, one.

If necessary, say: Three-get ready, two-with your eyes closed roll up your eyes, one-let your eyes open and take a deep breath.

REFERENCES

1. Rich AB. A right to pain: ethical, legal, and public policy considerations in The 25th Annual Scientific Meeting of the American Pain Society. 2006. San Antonio, TX.
2. Martin ML, Lennox PH. Sedation and analgesia in the interventional radiology department. J Vasc Interv Radiol, 2003;**14**:1119–28.
3. Martin ML, Lennox PH, Buckley BT. Pain and anxiety: two problems, two solutions. J Vasc Interv Radiol, 2005;**16**:1581–4.
4. Sanborn PA, Michna E, Zurakowski D, et al. Adverse cardiovascular and respiratory events during sedation of pediatric patients for imaging examinations. Radiology, 2005;**237**:288–94.
5. England A, Tam CL, Thacker DE, et al. Patterns, incidence and predictive factors for pain after interventional radiology. Clin Radiol, 2005;**60**:1188–94.
6. Bhananker AM, Posner KL, Cheney FW, Caplan RA, Lee LA, Domino KB. Injury and liability associated with monitored anesthesia care: a closed claims analysis. Anesthesiology, 2006;**104**:228–34.
7. Faymonville ME, Meurisse M, Fissette J. Hypnosedation: a valuable alternative to traditional anaesthetic techndques. Acta Chir Belg, 1999;**99**:141–6.
8. Dillard JN, Knapp S. Complementary and alternative pain therapy in the emergency department. Emerg Med Clin N Am, 2005;**23**:529–49.
9. Montgomery GH, Weltz GR, Seltz M, Bovbjerg DH. Brief presurgery hypnosis reduces stress and pain in excisional breast biopsy patients. Int J Clin Exp Hypn, 2002; **50**:17–32.
10. Patterson DR, Questad KA, deLateour BJ. Hypnotherapy as an adjunct to narcotic analgesia for the treatment of pain for burn debridement. Am J Clin Hypn, 1989; **31**:156–63.
11. Sinha M, Christopher NC, Fenn R, Reeves L. Evaluation of nonpharmacologic methods of pain and anxiety management for laceration repair in the pediatric emergency department. Pediatrics, 2006;**117**:1162–8.
12. Lang EV, Benotsch EG, Fick LJ, et al. Adjunctive non-pharmacologic analgesia for invasive medical procedures: a randomized trial. Lancet, 2000;**355**:1486–90.
13. Lang EV. Nonpharmacologic analgesia and anxiolysis for interventional radiological procedures. Sem Intervent Radiol, 1999;**16**:113–23.
14. Mandle CL, Domar AD, Harrington DP, et al. Relaxation response in femoral angiography. Radiology, 1990;**174**:737–9.
15. Horne DJ, Vatmanidis P, Careri A. Preparing patients for invasive medical procedures and surgical procedures 1: adding behavioral and cognitive interventions. Behav Med, 1994;**20**:5–13.

16. Schupp C, Berbaum K, Berbau M, Lang EV. Pain and anxiety during interventional radiological procedures. Effect of patients' state anxiety at baseline and modulation by nonpharmacologic analgesia adjuncts. J Vasc Intervent Radiol, 2005;**16**:1585–92.

17. Acute Pain Management Guideline Panel. Acute pain management: operative or medical procedures and trauma. Clinical practice guideline. AHCPR Pub. No.92–0032. (Rockville, MD: Agency for Health Care Policy and Research, Public Health Service, U.S. Department of Health and Human Services, 1992).

18. Faymonville ME, Mambourg PH, Joris J, et al. Psychological approaches during conscious sedation. Hypnosis versus stress reducing strategies: a prospective randomized study. Pain, 1997;**73**:361–7.

19. Syrjala KL, Donaldson GW, Davis MW, Kippes ME, Carr JE. Relaxation and imagery and cognitive-behavioral training reduce pain during cancer treatment: a controlled clinical trial. Pain, 1995;**63**:189–98.

20. Astin JA. Mind-body therapies for the management of pain. Clin J Pain, 2004;**20**:27–32.

21. Honda K, Jacobson JS. Use of complementary and alternative medicine among United States adults: the influences of personality, coping strategies, and social support. Prev Med 2005;**40**:46–53.

22. Liossi C, Hatira P. Clinical hypnosis in the alleviation of procedure-related pain in pediatric oncology patients. Int J Clin Exp Hypn, 2003;**51**:4–28.

23. Seskevich JE, Crater SW, Lane JD, Krucof MW. Beneficial effects of noetic therapies on mood before percutaneous intervention for unstable coronary syndromes. Nursing Res, 2004;**53**:116–21.

24. Zeltzer L, LeBaron S. Hypnosis and nonhypnotic techniques for reduction of pain and anxiety during painful procedures in children and adolescents with cancer. J Pediatr, 1982;**101**:1032–5.

25. Sindhu F. Are non-pharmacological nursing interventions for the management of pain effective? – a meta-analysis. J Adv Nursing, 1996;**24**:1152–9.

26. Saadat H, Drummond-Lewis J, Maranets I, et al. Hypnosis reduces preoperative anxiety in adult patients. Anesth Analg, 2006;**102**:1394–6.

27. National Center for Complementary and Alternative Medicine. http//nccam.nih.gov. Accessed on 05/30/2006.

28. Garrison DW, Foreman RD. Decreased activity of spontaneous and noxiously evoked dorsal horn cells during transcutaneous electrical nerve stimulation (TENS). Pain, 1994;**58**:309–15.

29. Mora B, Giorni E, Dobrouits M, et al. Trancutaneous electrical nerve stimulation: an effective treatment for pain caused by renal colic in emergency care. J Urol, 2006; **175**:1737–41.

30. Erdogan M, Erdogan A, Erbil N, Karakaya HK, Demircan A. Prospective, randomized, placebo-controllled study of the effect of TENS on postthoracotomy pain and pulmonary function. World J Surg, 2005;**29**:1563–70.

31. Forster EL, Kramer JF, Lucy SD, Scudds RA, Novick RJ. Effect of TENS on pain, medications, and pulmonary function following coronary artery bypass graft surgery. Chest, 1994;**106**:1343–8.

32. NIH Consensus Conference. Acupuncture. JAMA, 1998;**280**:1518–1524.

33. Kotani N, Hashimoto H, Sato Y, et al. Preoperative intradermal acupunture reduces postoperative pain, nausea and vomiting, analgesic requirement, and sympathoadrenal responses. Anesthesiology, 2001;**95**:349–56.

34. Vickers AJ, Rusch VW, Malhotra VT, Downey RJ, Cassileth R. Acupunture is a feasible treatment for post-thoracotomy pain: results of a prospective pilot trial. BMC Anesthesiol, 2006;**6**:5.

35. Dimond EG. Acupuncture anesthesia. Western Medicine and Chinese traditional medicine. JAMA, 1971;**218**:1558–63.

36. Lee H, Ernst E. Acupuncture analgesia during surgery: a systematic review. Pain, 2005;**114**:511–7.

37. Benson H, Klipper MZ. The relaxation response. 9th ed. (New York, NY: Avon, 1976), pp. 1–222.

38. Good M, Anderson GC, Ahn S, Cong X, Stanton-Hicks M. Relaxation and music reduce pain following intestinal surgery. Res Nursing Health, 2005;**28**:240–51.

39. Haase O, Schweak W, Hermann C, Muller JM. Guided imagery and relaxation in conventional colorectal resections: a randomized, controlled, partially blinded trial. Dis Colon Rectum, 2005;**48**:1955–63.

40. Bugbee ME, Wellisch DK, Arnott IM, et al. Breast core-needle biopsy: clinical trial of relaxation technique versus medication versus no intervention for anxiety reduction. Radiology, 2005;**234**:73–8.

41. Applied Psycholophisiology & Biofeedback. http://aapb.org. Accessed on 05/30/2006.

42. Hermann C, Kim M, Blanchard E. Behavioral and prophylactic pharmacological intervention studies of pediatric migraine: an exploratory meta-analysis. Pain, 1995;**60**:239–56.

43. Chiarioni G, Whitehead WE, Pezza V, Morelli A, Bassotti G. Biofeedback is superior to laxatives for normal transit constipation due to pelvic floor dyssynergia. Gastroenterology, 2006;**130**:657–64.

44. Scharff L, Marcus D, Masek B. A controlled study of minimal-contact thermal biofeedback treatment in children with migraine. J Pediatric Psychol, 2002;**27**:109–19.

45. Huth MM, Broome ME, Good M. Imagery reduces children's postoperative pain. Pain, 2004;**110**:439–48.

46. Krucoff MW, Crater SW, Green CL, et al. Integrative noetic therapies as adjuncts to percutaneous intervention during unstable coronary syndromes: monitoring and actualization of noetic training (MANTRA) feasibility pilot. Am Heart J, 2001;**142**:760–7.

47. Benson H, Dusek JA, Sherwood JB, et al. Study of the therapeutic effects of intercessory prayer (STEP) in cardiac bypass patients: a multicenter randomized trial of uncertainty and certainty of receiving intercessory prayer. Am Heart J, 2006;**151**:934–42.

48. Krucoff MW, Crater SW, Gallup D, et al. Music, imagery, touch, and prayer as adjuncts to interventional cardiac care: the monitoring and actualisation of noetic trainings (MANTRA) II randomised study. Lancet, 2005;**366**:211–7.

49. Rainville P, Carrier S, Hofbauer K, Bushnell M, Duncan GH. Dissociation of sensory and affective dimensions of pain using hypnotic modulation. Pain, 1999;**82**:159–71.

50. Butler LD, Symons BK, Henderson SL, Shortliffe LD, Spiegel D. Hypnosis reduces distress and duration of an invasive medical procedure for children. Pediatrics, 2005;**115**:77–85.

51. Esdaile J. Mesmerism in India and its practical application in surgery and medicine. London. Reissued as Hypnosis in medicine and surgery. (New York, NY (1957): Julian Press, 1846).

52. Crasilneck HB, McCranie EJ, Jenkins MT. Special indications for hypnosis as method of anesthesia. JAMA, 1956;**126**:1606–8.

53. Blankfield RP. Suggestion, relaxation, and hypnosis as adjuncts in the care of surgery patients: a review of the literature. Am J Clin Hypn, 1991;**33**:172–86.

54. Stewart JH. Hypnosis in contemporary medicine. Mayo Clin Proc, 2005;**80**:511–24.

55. Montgomery GH, David D, Winkel G, Silverstein JH, Bovbjerg DH. The effectiveness of adjunctive hypnosis with surgical patients: a meta-analysis. Anesth Analg, 2002;**94**:1639–45.

56. Hippel CV, Hole G, Kaschka WP. Autonomic profile under hypnosis as assessed by heart rate variability and spectral analysis. Pharmacopsychiatry, 2001;**34**:111–3.

57. Baglini R, Sesana M, Capuano C, Gnecchi-Ruscone T, Ugo L, Danzi GB. Effect of hypnotic sedation during percutaneous transluminal coronary angioplasty on myocardial ischemia and cardiac sympathetic drive. Am J Cardiol, 2004;**93**:1035–8.

58. Krauss B, Green SM. Procedural sedation and analgesia in children. Lancet, 2006;**367**:766–80.

59. Morgan AH, Hilgard ER. Age differences in susceptibility to hypnosis. Int J Clin Exp Hypn, 1972;**21**:78–85.

60. Corah NL, Gale EN, Illig SJ. The use of relaxation and distraction during dental procedures. J Am Dent Assoc, 1979;**98**:390–4.

61. Ghoneim MM, Block RI, Sarasin DS, Davis CS, Marchman SN. Tape-recorded hypnosis instructions as adjuvant in the care of patients scheduled for third molar surgery. Anesth Analg, 2000;**90**:64–8.

62. Wilson JF, Moore RW, Randolph S, Hanson BJ. Behavioral preparation of patients for gastrointestinal endoscopy: information, relaxation and coping style. J Hum Stress, 1982;**8**:13–23.

63. Smith JT, Barabasz A, Barabasz M. Comparison of hypnosis and distraction in severely ill children undergoing painful medical procedures. J Counseling Psychol, 1996;**43**:187–95.

64. Spiegel H. Nocebo: the power of suggestibility. Prevent Med, 1997;**26**:616–21.

65. Lang EV, Hatsiopoulou O, Koch T, et al. Can words hurt? Patient-provider interactions during invasive medical procedures. Pain, 2005;**114**:303–9.

66. Lang EV, Berbaum KS. Educating interventional radiology personnel in nonpharmacologic analgesia: effect on patients' pain perception. Acad Radiol, 1997;**4**:753–7.

67. Lang EV. Empathic attention and self-hypnotic relaxation for interventional radiological procedures. (Iowa City, IA: The University of Iowa, 1996).

68. Lang EV, Rosen M. Cost analysis of adjunct hypnosis for sedation during outpatient interventional procedures. Radiology, 2002;**222**:375–82.

69. Faintuch S, Lang EV, Rosen MP. Cost-effectiveness of self-hypnosis during outpatient interventional radiologic procedures: update and impact. Sociedad Iberoamericana de Informacion Cientifica.

70. Lang EV, Laser E, Anderson B, et al. Shaping the experience of behavior: construct of an electronic teaching module in nonpharmacologic analgesia and anxiolysis. Acad Radiol, 2002;**9**:1185–93.

71. Lynn SJ, Martin DJ, Frauman DC. Does hypnosis pose special risks for negative effects? A master class commentary. Int J Clin Exp Hypn, 1996;**44**:7–19.

72. MacHovec F. Hypnosis, complications, risk factors and prevention. Am J Clin Hypn, 1988;**31**:40–9.

73. Page RA, Handley GW. In search of predictors of hypnotic sequelae. Am J Clin Hypn, 1996;**39**:93–6.

74. Barber J. When hypnosis causes trouble. Int J Clin Exp Hypn, 1998;**46**:157–70.

75. Spiegel D, Detrick D, Frischolz E. Hypnotizability and psychopathology. AJ Psychiatry, 1982;**139**:431–7.

Postprocedural Pain Control

Stan Zipser

INTRODUCTION

A sound knowledge of postprocedural pain control is essential as interventional radiologists take the lead in managing their patients and as interventional radiology continues to grow as a clinical service. Not only do patients deserve to receive adequate postprocedural pain management but also regulatory and other quality control bodies, such as the Joint Commission on Accreditation of Healthcare Organizations (1) and at least one medical malpractice insurance carrier (2), critically evaluate a practitioner's and hospital plan for pain control after a procedure.

Postprocedural pain is clearly an important issue for interventional radiology and in medicine in general. Consider that in a sample of 250 patients who had recently had surgery, 80% of patients actually experienced acute postoperative pain, 86% of these patients had moderate-to-extreme pain, and 59% cited experiencing postoperative pain as their most common concern (3). Specifically concerning interventional radiology, many multicenter trials examining uterine fibroid embolization (UFE) have found postprocedural pain the most common side effect after the procedure (4) and inadequate pain relief as the most common adverse event after discharge necessitating readmission (5,6,7).

This chapter will review the management of postprocedural pain. A brief summary of the physiological mechanism of pain will be followed by a general treatment strategy, a review of pertinent medications and different techniques for pain control, and then an examination of postprocedural pain strategies for specific procedures, namely, UFE, transarterial hepatic chemoembolization, percutaneous biliary procedures, and various other procedures.

With the exception of pain control after UFE, there is little on the subject of postoperative pain management in the interventional radiology literature. Therefore, much of the information for this chapter was obtained from the anesthesiology and surgery literature.

GENERAL CONSIDERATIONS

Mechanisms of Postprocedural Pain

Nocioception refers to central nervous system signal reception evoked by activation of specialized peripheral sensory receptors (nociceptors) that are activated by tissue injury (8). Tissue injury, iatrogenic or otherwise, causes release of inflammatory mediators such as histamine, prostaglandins, bradykinin, and serotonin at the site of injury. These inflammatory substances activate peripheral nociceptors that transduce afferent information to the dorsal horn of the spinal cord, and then to centers in the reticular formation, thalamus, and cerebral cortex, leading to the sensation of pain. The nocioceptor has an efferent function as well, releasing neurotransmitters such as substance P and calcitonin-gene-related peptide that induce vasodilatation and plasma extravasation, as well as activation of many nonneuronal inflammatory mediating cells including mast cells and neutrophils, furthering the inflammatory and pain process (9).

Treatment Strategy

Although there are general concepts that should be followed in postprocedural pain management, treatment plans should be individualized to each patient. Before the procedure, patients should be educated on the upcoming procedure, the pain medications and routes of administration that will be utilized, and the patients' role in reporting pain (11). In addition, treatment of preexisting pain and adjustments of current medications should be made to prevent an abstinence syndrome (21). Following the procedure, patients should be intermittently reassessed to evaluate their response to the pain management. Adjustments need to be made for the individual's level of pain tolerance and individualized symptoms, response to medication, and comorbidities such as renal or hepatic dysfunction, respiratory disease such as chronic obstructive pulmonary disease, or underlying mental incapacity or dementia.

Immediately following the procedure, residual effects from the intraprocedural analgesic and sedation medication require continued monitoring of the patient. The American Society of Anesthesiologists has established guidelines (10) for postprocedural recovery care that states in part that the level of consciousness, vital signs, and oxygenation should be recorded at regular intervals and resuscitation equipment should be present in the recovery area; a nurse or other individual trained to monitor patients and complications should be in attendance, and an individual who can manage complications should be immediately available, until discharge criteria are fulfilled; up to two hours should be allowed to pass until discharge if reversal agents have been given; and patients should be provided with written instructions regarding diet, medication, activity restrictions, and a phone number to call in case of emergency (10).

There are multiple medications and techniques to control pain after an interventional radiology procedure. Medications include opioids, nonsteroidal anti-inflammatory medications, sedatives, antinausea agents, and antiemetics. Other analgesic techniques include regional anesthesia such as epidural anesthesia and peripheral nerve blocks. Whatever treatment plan is decided on for a patient, using a multimodal (balanced) approach – using different classes of drugs to optimize pain control – should be utilized (21). In general, an opioid sparing strategy should be employed whenever possible (11).

Multimodal Analgesia

Multimodal, or "balanced," anesthesia refers to using different classes of analgesics with different mechanisms of action to optimize pain control. There are many benefits to this approach for analgesia, including achieving more effective pain control by creating an additive or synergistic effect among analgesics with different mechanisms of action, and using lower doses of each agent that help avoid the each medications side effects (12,27). Multiple studies have demonstrated the benefit of a multimodal approach to postoperative pain control in reducing the doses of specific agents, increased analgesia (13,14), and decreasing side effects (14). Not only is the combination of oral and intravenous (IV) medications beneficial but other forms of pain control such as regional nerve block, specific site infiltration with local anesthetics, and epidural anesthesia are also used in various combinations with oral or parenteral medication to achieve optimal pain control with fewer side effects (13). The American Society of Anesthesiologists Task Force on Acute Pain Management specifically recommends multimodal pain management therapy whenever possible (21).

In their extensive review on multimodal analgesia for postoperative pain control, Jin and Chung concluded the following: combined use of systemic opioids and nonsteroidal anti-inflammatory drugs (NSAIDs) relieved postoperative pain more effectively than single drug regimens in outpatients and inpatients, epidural combinations of local anesthetics and opioids were efficacious in controlling postoperative pain, and multimodal anesthesia with combined local anesthesia or nerve block and systemic opioids or NSAIDs provided better analgesic effect for major surgical procedures. In general, patients have been shown to have lower pain scores, need fewer analgesics, and have a prolonged time to requiring analgesics after surgery if they are given analgesia in a multimodal manner (13).

Regarding side effects, a meta-analysis was published recently of randomized control trials comparing postoperative morphine patient-controlled analgesia (PCA) use, with and without concurrent NSAID use, to evaluate the risk of morphine adverse effects (14). In patients who received NSAIDS along with a morphine PCA, a significant decrease in postoperative nausea and vomiting and sedation was noted, as well as a slight decrease in pruritus. No decrease in respiratory depression was found, perhaps due to the very low overall incidence of respiratory depression in the trials (14).

POSTPROCEDURAL MEDICATIONS

Analgesic Medications

Analgesic medications are a diverse group of medications that control pain through different mechanisms of action. This group of medications includes opioids, NSAID, and local anesthetic agents. Their potency and analgesic effect often varies with the route of administration, and the patient's underlying hepatic and renal function.

OPIOIDS

Opioid analgesics are a mainstay of postprocedural pain control, especially for moderate to severe pain (13,20,27). Opiates bind to μ-receptors in the CNS providing their analgesic and other major therapeutic effects. They are commonly used during the postprocedural period because of their rapid onset, ability to provide analgesia without loss of consciousness, reversibility, lack of analgesic ceiling, and diverse routes of administration (15).

Side effects of opiates include respiratory depression, due at least in part to a direct effect on the brainstem. Maximal respiratory depression occurs 5–10 minutes after IV administration of morphine, or 30–90 minutes post-intramuscular (IM) or subcutaneous administration. Other side effects include decreased stomach and bowel motility with increased fluid reabsorption, sphincter of Oddi constriction, nausea and vomiting, urinary retention, pruritis, miosis, vasodilatation, and muscle rigidity and seizures in high doses.

All opioid analgesics are metabolized in the liver and should be used cautiously in patients with hepatic insufficiency. Elderly patients have been shown to be more sensitive to opioids, which may be due to decrease renal clearance rates or from another mechanism that has yet to be elucidated (16).

SPECIFIC OPIOIDS

Morphine

Morphine is the prototype and most widely used opioid. It is a very effective analgesic and is reversible. The bioavailability of the oral preparation is 25% due to significant first-pass metabolism in the liver, which should be considered in patients with hepatic insufficiency, because cumulative effects or increased bioavailability may occur after oral administration (15). It has a renally excreted active metabolite that can accumulate in patients with renal insufficiency, increasing the risk of respiratory depression. It is safe in low doses in patients with liver dysfunction (20). Morphine can be administered in oral, IM, IV, or epidural preparations. Dosing is usually 2–10 mg IV and 5–30 mg every four hours orally.

Fentanyl

Fentanyl citrate (Sublimaze) has many favorable properties making it a popular analgesic: rapid onset and short duration of action, no active metabolites, reversibility, and can be used safely in patients with hepatic and renal dysfunction (20). It is 100 times as potent as morphine as an analgesic, and its congener, sufentanil citrate (Sufenta), is 1,000 times more potent than morphine. Fentanyl has similar side effects as the other opioids. Fentanyl has parenteral, transdermal (Duragesic), and transmucosal routes of administration. The transdermal patch is appropriate for chronic pain but not indicated for acute pain because it is not titratable.

Hydromorphone

Hydromorphone (Dilaudid) has five to eight times the potency of morphine. It has no metabolites and may have fewer side effects than other narcotics.

Codeine

Codeine is 60% as effective orally as parenterally due to less first-pass metabolism in the liver. Codeine is an effective analgesic and antitussive agent.

Its analgesic effect is due to its conversion to morphine. Codeine is available in injectable, suspension, and oral tablet forms. It can also be taken in combination with acetaminophen (Tylenol 3). Codeine is typically dosed at 15–60 mg every 4–6 hours, whereas codeine with acetaminophen is given at a dose of acetaminophen 300–1000 mg/codeine 15–60 mg every four hours.

Tramadol

Tramadol (Ultram) is a synthetic codeine analog that exhibits weak μ-agonist activity and is effective for treating moderate postoperative pain. Its benefit is its relative lack of respiratory depression, lack of major organ toxicity, lack of depression of gastrointestinal motility, and low potential for abuse. Tramadol is available in tablet form and is orally dosed 50–100 mg every 4–6 hours. Side effects include dizziness, drowsiness, sweating, nausea, vomiting, dry mouth, and headache (27).

Meperidine

Meperidine (Demerol) has an active metabolite, normeperidine, with a long half-life of 15–20 hours. It can cause CNS excitation characterized by tremors, shakiness, and seizures (15,20). Because of these side effects it is not recommended for elderly patients (17), or for use in PCAs (20). However, it is an efficient agent to treat shivering, though the mechanism is not well understood (18).

Hydrocodone

Hydrocodone is contained in combined oral preparations such as Vicodin and Lortab where it is combined with acetaminophen, and Vicoprofen where it is combined with ibuprofen. It is available in elixir and tablet form, with varying dose strengths of both hydrocodone and the anti-inflammatory medication. Normal dosing regimens are hydrocodone 2.5–10 mg/acetaminophen 500–750 mg, taken every 4–6 hours.

Oxycodone

Oxycodone is another opioid analgesic commonly given for postprocedural pain control. It is available in isolated form (OxyFast, Oxycontin) or in combination with acetaminophen (Percocet, Tylox). All combinations are available in oral form only. Typcial dosing regimens are 2.5–10 mg oxycodone/ 325–500 mg acetaminophen every six hours. Extended release forms are also available, which decreases the need for six-hour dosing.

Opiods are highly variable in their potency, and individuals must be aware that the dosing regimens of opioids vary widely. Table 1 presents equianalgesic doses for various commonly used opiods.

Patient-controlled Analgesia

A commonly used method of delivery of opioids is a PCA pump. This route of delivery may be used for intravenous or epidural administration, but intravenous administration is used much more commonly. The advantages of administering opioids through a PCA include avoiding delays in analgesic administration, immediate pain relief, allowing for the patients variability in

Table 1. Equianalgesic Doses of Opioids		
	IV	*PO*
Morphine	10	30
Fentanyl (Sublimaze)	0.1	—
Hydromorphone (Dilaudid)	1.5–2.0	6–7.5
Codeine	130	200
Meperidine (Demerol)	75	300
Oxycodone	15	20–30

response to opioids, and a greater sense of control for the patient (15,20). A systematic review of trials comparing PCAs to conventional opioid therapy showed that PCAs improve analgesia, decrease the risk of pulmonary complications, and that patients prefer them over other routes of administration (20,19). PCAs are not appropriate for patients who cannot ably use the device, such as mentally incapacitated or demented patients.

Basal (background) doses are not recommended in opioid naive patients as it has been shown to increase the incidence of respiratory depression and other side effects without providing increased analgesia (20,27). Providing for a supplemental nurse-activated dose is important in case of breakthrough pain (20).

Opioid Reversal Agents

NALAXONE

Nalaxone (Narcan) is an opioid antagonist and reversal agent. In the setting of monitored analgesia, it is administered intravenously in 0.04- to 0.08-mg doses. For acute opioid overdose, a dose of 0.4 mg IV is given. An increase in respiratory rate should be seen in 1–2 minutes; if not, repeat doses may be given at intervals of 2–3 minutes. Rapid, large boluses should not be given to avoid a surge of catecholamines causing hypertension, tachycardia, and cardiac arrthymias, as well as anxiety and pain. The duration of naloxone effect is 1 4 hours. After a reversal agent is administered, the patient should be monitered up to two hours to avoid continued effects of the opioid medication outlasting the reversal agent (10).

NONSTEROIDAL ANTI-INFLAMMATORY DRUGS

NSAIDS are a diverse group of medications that include aspirin, ibuprofen, acetaminophen, and cyclooxygenase-2 (COX-2) inhibitors. These medications act as analgesic, antipyretic, and anti-inflammatory agents; one important exception is acetaminophen, which has analgesic and antipyretic properties, and only weak anti-inflammatory effects.

NSAIDS are effective in treating low-to-moderate pain (22), and are also an important complement to opioids for pain control and to decrease opioid side effects. A recent meta-analysis found that NSAID administration decreased postoperative nausea by 30 %, most likely due to decreased opioid

Table 2. Available Forms and Typical Doses for Commonly Used Postprocedural Medications

Drug	Form	Common Dosage
Analgesic		
Opioids		
Morphine	IM, IV, PO	2–10 mg IV or 5–30 mg PO q4hr
Fentanyl	IV, PO, TD	50 mcg IV: titrate to effect; 200 mcg PO over 15 min; 25 mcg/hr TD
Hydromorphone	IM, IV, PO	1–2 mg IM/IV/SQ q4-6hr
Codeine	IM, IV, PO	300–1000 mg acetaminophen/15–60 mg codeine PO q4hr
Tramadol	PO	50–100 mg PQ q4-6hr
Meperidine	IM, IV, PO	50–150 mg PO/IM/SQ q3-4hr
Hydrocodone	PO	2.5–10 mg hydrocodone/500–750 mg acetaminophen POq4–6hr
Oxycodone	PO	2.5–10 mg oxycodone/325–500 mg acetaminophen POq6hr
NSAID		
Aspirin	PO	81–650 mg PO q4-6hr
Acetaminophen	PO	325–1000 mg PO q4-6hr
Ketorolac	IM, IV, PO	15–30 mg IV or 30–60 mg IM q6hrs; 5–30 mg PO q4-6hr
COX-2	PO	200 mg q24hr
Sedative		
Benzodiazepine		
Diazepam	IM/IV/PO	2–10 mg IM/IV/PO q6–12hr
Midazolam	IM/IV/PO	0.5–2 mg IV – titrate to effect; 0.07mg/kg IM x 1
Lorazepam	IM/IV/PO	2–6 mg q24hr
Antiemetic		
Promethazine	IM/IV/PO	12.5–25 mg q4–6hr
Droperidol	IM/IV	1 mg/25 lbs IV
Scopolamine	TD	1 patch x 24 hr postprocedure
Odansetron	IV/PO	4–8 mg IV x1 dose; 8 mg PO q12hr
Metoclopramide	IM/IV/PO	10–20 mg IV q3hr

Note: IV – intravenous; IM – intramuscular; PO – oral; SQ – subcutaneous; TD – transdermal.

requirements (20,14). They also lack the neurological, respiratory depressant, constipating, or withdrawal side effects associated with opioid analgesics. In general, there should be scheduled, around-the-clock dosing for NSAIDs, acetominophen, or COX-inhibitors if there are no contraindications (12,21).

The principal therapeutic effect of NSAIDS derives from their ability to inhibit prostaglandin production (22). Prostaglandins are mediators in pathways of pain and inflammation. The precursor to prostaglandins is arachadonic acid, which is converted to prostaglandin precursors, PGG2 and PGH2, by the enzyme cyclooxygenase. There are two forms of cyclooxygenase, cyclooxygenase-1 (COX-1) which is found in most normal cells and tissue, and COX-2, which is found in the setting of inflammation. COX-2 is also found in normal kidney and brain but not the stomach, which accounts for COX-2 inhibitor's decreased gastric side effects when compared to other NSAIDS. The many different NSAIDs operate at different steps along the cyclooxygenase pathway.

ASPIRIN

Aspirin's anti-inflammatory effects derive from modifying COX-1 and COX-2, irreversibly inhibiting cyclooxygenase activity. In addition, inactivation of cyclooxygenase causes aspirin's antiplatelet effects by inhibiting platelet cyclooxygenase for the life of the platelet and thromboxane, a proplatelet aggregrate enzyme (22). Aspirin is dosed 325–650 mg every 4–6 hours.

OTHER NSAIDs

Most other NSAIDs, including ibuprofen, naproxen, and ketorolac, are reversible cyclooxygenase inhibitors and therefore have shorter durations of action both in their anti-inflammatory effects and their antiplatelet aggregating effects. These are primary oral agents, except ketorolac and diclofenac that can be administered intravenously. Side effects include bleeding, gastric upset and ulceration, and renal injury. Renal injury most often occurs in patients with preexisting renal dysfunction (12).

ACETAMINOPHEN

Acetominophen is primarily an analgesic and antipyretic agent with minimal anti-inflammatory properties due to weak anticyclooxygenase activity. It does not share the side effects of other NSAIDs such as impaired platelet aggregation, cardiac and renal effects, and gastric upset. The oral dose is 325–1000 mg, with a total daily dose of 4,000 mg. There are parenteral forms now available as the prodrug, propacetamol and paracetamol (12). Single doses over 10 g are hepatotoxic (22).

KETOROLAC

Like acetaminophen, ketorolac (Toradol) is a potent analgesic but weak anti-inflammatory agent. It is one of the few NSAIDs that can be administered parenterally and is therefore useful in intraprocedural administration and for nauseous patients, or those who are unable to take anything orally. Dosing is 5–30 mg orally every 4–6 hours, and 15– 30 mg IV or 30–60 mg IM every six hours. Side effects include dizziness, headache, gastrointestinal upset, and nausea. Due to potential renal toxicity, ketorolac must be discontinued after five days of use.

CYCLOOXYGENASE-2 INHIBITORS

COX-2 inhibitors act by selective inhibition of COX-2 found in inflammatory sites. They have an advantage over other NSAIDs because they do not inhibit other prostaglandin synthesis reducing the risk of gastric upset and ulcer disease. However, recently, rofecoxib (Vioxx) and valdexoxib (Bextra) were withdrawn from the market due to their cardiovascular and gastrointestinal risks (24). Celecoxib (Celebrex) is the only remaining COX-2 inhibitor available today but carries an FDA warning about increased risk for adverse cardiovascular events (23,24).

OTHER ANALGESIC MEDICATIONS

Because N-methyl-d-aspartate (NMDA) receptors are involved in the pain pathway, NMDA receptor antagonists such as ketamine and dextromethorphan are increasingly being used in postoperative analgesia (12,33,25). Subanesthetic doses of ketamine have been shown to decrease pain scores and opioid requirements, and possibly prevent the development of opioid tolerance (20). Alpha-2 agonists such as clonidine and dexmedetomidine, and corticosteroids are also being used (12). Although these medications are used in the perioperative period, the role of these agents in postinterventional procedural pain control is yet to be defined.

OTHER PAIN CONTROL

Regional Analgesic Techniques: Epidural Anesthesia and Peripheral Nerve Blocks

The use of regional analgesia techniques both during and after an interventional procedure can aid in intraprocedural and postprocedural pain control. Epidural anesthesia is a widely used and effective analgesic technique in surgery and anesthesia that is associated with a high degree of patient satisfaction (26). Epidural anesthesia involves administering analgesic medications, such as opioids, local anesthetic agents, clonidine, or ketamine, through a catheter into the epidural space. Variables affecting the epidural technique include the timing of epidural administration, duration of the epidural analgesia, the location of the epidural catheter, and infusion drug composition (26,27). Not surprisingly, epidural analgesia has been shown to provide statistically significant superior pain relief when compared to IV PCA with opioids but with higher incidence of motor block, nausea, and vomiting (28). Other side effects include hypotension from sympathetic blockade, urinary retention, pruritus, and respiratory depression (27). Also, this analgesic technique can be labor intensive to manage and causes safety issues when using anticoagulation and other antiplatelet medications (20,26); newer medications used in epidural anesthesia may help alleviate some of these side effects (26).

Peripheral nerve block is performed by infiltrating the area around a ganglion, nerve plexus, or nerve root with anesthetic agent, usually bupivicaine. This approach has the advantage of excellent pain relief and reduced opioid requirements.

The successful use of these techniques in interventional radiology has been employed during uterine fibroid embolization (52,29), hepatic chemoembolization (56), and percutaneous biliary procedures (60). They are not commonly used during interventional radiology procedures, however, which may be due to any one of a number of factors: intraprocedural and postprocedural pain control with IV medications may be considered adequate and therefore there is no need for more invasive pain control; interventionalists, most often performing less invasive, less painful procedures, are less familiar with these techniques and what they can offer; or because they may add considerable time and complexity to a procedure that is intended to be minimally invasive.

ACUPUNCTURE

Acupuncture and other less conventional therapies have been gaining in popularity in recent years. In their thorough and excellent review of perioperative acupuncture and related techniques, Chernyack and Sessler concluded that, although it has been practiced for more than 2,500 years, and with over 30 years of research, the exact mechanism of action and efficacy of acupuncture have yet to be clearly elucidated. Acupuncture may be effective for postoperative pain control but likely requires application by a practitioner with a high level of training and experience. Acupuncture has been shown to effectively treat postoperative nausea and vomiting in routine clinical practice in combination with, or as an alternative to, conventional antiemetics when administered before induction of general anesthesia (30).

Please see Chapter 19 for a review of nontraditional intraprocedural pain control methods.

Sedatives

BENZODIAZEPINES

Benzodiazepines are a group of medications that exert a sedative, hypnotic, and anxiolytic effect by binding to sites near gamma-aminobutyric acid (GABA) receptors in the CNS, increasing the receptors affinity to GABA. Benzodiazepines have no analgesic properties, and they are metabolized by different hepatic microsomal enzyme systems. At high doses, they may cause respiratory depression, especially in patients with underlying respiratory disorders such as COPD and obstructive sleep apnea (31). There are many types of benzodiazepines, each with a different duration and onset of action. Shorter-acting agents [midazolam (Versed)], medium-acting agents [lorazepam (Ativan)], and longer acting agents [diazepam (Valium)] are all widely available and may be used according to the patients needs.

Flumazenil (Romazicon) is a specific benzodiazipine antagonist and is used as a reversal agent. Small aliquots of 0.2–0.5 mg can be given to reverse benzodiazepines effects. As when using naloxone, the opioid antagonist, the dose should be given slowly to avoid a rebound reaction, and the patient should be monitored for up to two hours to ensure repeat sedation does not occur after the effects of flumazenil diminish.

Antiemetic Medications

PROMETHAZINE

Promethazine (Phenergan) is a phenothiazine that acts by blocking dopamine receptors in the chemoreceptor trigger zone of the brain. It has antiemetic and neuroleptic effects. It can be administered orally, intravenously, or rectally. Side effects include extrapyramidal effects ranging from restlessness to oculgyric crisis, and anticholinergic effects such as sedation, dry mouth, and confusion (32). Because of its side effect profile it is not recommended as an outpatient antiemetic (33).

DROPERIDOL

Droperidol (Inapsine) is a butyrophenone and is also a neuroleptic agent that acts by blocking central dopamine receptors. It is an effective antiemetic in low doses (<10 µg/kg). Side effects include dyskenisia, restlessness, and dysphoria. Prolongation of the QT interval can occur with higher doses, leading to sudden death in some cases (33). In 2001, this complication led to a "black box" warning (the most serious warning, named because of the black background color of the warning statement on medication inserts) by the FDA for droperidol.

SCOPOLAMINE

Scopolamine is a centrally active anticholinergic with antiemetic properties. The transdermal patch can be placed preprocedurally to achieve a therapeutic level in the postprocedure period. Anticholinergic side effects of this medication include dry mouth, somnolence, dizziness, and mydriasis (33).

ODANSETRON

Odansetron (Zofran) is a serotonin (5-HT3) receptor antagonist antiemetic. It is nonsedating and is often used for oncology patients during chemotherapy administration. It can be administered intravenously or orally and has a plasma half-life of 3–4 hours. There is a 32-mg total daily dose limit that can be given in divided doses. It is usually well tolerated, with only transient mild side effects of headache, constipation, and dizziness. Another serotonin antagonist is granisetron (Kytril) (32).

METOCLOPRAMIDE

Metoclopramide (Reglan) is a gastric and small-bowel promotility agent with antiemetic effects. It also increases lower-esophageal sphincter tone. It is dosed 20 mg IV or 0.2 mg/kg IV, and its half-life is 4–6 hours. Its side effects include extrapyramidal symptoms, anxiety, and depression (32).

POSTPROCEDURAL PAIN CONTROL IN INTERVENTIONAL RADIOLOGY

There are very few studies on postprocedural pain control in interventional radiology. The majority of studies examining the subject center on uterine fibroid embolization, which will be discussed in detail separately in this chapter.

In one study specifically addressing postprocedural pain, England et al. investigated the incidence of pain and the positive predictors of pain in 150 patients undergoing nine different nonarterial interventional radiology procedures (34). They found significant increases in patients' pain scores eight hours after percutaneous biliary procedures, six hours after central venous access placement and gastrostomy tube insertion, and four hours after esophageal stenting. There was a significant reduction in pain following percutaneous nephrostomy. No increase in pain was reported with colonic and duodenal stenting. The study further found that the only two positive predictors for postprocedural pain were the patients' preprocedural pain score and preprocedural analgesia; patients who had no pain before their procedure, or had no preprocedural analgesia, reported significant increases in their pain score after the procedure. There was no correlation between pain score and length of procedure, age, or gender. They concluded that patients who were to undergo a painful interventional radiology procedure should have preprocedural anesthesia, that longer acting local anesthesia should be used instead of lidocaine, and that postprocedural analgesia should be integrated into the postprocedure care of the interventional radiology patient.

PREEMPTIVE ANALGESIA

The concept of preemptive analgesia, treating postoperative pain by preventing the establishment of central sensitization, has proven effective in experimental studies but has had mixed results in clinical studies before surgery (25,27,35). Preemptive analgesia should be differentiated from pain existing before the procedure, which should always be treated (21). Preemptive analgesia is a controversial area due to many factors including the design of the studies examining the topic and even the basic definition of preemptive analgesia (25,27,36). Despite the current lack of convincing clinical evidence many authors advocate its use (25,27,36,34). In the interventional radiology literature, one author specifically recommends that all patients undergoing painful procedures should receive acetaminophen 1 g orally and an NSAID 30–60 minutes prior to initiating the procedure (36).

Specific Procedures

UTERINE FIBROID EMBOLIZATION

Postprocedural pelvic pain is to be expected after UFE (29,37), and achieving adequate postprocedural pain control is a vital part of the procedure contributing to a successful outcome and patient satisfaction. Many multicenter trials examining UFE have found postprocedural pain as the most common side effect after the procedure (38) and inadequate pain relief the most common adverse event after discharge necessitating readmission (39,40). Indeed, the importance of procedural and postprocedural pain control is highlighted by the high incidence of postprocedural pain and readmission when little pain medication was prescribed to the patients evaluated in a recent multicenter trial comparing UFE versus hysterectomy (40).

The most likely cause of pain after UFE is thought to be ischemic pain in normal myometrium (41). However, large fibroid size has also been found to correlate with increased postprocedural pain (40), possibly indicating that ischemia of the fibroid itself causes pain (37).

PROCEDURAL TECHNIQUE AND EMBOLIC AGENTS AFFECTING POSTPROCEDURAL PAIN

The procedural technique employed and type of embolic agent used has been shown to impact the amount of postprocedural pain. First, multiple studies have shown that the degree of embolization of the uterine arteries has been shown to correlate with the amount of patient's postprocedural pain. Embolizing to stasis and with multiple agents has been shown to increase postprocedural pain, whereas less aggressive embolization – to near stasis or just of the perifibroid vascular plexus – does not result in the same amount of pain (42). In a dedicated study of 99 patients that examined pain after UFE, the authors conjectured that their lower rate of postprocedural pain when compared to prior studies was due to using a less extensive embolization technique and more complete pain management technique (43). Similarly, a recent multicenter study found that there was a direct dose-effect relationship between the amount of polyvinyl alcohol (PVA) used and postprocedural pain and fever (40).

The type of embolic agent used has also been shown to correlate with the amount of postprocedural pain. One study found elevated pain scores reported in patients who were treated with Gold Embospheres (Embogold; Biosphere Medical, Rockland, MD) compared to Contour SE (Boston Scientific, Natick, MA) and Embospheres (Biosphere), and that patients treated with Contour SE tended to use a lesser amount of supplemental narcotics compared to the other two agents (49). Another study comparing Embogold and Embospheres showed similar findings with patients treated with Embogold requiring more days to return to routine daily activities and increased skin rash post-UFE than those treated with Embospheres (44). A high incidence of post-UFE endometritis has also been reported when using Embogold (45). No difference in postprocedural pain was found in a study comparing Embospheres and PVA particles (46).

POST-UFE PAIN CONTROL MEDICATIONS

Forming a coherent and manageable postprocedural protocol is the first step in delivery of adequate pain medications after UFE. The treatment plan should be in place before the procedure takes place and should be ready to be implemented after the procedure (41).

Although there is no single universal medication protocol utilized for postprocedural pain control, there are many commonly used medications. The most frequently used medications are opiates (typically delivered through a PCA), NSAIDs, and antiemetics. The pain control protocol reported by Bruno et al. (43) is typical: intravenous opioid medication through a PCA is given until the next morning with the conversion to oral opioid analgesic, and ketorolac is given around the clock. Antiemetics (odansetron or phenergan) are given on as needed basis. Most often patients can be discharged the day following the procedure on scheduled NSAIDs followed by oral opioid analgesics and antiemetics as needed. Variations on this protocol include continuous IV opioid administration during the procedure, which are decreased postprocedure with an as-needed additional dose (47) and scheduled antiemetics.

Siskin et al. developed a pain and symptom relief regimen to be used to perform UFE on an outpatient basis (48). They found that 96% of patients experienced adequate pain and symptom relief after being discharged no less than 5.5 hours post-UFE. Their regimen included ketorolac (60 mg IV) along with fentanyl and midazolam during the procedure; meperidine, hydroxyzine, ketoralac, and lortab (all as needed) immediately postprocedure; and prochlorperazine, meperidine, lortab, hydrocodone, ketorolac followed by ibuprofen (all as needed), and routine levfloxacin as discharge medications (48).

One study found no difference in the efficacy of ibuprofen and the COXIB rofecoxib (Vioxx) in reducing postprocedural pain or in their side effects (49). The COXIB has the theoretical benefit of single-day dosing and decreased stomach upset when compared to ibuprofen. However, rofecoxib has been removed entirely from the market due to its risk of stroke and myocardial infarction (24). It is not known whether the only remaining commercially available COX-2 inhibitor, celecoxib, is equally as effective as rofecoxib in postprocedural pain control.

OTHER PAIN CONTROL TECHNIQUES

A variety of other pain control techniques have been used to control post-UFE pain. Spinal and epidural anesthesia is used in some centers (29); however, perhaps because other less invasive pain control protocols have proven effective, these techniques are not widely used. In 46 patients, Zhan et al. reported a significant reduction in post-UFE pain for up to 48 hours by administering 6 ml of 0.067% dilute lidocaine in divided doses into each uterine artery after embolization was completed (50). These results were superior to an approach by Keyoung et al., who administered 10 ml 1% lidocaine intraarterially prior to embolization (51) as this approach caused significant vasospasm of the uterine artery complicating administration of embolic agents. Lastly, a recent study evaluating superior hypogastric nerve blocks performed during UFE in 139 patients, who also received supplementary pain control post-UFE, resulted in all patients being discharged on the day of the procedure with only seven being readmitted for pain control (52). However, because this technique involves another invasive procedure with own risks of complications it may not achieve widespread use in UFE.

SUMMARY OF POST-UFE PAIN CONTROL

In summary, postprocedural pain control is a vital part of UFE. Lack of adequate pain control is the most common complication following UFE. Less aggressive embolization has been shown to result in less postprocedural pain. Additionally, certain embolic agents have been shown to increase postprocedural pain. A comprehensive pain management protocol must be in place utilizing complementary pain medications as well as antiemetic medications. Other approaches such as epidural anesthesia or regional nerve block are available for patients with an increased need for analgesia.

Transarterial Hepatic Chemoembolization

Transarterial hepatic chemoembolization is a commonly performed procedure for treatment of hepatic masses that often causes postprocedural pain and other symptoms such as fever, nausea, and vomiting (53–56). The pain is thought to arise from tissue ischemia and an inflammatory response to chemoembolization (53). Variables that have been found to increase postprocedural pain include inadvertent embolization of the gallbladder, the amount of administered chemoembolic agents (possibly solely due to the amount of the embolic agent used, rather than the chemotherapeutic agent), and first-time embolization procedures (53). Another investigation found no difference in pain among patients receiving chemoembolization for the first time versus repeat chemoembolization, nor a correlation with age or preprocedure laboratory values (55). In the author's experience, the amount of postprocedural pain correlates with the amount of embolization performed: the greater the amount of embolic agent used, the greater the postoperative pain. In addition, in our patients who receive chemotherapy mixed with only lipiodol, most often causes only a small amount of postprocedural pain.

One relatively simple technique for decreasing postprocedural pain is the administration of intra-arterial lidocaine during chemoembolization procedures (57). Lee et al. found that administering 100 mg of 2% lidocaine intra-arterially 30 seconds prior to chemoembolization was very effective in reducing patients' postprocedural pain and pain medication requirements when compared to patients who received the same dose of intra-arterial lidocaine after the chemoembolic agents, or no intra-arterial lidocaine at all (58). Another successful method of pain control is celiac plexus block, which has been shown to reduce both intraprocedural and postprocedural pain following hepatic chemoembolization (56).

Postchemoembolization pain control usually employs an approach similar to UFE: intravenous opioids until the patient is able to take medications orally, NSAIDs, antiemetics on an as-needed basis, and IV hydration (54,59).

PERCUTANEOUS TRANSHEPATIC CHOLANGIOGRAPHY AND DRAINAGE

Percutaneous transhepatic cholangiography (PTC) and drainage is among the most painful procedures performed in interventional radiology, with pain often extending into the postprocedural period (34). The procedure is most often performed with moderate sedation, with analgesic medication given after the procedure. Other pain control techniques include epidural anesthesia, celiac plexus, and intercostal nerve block. Culp et al. reported successful results using a thoracic paravertebral block for pain relief during PTC and drainage (60). The anesthetic effect lasted throughout the night and the next morning, and the patient required no analgesia and only reported pain except with deep inspiration (60). An older study comparing intraprocedural intravenous sedation versus epidural anesthesia found a significant decrease in patients' pain scores when epidural anesthesia was used (61). However, administering the epidural added cost and time to the procedure, and required the help of the anesthesia service (61). Postprocedural pain was not addressed in this study.

Intercostal nerve blocks (INB) are simple procedures that may be performed on the majority of patients undergoing PTC and are particularly effective when the PTC is placed in an intercostal space. Once the skin site for the PTC is identified, the rib superior to the site is followed dorsally for 5–10 cm (because most PTC are placed in the right mid axillary line, the editor uses the posterior axillary line as the location for INB). A 25-gauge needle is advanced to the rib, which is intentionally hit with the needle. Because the goal is to inject the local anesthetic adjacent to the intercostals nerve, the needle is directed inferior to the rib margin. As the needle slides under the rib, aspiration on the syringe is performed – if a flash of blood is noted in the needle hub, the needle is redirected to avoid direct injection of anesthetic into the vascular system. Once the needle is in good position, an injection of 5–10 ml of 0.25% bupivicaine is performed. The procedure is performed one rib space above and one rib space below the inercostal space into which the PTC will be placed (three levels in total).

REFERENCES

1. http://www.jointcommission.org/AccreditationPrograms/Office-BasedSurgery/Standards/standards_sampler.htm?HTTP___JCSEARCH.JCAHO.ORG_CGI_BIN_MSMFIND.EXE?RESMASK=MssResEN.mskhttp%3A//jcsearch.jcaho.org/cgi-bin/MsmFind.exe%3Fhttp%3A//jcsearch.jcaho.org/cgi-bin/MsmFind.exe%3FRESMASK%3DMssResEN.msk. Accessed May 21, 2007.

2. NORCAL Mutual Insurance Company, Claims Rx, June 2006 – CME Edition, Pain management in the ICU.

3. Apfelbaum, JL, Chen, C, Mehta, SS, Gan, TJ. Postoperative pain experience: results from a national survey suggest postoperative pain continues to be undermanaged. Anesth Analg (2003);97:534–40.

4. Bucek, RA, Puchner, S, Lammer. Mid- and long-term quality-of-life assessment in patients undergoing uterine fibroid embolization. AJR Am J Roentgenol (2006);186:877–82.

5. Worthington-Kirsch, R, Spies, JB, Myers, ER, et al. The fibroid registry for outcomes data (FIBROID) for uterine embolization, short-term outcomes. Obstet Gynecol (2005);106(1):52–9.

6. Volkers, NA, Hehencamp, JK, Birnie, E, et al. Uterine artery embolization in the treatment of symptomatic uterine fibroid tumors (EMMY trial): periprocedural IR and complications. J Vasc Interv Radiol (2006);17(3):471–80.

7. Pron, G, Mocarski, E, Bennett, J, et al. Tolerance, hospital stay and recovery aftery uterine artery embolization for fibroids: the Ontario uterine fibroid embolization trial. J Vasc Interv Radiol (2003);14:1243–50.

8. Jessel, TM, Kelly, DD. Pain and analgesia. In Principles of Neural Science, 3rd ed. (Kandel ER, Schwartz Jessel eds.), TM, Elsevier Science: New York, 1991; pp. 385–99.

9. Julius, D, Basbaum, AI. Moecular mechanisms of nociception. Nature (2001);413:203–10.

10. Practice Guidelines for Sedation and Analgesia by Non-Anesthesiologists: An updated, report by the American Society of Anesthesiologists Task Force on Pain Management on Sedation and Analgesia by Non-Anesthesiologists. Anesthesiology (2004);96(4):1004–17.

11. Hatssiopoulou, O, Cohen, RI, Lang, EV. Postprocedure pain and management of interventional radiology patients. J Vasc Interv Radiol (2003);14:1373–85.

12. Joshi, GP. Multimodal analgesia techniques for ambulatory surgery. Int Anesth Clin (2005);43(3):197–204.

13. Jin, F, Chung, F. Multimodal analgesia for postoperative pain control. J Clin Anesth (2001);13:524–39.

14. Marret, E, Kurdi, O, Zufferey, P, Bonnet, F. Effects of nonsteroidal anti-inflammatory drugs onpatient controlled analgesia morphine side effects: meta-analysis of randomized controlled trials, Anesthesiology (2005);102:1249–60.

15. Resine, T, Pasternak, G. Opioid analgesics and antagonists. In Goodman and Gilman's The Pharmacological Basis of Therapeutics (Hardman, JG, Goodman Gilman, A, Limbird, LE, eds.), McGraw Hill, New York; NY, 2001; pp. 521–56.

16. Austrup, ML, Korean, G. Analgesic agents for the postoperative periods: opioids. Surg Clin N Am (1999);79(2):253–73.

17. Palmer, RM. Perioperative care of the elderly patient. Cleveland Clin J Med (2006);73 (Supp 1):S106–10.

18. Dewitte, J, Sessler, DI. Perioperative shivering: physiology and pharmacology. Anesthesiology (2002);96(2):467–84.

19. Walder, B, Schafer, M, Henzi, I, Tramer, MR. Efficacy and safety of patient-controlled opioid analgesia for acute postoperative pain. A quantitative systematic review. Acta Anaesthesiol Scand (2001);45(7):795–804.

20. Ritchey, RM. Optimizing postoperative pain management. Cleveland Clin J Med (2006);73 (Supp 1);S72–76.

21. Practice guidelines for acute pain management in the perioperative setting: an updated, report by the American Society of Anesthesiologists Task Force on Pain Management on Acute Pain Management. Anesthesiology (2004);100:1573–81.

22. Roberts LJ II, Morrow, JD. Analgesic-antipyretic and anti-inflammatory agents and drugs employed in the treatment of gout. In Goodman and Gilman's The Pharmacological Basis of Therapeutics, 10th ed. (Hardman, JG, Goodman Gilman, A, Limbird, LE, eds.), McGraw Hill, 2001; pp. 687–731.

23. Ardoin, SP, Sundy, JS. Update on nonsteroidal anti-inflammatory drugs. Curr Opin Rheumatol (2006);18:221–6.

24. http://www.fda.gov/cder/drug/infopage/COX2/default.htm. Accessed May 2005.

25. White, PF. The role of non-opioid analgesic techniques in the management of pain after ambulatory surgery. Anesth Analg (2002);94:577–85.

26. Vicussi, ER. Emerging techniques in the management of acute pain: epidural anesthesia. Anesth Analg (2005);101:S23–9.

27. Wu, CL. Acute postoperative pain. In Miller's Anesthesia, 6th ed. (Miller RD, ed.), Elsevier, Philadelphia, 2005; pp. 2729–62.

28. Wu, CL, Cohen, SR, Richman, JM, et al. Efficacy of postoperative patient-controlled and continuous infusion of epidural analgesia versus intravenous patient patient–controlled analgesia with opioids: a meta-analysis. Anesthesiology (2005);103:1079–88.

29. Andrews, RT, Spies, JB, Sacks, D, et al. Patient care and uterine artery embolization for leiomyomata. J Vasc Interv Radiol (2004);15:115–20.

30. Chernyack, GV, Sessler, DI. Perioperative acupuncture and related techniques. Anesthesiology (2005);102:1031–49.

31. Hobbs, WR, Ral, TW, Verndoorn, TA. Hypnotics and sedatives; ethanol. In Goodman and Gilman's The Pharmacological Basis of Therapeutics, 10th ed. (Hardman, JG, Goodman Gilman, A, Limbird, LE, eds.), McGraw Hill, 2001; pp. 399–427.

32. Brunton, LL. Agents affecting gastrointestinal water flux and motility; emesis and antiemetics; bile acids and pancreatic enzymes. In Goodman and Gilman's The Pharmacological Basis of Therapeutics, 9th ed. (Hardman, JG , Goodman Gilman, A, Limbird, LE, eds.), McGraw Hill, New York: NY, 1996, pp. 917–36.

33. White, PF, Freire, AR. Ambulatory (outpatient) anesthesia. In Miller's Anesthesia, 6th ed. (Miller, RD, ed.), Elsevier, Philadelphia, 2005; p. 2589.

34. England, A, Tam, CL, Thacker, DE, et al. Patterns, incidence and predictive factors for pain after interventional radiology. Clin Radiol (2005);60:1188–94.

35. Kehlet, H, Jensen, TS, Woolf, CJ. Persistent postsurgical pain: risk factors and prevention. Lancet (2006);367:1618–25.

36. Martin, ML, Lennox, PH. Sedation and analgesia in the interventional radiology department. J Vasc Interv Radiol (2003);14:1119–28.

37. Hovsepian, DM, Siskin, GP, Bonn, J, et al. Quality improvement guidelines for uterine artery embolization for symptomatic leiomyomata. J Vasc Interv Radiol (2004);15:535–42.

38. Bucek, RA, Puchner, S, Lammer J. Mid- and long-term quality-of-life assessment in patients undergoing uterine fibroid embolization. AJR Am J Roentgenol (2006);186: 877–82.

39. Worthington-Kirsch, R, Spies, JB, Myers, ER, et al. The fibroid registry for outcomes data (FIBROID) for uterine embolization, short-term outcomes. Obstet Gynecol, 2005;106(1):52–9.

40. Volkers, NA, Hehencamp, JK, Birnie, E, et al. Uterine artery embolization in the treatment of symptomatic uterine fibroid tumors (EMMY trial): periprocedural IR and complications. J Vasc Interv Radiol (2006);17(3):471–80.

41. Spies, JB. Commentary, Recovery after uterine artery embolization: understanding and managing short term outcomes, J Vasc Interv Radiol (2003);14:1219–22.

42. Pelage, JP. Commentary, Polyvinyl alcohol particles and tris-acryl gelatin microspheres for uterine artery embolization for leiomyomas. J Vasc Interv Radiol (2004);15(8):789–91.

43. Bruno, J, Sterbis, K, Flick, P, et al. Recovery after uterine artery embolization for leimyomas: a detailed analysis of its duration and severity. J Vasc Interv Radiol (2004);15(8):801–7.

44. Lohle, PNM, Boekkooi, FP, Smeets, AJ, et al. Limited uterine artery embolization for leimyomas with tris-acryl gelatin microspheres: 1-year follow up. J Vasc Interv Radiol (2006);17(2 Part 1):283–7.

45. Richard, H, Siskin, G, Stainken, B. Endometritis after uterine artery embolization with gold-colored gelatin microspheres. J Vasc Interv Radiol (2004);15:406–7.

46. Spies, JB, Allison, S, Flick, P, et al. Polyvinyl alcohol particles and tris-acryl gelatin microspheres for uterine artery embolization for leiomyomas: results of a randomized comparative study. J Vasc Interv Radiol (2004);15(8):793–800.

47. Ryan, JM, Gainey, M, Glasson, J, et al. Simplified pain-control after uterine artery embolization. Radiology (2002);224:610–3.

48. Siskin, GP, Stainken, BF, Dowling, K, Meo, P, Ahn, J, Dolen, EG. Outpatient uterine artery embolization for symptomatic uterine fibroids: experience in 49 patients. J Vasc Interv Radiol (2000);11:305–11.

49. Hovsepian, DM, Mandava, A, Pilgram, TK, et al. Comparison of adjunctive use of rofecoxib versus ibuprofen in the management of postoperative pain after uterine artery embolization. J Vasc Interv Radiol (2006);17(4):665–70.

50. Zhan, S, Li, Y, Wang, G, et al. Effectiveness of intra-arterial anesthesia for uterine fibroid embolization using dilute lidocaine. Eur Radiol (2005);15:1752–6.

51. Keyoung, JA, Levy, EB, Roth, ER, et al. Intraarterial lidocaine for pain control after uterine artery embolization for leiomyomata. J Vasc Interv Radiol (2001);12: 1065–73.

52. Rasuli, P, Jolly, EE, Hammond, I, et al. Superior hypogastric nerve block for pain control in outpatient uterine artery embolization. J Vasc Interv Radiol (2004);15:1423–9.

53. Ramsey, DE, Kernagis, LY, Soulen, MC, Geschwind, JFH. Chemoembolization of hepatocellular carcinoma. J Vasc Interv Radiol (2002);13:S211–21.

54. Leung, DA, Goin, JE, Sickles, C, Raskay, BJ, Soulen, MC. Determinants of postembolzation synfrome and hepatic chemoembolization. J Vasc Interv Radiol (2001); 12:321–6.

55. Patel, NH, Hahn, D, Rapp, S, Bergan, K, Coldwell, DM. Hepatic artery embolization: factos predisposing to postembolization pain and nausea, J Vasc Interv Radiol (2000);11:453–60.

56. Coldwell, DM, Loper, KA. Regional anesthesia for hepatic arterial embolization. Radiology (1989);172:1039–40.

57. Hartnell, GG, Gates, J, Stuart, et al. Hepatic chemoembolization; effect of intra-areterial lidocaine on pain and postprocedure recovery. Cardiovasc Interv Radiol (1999);22:293–7.

58. Lee, SH, Hahn, ST, Park, SH. Intraarterial lidocaine administration for relief of pain resulting from transarterial chemoembolization of hepatocellular carcinoma: its effectiveness and optimal timing of administration. Cardiovasc Interv Radiol (2001);24:368–71.

59. Brown, DB, Geschwind, JFH, Soulen, MC, Millward, SF, Sacks, D. Society of Interventional Radiology position statement on chemoembolization of hepatic malignancies. J Vasc Interv Radiol (2006);17:217–23.

60. Culp WC Jr.,Culp, WC. Thoracic paravertebral block for percutaneous transhepatic biliary drainage. J Vasc Interv Radiol (2005);16:1397–1400.

61. Harshfield, DL, Teplick, SK, Brandon, JC. Pain control during interventional biliary procedures: epidural anesthesia vs. IV sedation. AJR Am J Roentgenol (1993);161: 1057–9.

Index

315